NO MORE
DIGESTIVE
PROBLEMS

AGA ADVISORY BOARD

NO MORE DIGESTIVE PROBLEMS

The Answers Every Woman Needs—
Real Solutions to Stop the Pain
and Achieve Lasting Digestive Health

by CYNTHIA YOSHIDA, M.D.

with DEBORAH KOTZ

BANTAM BOOKS

NO MORE DIGESTIVE PROBLEMS
A Bantam Book

PUBLISHING HISTORY
Bantam trade paperback edition published April 2004
Bantam mass market edition / January 2006

Published by
Bantam Dell
A Division of Random House, Inc.
New York, New York

All rights reserved
Copyright © 2004 by American Gastroenterological Association
Illustrations by Scott Bodell
Book design by Ox and Company, Inc.
Cover photo by Town & Country Photography

Library of Congress Catalog Card Number: 2003063682

Bantam Books and the rooster colophon are registered trademarks
of Random House, Inc.

ISBN-10: 0-553-58875-3
ISBN-13: 978-0-553-58875-0

Printed in the United States of America
Published simultaneously in Canada

www.bantamdell.com

OPM   10 9 8 7 6 5 4 3 2 1

For my mother, Marian, who planted the seed of achievement.
To Tom, TJ, and Lauren for their patience and unconditional love.

—Cindy Yoshida

To David, my enduring love.
To Shira, Joshua, and Ruven, who make life worth living.

—Debbie Kotz

The material in this book is for informational purposes only. It is not intended to serve as a diagnostic tool or prescription manual, or to replace the advice and care of your medical doctor. Although every effort has been made to provide the most up-to-date information, the medical science and information in this field are rapidly changing. Therefore, we strongly recommend that you consult with your physician before attempting any of the treatments or programs discussed in this book.

The authors, the publisher, and the American Gastroenterological Association (AGA) expressly disclaim responsibility for adverse effects that may result from the use or application of the information contained in this book. AGA does not endorse or favor any specific commercial product or company. Trade, proprietary, or company names appearing in this document are used only because they are considered necessary in the context of the information provided. If a product is not mentioned, this does not mean or imply that the product is unsatisfactory.

ACKNOWLEDGMENTS

In May 2001, while serving my last year as Chair of the AGA's Committee on Women, I was approached by the American Gastroenterological Association about writing this book. Only two years prior, I had started the Women's GI Clinic at the University of Virginia. I had the good fortune of working with a fabulous staff of women who shared their knowledge and my passion for women's GI health. This book is my opportunity to give back, to be able to share my patients' stories and hopefully to impart some of the wisdom that I learned along my journey.

I first need to thank the leaders of the American Gastroenterological Association for entrusting me with this project. I am proud to be a member of this prestigious organization that remains committed to the latest GI research, excellence in patient care, and educational efforts for their membership and for the public. Their vision and support of projects like this book promise that they will be an enduring, influential force in gastroenterology.

Within the AGA, I am appreciative of Dr. Jacqueline Wolf, who initiated this project and who continues to work tirelessly within the AGA and other organizations to advocate sex-based GI research. She, along with all other past and present members of the AGA's Committee on Women in Gastroenterology, deserves special commendation for her continued efforts to promote women's GI issues and to mentor young women gastroenterologists. From this group, I would especially like to recognize Drs. Joanne Wilson, Rosemarie Fisher, Joanne Donovan, Dayna Early, Sunanda Kane, Theresa Pizarro, and Deborah Rubin. I am, as is the AGA and its Foundation for Digestive Health and Nutrition, deeply indebted to Ms. Jacqueline Simkin, whose generous support helped to make this book a reality. Jacqueline is a director of AGA's Foundation for Digestive Health and Nutrition, a successful businesswoman, and lawyer. She is also a grateful Crohn's patient. Her support of and commitment to gastroenterology research have contributed greatly to our field and reflect both her innate generosity and gratitude to the gastroenterologists who have improved her health and helped make her life more comfortable. Heartfelt thanks goes to Amy Manela and Kay Twomey for their vision for this book and their belief in me. I owe my eternal gratitude to Kay for her tireless energy to see this book to completion. She read through numerous drafts of this book, helped me to look at it objectively, assured that I always had the most current information, and provided me with wise editorial comments. Most of all I cherish her friendship. I am also extremely grateful to Dr. Michael Stolar for his attention to detail, his wit, and his precious time to read through the manuscript.

I am extremely grateful to my co-author, Deborah Kotz. As a physician, I'm used to writing and speaking in scientific terms. Debbie grasped the medical science that I brought to her and was able to give it warmth, readability, and understanding. Through our exchanges, Debbie was also able to bring a lot of my voice and personality into this book. It was easy for me to write about others' stories and health problems, but it took a lot of nudging by her to add the personal touches that I may have otherwise been reluctant to share.

My education in writing this book was significantly enhanced by my fantastic editor at Bantam Dell, Toni Burbank. Her expertise in women's health books assured that we would provide a well-rounded, complete source of information for women. I am grateful to her for her attention to detail and for her patience in guiding me through this initial effort. The team of experts at Bantam Dell is also owed my deepest gratitude; these include Melanie Milgram, Theresa Zoro, Glen Edelstein, and Janet Biehl. I want to also thank Mr. Scott Bodell for his beautiful artwork that graces the pages of the book, and for his passion for excellence in his work. I am indebted to my agent, Barbara Lowenstein, for her belief in the concept of this book and for her practical, wise advice throughout the writing of the book. Thank you to my expert advisory board, Dr. Dayna Early, Dr. Sunanda Kane, Dr. Kathie Hullfish, Dr. Paul Lebovitz, Dr. Anthony Lembo, Dr. Steven Peikin, Dr. Donna Stewart, Dr. Norah Terrault, and to Dr. Douglas Drossman, Anna Miller, RN and Dr. Bruce Schirmer for generously sharing their expertise with me.

I would not be where I am today without my mentors and teachers. I am tremendously grateful to Dr. David Peura. He is a caring and competent clinician, excellent teacher, and wonderful role model. I cannot thank him enough for his encouragement and wise counsel throughout the years. I would also like to acknowledge Dr. David Stone, Dr. Norton Greenberger, and

Dr. Allan Cooke. They, through their own passion for our field and through their generous teachings, instilled in me an enduring gratification of gastroenterology.

I could never have written this book without my experiences with the Women's GI Clinic at UVA. The concept of this clinic was to provide GI health care for women by women and I am incredibly fortunate to have worked with so many exceptional women. I am most indebted to my beautiful nurse and partner in patient care, Beth Dierdorf. My practice could not function without her. She has keen clinical common sense, brilliant self confidence, fierce loyalty, and shares my genuine concern for all of our patients. I am also grateful to my incredibly caring secretary, Susan Fitzgerald. She has been my ambassador, she assures that my practice shines and she shares a tireless dedication to our patients.

When I started the Women's GI Clinic, I had the good fortune to work with three fabulous gastroenterology fellows, Dr. Vanessa Shami, Dr. Suzanne Miller, and Dr. Cheryl Cox. Completing our core team was an outstanding physician's assistant, Karen Finke. These four young women had no choice but to join me in this new venture and they did so with great enthusiasm. Their warm, competent medical care of our patients in those first years assured that the Women's GI Clinic would continue to succeed. I am indebted to them.

When I first envisioned the concept of the Women's GI clinic, I saw it as a multidisciplinary clinic that could provide well-rounded care. To this end, I was able to surround myself with a team of extraordinary women specialists. Psychologist Dr. Dania Chastain started the clinic with me and most recently I have been fortunate to work with Dr. J. Kim Penberthy, who graciously shared her expertise with me for this book. I would also like to thank our dietitians, Nicole Flaherty, Andrea Yoder, and especially Theresa Anderson, who shared their practical tips for good nutrition for the book. My dear friend Carol Parrish is nationally renowned in nutrition support. I am grateful for her incredible enthusiasm, for all she has taught me, and for so much that she continues to share. I am also deeply indebted to two fantastic gynecologists, Dr. JoAnn Pinkerton and Dr. Kathie Hullfish. Kathie and I collaborate to treat women with pelvic floor dysfunction and fecal incontinence. She has taught me so much about these important problems. JoAnn has a successful practice in midlife-health gynecology. She sees the importance of colo-rectal cancer screening and strongly encourages her patients to have colonoscopies. She has saved numerous lives.

On a special note, I also want to thank my patients for entrusting me with their health, for teaching me so much about women's unique gastrointestinal health issues, and for eagerly agreeing to have their stories told in this book.

I worked with an exceptional group of people at the Digestive Health Center of Excellence at UVA. I am fortunate to count this talented group of dedicated practitioners as friends. I would like to thank the chief of the division, Dr. Fabio Cominelli, for believing in the concept of the Women's GI Clinic. A special thank-you to: Drs. Paul Yeaton, Mark Worthington, Jeffrey Tokar, Khalouk Abdrabbo, Carl Berg, Stephen Bickston, Stephen Caldwell, Steven Cohn, Larry Comerford, Sheila Crowe, Peter Ernst, Michel Kahaleh, Abdullah Al-Osaimi, Steven Powell, Antoinette Saddler, Reid Adams, Eugene Foley, Charles Friel, and physician's assistants Karen Finke and Colleen Green. I would also like to thank my research nurse, Brigid Wonderly, and all of the wonderful endoscopy and clinic nurses and personnel that I worked with on a daily basis, most especially Irene Melo, Beth White, Patricia Cuadros, Kathy Tapscott, and Robin Hamlin. Practice at an academic university would not be complete without GI fellows and residents. I have had the great fortune to work with so many wonderful trainees whose enthusiasm inspires me and whose hard work and dedication assure excellent patient care.

The Nurses' Health Study from Harvard Medical School found that the more friends women have, the more likely they are to lead joyful lives. Thank you to my good friends, Dr. Sylvia Hendrix, Eileen Park, Dr. Laurel Rice, and Rebecca West, who are a constant source of strength and support.

Finally, I want to thank my family. My parents, Minoru and Marian, and my siblings, Kathy, Michael, and Michelle, have always encouraged and supported me. Most importantly, I am forever grateful to my wonderful husband, Tom Gampper, and my two children, TJ and Lauren, who bring love and balance to my life.

—Cynthia Yoshida

CONTENTS

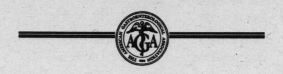

NO MORE
DIGESTIVE
PROBLEMS

Part I

DIGESTIVE ISSUES FOR WOMEN

THE GUTS BEHIND
THE WOMAN

It's no secret that women are different from men. We think differently, we feel differently, we communicate differently. And women live longer than men—an average of 5.4 years, to be exact. To some extent, women and men even have different digestive systems.

In fact, the two sexes seem to be separate subspecies when it comes to gastrointestinal health problems. Menstruation, pregnancy, and menopause all put a distinct feminine stamp on your digestive tract. So although you may have the same digestive symptoms as a man, you may not be suffering from the same digestive health problem.

After all, men don't experience the nine months of digestive disturbances that can come with pregnancy. Nor do they cope with the bloating, diarrhea, or constipation that waxes and wanes with menstrual cycles. And men certainly don't get painful hemorrhoids after delivering a baby.

These are just a few of the reasons why you, as a woman, need a digestive health book that you can call your own. Although you might reach for the Pepto-Bismol that your husband or boyfriend uses, the cause of your symptoms may be completely different. You may require a different diagnostic workup and a different course of treatment.

It's for this very reason that I, as a gastroenterologist, decided to focus my practice on women's health. I wanted to address the special concerns of women like you.

I really came to understand the importance of gender differences in gastrointestinal (GI) disorders after medical school, during my gastroenterology fellowship training in the early 1990s. I began to see so many women with diverse digestive problems that stemmed from a wide range of sources such as eating disorders, pregnancy, hormone replacement therapy, and childbirth. At that time sex-based differences in disease weren't included in my medical school or specialty training. I knew, of course, that when it came to digestive problems, women had unique issues that set them apart from men. But I really gleaned my knowledge from experience and by digging up GI research studies that highlighted women's health issues.

A decade ago women weren't included in clinical trials. It was assumed that diseases in men and women were the same and that women would react to medications the same way men did. This was a very wrong assumption to make, as researchers found out when they began including women in studies.

The National Institutes of Health now have an Office of Research on Women's Health that funds studies performed exclusively on women. As a result of these pioneering efforts, researchers have gathered a significant amount of evidence delineating differences in GI function in men and women. Women are unique. And there is a definite connection between a woman's reproductive tract and her digestive tract.

One study published in *Gastroenterology,* the official journal of the AGA, found that women with gastrointestinal disorders like irritable bowel syndrome (IBS) and inflammatory bowel disease are far more likely to experience premenstrual syndrome (PMS) than healthy women. The study also found that women who had digestive disorders and PMS often reported that their symptoms—like diarrhea, constipation, and abdominal

PARTICIPATING IN A CLINICAL TRIAL

The importance of clinical research trials goes without question, and much more research still needs to be done in the field of women's gastrointestinal health. Of course, these studies require participants, women like you to volunteer in the effort to help advance medical knowledge. Without female volunteers, two new drugs that were recently approved to treat IBS exclusively in women would never have made it on the market.

The Society for Women's Health Research can provide you with information and links to current clinical trials in women's digestive health and other areas. They've partnered with the AGA and other prominent medical organizations to launch a campaign to educate women on the importance of medical research and participation in clinical trials. Log on to their website www.womens-health.org, or call (877) 332-2626.

pain—got better and worse during the course of their menstrual cycle.

The latest research shows that female hormones, such as estrogen and progesterone, affect the function of your GI tract. Here's just one example: A 2002 finding from the landmark Heart and Estrogen/Progestin Replacement Study (HERS) found that postmenopausal women who used hormone replacement therapy for six years had a 45 percent increased risk of developing gallbladder disease compared to their counterparts who did not take hormones.

Some exciting research findings have dramatically altered the way digestive problems are diagnosed and treated in women. In recent years several myths have been shattered. For example, little more than a decade ago women with IBS were told that their symptoms were all in their head or were caused by too much mucus in their gut. Today gastroenterologists know that both of these assumptions were wrong: IBS has been shown to be caused by a breakdown in the way food moves through the intestines or by a heightened sensitivity of the intestines to the normal movement of food. Our diet and even our emotional state can be aggravating factors in this syndrome. Another myth that's gone by the wayside is that ulcers are caused by too much stress or spicy foods. We now know they're caused by the bacteria *Helicobacter pylori* or by the chronic use of nonsteroidal anti-inflammatory drugs like aspirin or ibuprofen (Advil, Nuprin)—taken by millions of women who suffer from chronic back pain, headaches, or arthritis.

Physicians have also become more aware of GI diseases that are more common in women than men. These include constipation, pelvic floor dysfunction, and certain liver diseases such as primary biliary cirrhosis, which can cause liver failure. One research study found that women who need liver transplants due to severe liver disease have much higher rates of bone fractures. This led to additional research, which found that women who had liver problems were at much higher risk of developing osteoporosis than men with liver problems. Further research found that women with other GI problems like inflammatory bowel disease also have a higher risk of osteoporosis. As a result of this work, women with these conditions now have bone density tests routinely and are given appropriate medications to prevent bone loss.

New findings also suggest that medications don't always work the same in women as in men. Researchers have discovered that men and women metabolize drugs differently because some of the liver enzymes that break down drugs are more active in women than in men. At least four of ten drugs removed from the market in recent years, due to unacceptable side effects, posed greater health risks to women than to men.

The field of women's digestive health is no passing fad. Female medical school students are entering gastroenterology in greater and greater numbers, often becoming subspecialists in women's health. During the last few years the number of women entering gastroenterology fellowship training increased dramatically. In 2002 one in four GI "fellows" was a woman! And many GI practices are specifically seeking out women to join their practice.

What's more, this past year the American Gastroen-terological Association (AGA) along with the American College of Gastroenterology, the American Society for Gastrointestinal Endoscopy, and the American Associa-tion for the Study of Liver Disease, updated the GI training curriculum used for all gastroenterology fel-lows to include women's health issues. This training will focus on digestive disease issues specific to women, such as how menstruation, pregnancy, and menopause affect our digestive tract. It also touches on the use of stress management, herbal therapies, and other alterna-tive therapies to relieve GI symptoms.

All of these issues are vital to getting the solutions you need to cure your digestive problems. They are all addressed in this book and really form the basis for why you, as a woman, need a digestive health book that's tai-lored for your unique health needs. Through this book I want to pass on the knowledge that I've learned by serving for more than ten years as an attending physi-cian in the gastroenterology department at the Univer-sity of Virginia (UVA) Hospital in Charlottesville. As founder of the Women's GI Clinic at UVA, I have fo-cused my own clinical and research interests in women's digestive health.

WHY I STARTED A WOMEN-ONLY GI CLINIC

By and large, research studies on women's digestive health were just coming to light when I first made my decision to open a women's GI clinic four years ago. The basis for my decision was—pardon the pun—a gut instinct. My interest in women's health began several years ago when a colleague of mine, a midlife-health gynecologist, started referring all her patients over fifty to me for colon cancer screening. At that time flexible sigmoidoscopy was the most common scoping procedure to screen for colon cancer. During this procedure patients don't need to be sedated because the scope only goes part of the way up the colon. (Colonoscopy, which usually requires sedation, has begun to replace sigmoidoscopy because the colonoscope can reach through the entire span of the colon instead of just the lower one-third portion reached by the sigmoidoscope.)

As I performed sigmoidoscopies on these women, I found that many took the opportunity to ask me—in a confidential tone—about their GI woes. "I have diarrhea at certain times of the month. Is this normal?" asked one patient. "Why do I sometimes leak stool?" asked another. Another woman wanted to know, "Is it normal to have my bowel movements feel like they're getting stuck at the end of my rectum?"

I was peppered with questions about bloating, gas, hemorrhoids, and chronic indigestion and soon discovered that these women hardly ever discussed these problems with their primary care physicians. Most were too embarrassed to bring up their bowel habits during an annual exam. Many women told me they felt more comfortable talking to me because I was a woman. None had considered seeking out a gastroenterologist for help.

After talking with patient after patient during their routine colon screenings, I really felt that I had something to offer to the women of our community. I wanted to create an environment where women would feel comfortable opening up about their GI problems. I also knew from my experience that far too many women had digestive problems that ran much deeper than their symptoms. I've seen women whose constipation was caused by lingering memories of childhood incest or by years of sexual abuse by their husbands. Mothers have brought their daughters to me with unexplained diarrhea and vomiting and were shocked to hear that their daughters had an eating disorder and were inducing the diarrhea (by taking laxatives) and vomiting.

I knew there was a void in the area of women's digestive health that needed to be filled. My boss, Fabio Cominelli, the head of the gastroenterology department, agreed with me 100 percent. He backed my idea to start a women-only GI clinic staffed with women health professionals.

Mary, a fortyish mother of two, was one of my first patients. She suffered from such severe attacks of abdominal pain and diarrhea that she had trouble holding down a job and caring for her family. In fact, she told me, she knew the location of every public bathroom between her home and her workplace and found herself making frequent stops along the way. Mary saw several doctors in town but was never able to get relief from her symptoms. She began to think her doctors didn't believe she was actually in severe pain. Finally, her family physician called me and asked me to see her.

Mary and I spent the entire appointment talking about her symptoms and their triggers. I believed that she had IBS, and a few tests to rule out other conditions confirmed my diagnosis. On our next visit Mary paced around my office and told me that the last year had been incredibly stressful because of a troubled relationship with her daughter and her increased responsibility caring for her aging mother. I told her that I understood what she was going through and that I believed that her symptoms were very real. I also reassured her that her condition wasn't life threatening. Suddenly, I saw her shoulders relax. She stopped pacing and sat in a chair. She turned to me and for the first time really began to listen as I gave her details about a medical condition that had been plaguing her for many years.

We mapped out a plan of action. Mary agreed to keep a symptom diary, and I discussed several treatment options for her diarrhea and abdominal pain. I referred Mary to our pain psychologist to help her cope with her anxiety. I also encouraged her to take better care of herself. "IBS is most likely to strike when you're at your weakest, so if you exercise, cut the fat in your diet, and take time to do the things you enjoy, you'll be safeguarding yourself against another attack." At first I saw Mary every week, then once a month as her symptoms improved.

Now years later Mary still checks in with me every once in a while. She still has occasional bouts of IBS, but she now has control over her symptoms and has regained a full quality of life. Best of all, she has the awareness of why her attacks are occurring. She can usually pinpoint the stress trigger or knows when she's strayed from her healthy habits like walking every day or eating ample servings of fruits and vegetables.

If I had to sum up the goal of the Women's GI

Clinic, I would use four words: *Put women at ease.* I want patients to feel as comfortable as possible so that they can freely discuss all those strange bodily functions that make us all squeamish. I have definitely found that communication is the absolute key to getting treatment. Even the best doctors can't diagnose and treat you if they don't know the full extent of your symptoms.

I hold the philosophy—as do many doctors—that you have to treat the whole person in order to effectively manage the medical problems. Too often we're tempted to just write a prescription and send patients on their way. But this is doing an extreme disservice. The Women's GI Clinic is based on a team approach. I am fortunate to work with some incredible women. From my secretary, Susan, to my invaluable nurse, Beth, we try hard to listen, care, and nurture. We know that medical conditions are usually triggered by a combination of factors—not one single thing.

In addition to nurses and medical residents, I wanted psychologists and nutritionists on hand to deal with the deeper issues that cause GI problems. I envisioned a holistic health center that would deal with a woman's digestive health problems on all levels—from psychological issues to nutrition planning.

Let's say you came to me because you were severely bloated, and part of the reason for your problem was that you were embarrassed to pass gas in a public place. I might refer you to a female psychologist that I work with who would suggest behavioral strategies for overcoming your problem. (I outline these strategies in Chapter 5.)

But I'm not here to tell you that you need to find a women's GI clinic in order to achieve relief from your symptoms. That would be hard to do if you don't live near one, and there are only a handful of clinics like mine scattered throughout the United States. You can still get the optimal care you deserve by finding the right doctor who will take all your symptoms seriously and treat you as a whole patient and by using this book as a supplement.

The advice doled out by the various professionals at the clinic is found throughout this book. You'll find dietary approaches recommended by the nutritionist and breathing and relaxation exercises for stress reduction that the clinic psychologist uses. Basically, I've tried to include everything in this book that my patients always ask me about, from herbal remedies to gastric bypass weight-loss surgery to colonics.

I have also relied on a team of experts who served on the AGA advisory board for this book. These physicians have their own areas of expertise, such as nutrition, alternative health, IBS, and women's health. Many of them have broken new ground through their own research studies and contributed their knowledge of cutting edge treatments and diagnostic techniques to his book.

What's amazing to me is that my initial "gut instinct" to open a women's GI clinic now has the medical research to back it up. We now know from accumulated research that your menstrual cycle does play a role in your digestive function. We know a lot more about the role that pregnancy and menopause play in gastrointestinal symptoms. And of course, women and men aren't built the same anatomically and have different ways of dealing with emotions and handling stress. All of this comes into play when it comes to your digestive health. Let's begin the journey to see how.

DIGESTION 101

First You Chew

From the moment you bite into biscotti or sip a café au lait, your digestive tract kicks into gear. Salivary glands in your mouth squirt out enzymes to start the digestion of sugar, whether it's in your biscotti, coffee, or some other food being savored by your tongue. As you chew and push the morsels around in your mouth, your brain sends a signal to your digestive system to prepare itself for an onslaught of incoming food. Organs like your stomach and gallbladder begin to release digestive juices, so food will be better digested along the way.

Then You Swallow

Once you swallow, your gut's own nervous system takes over. Functioning on automatic pilot, nerves in your GI tract now take full control of the food you've just eaten. It takes anywhere from thirty seconds to a minute for food to travel down the foot-long tube, called the *esophagus,* into your stomach. Nerve cells that surround your digestive tract cause digestive muscles to contract in syncopated pulses, sort of like the steady rhythm of your heartbeat. These wavelike movements are called *peristal-*

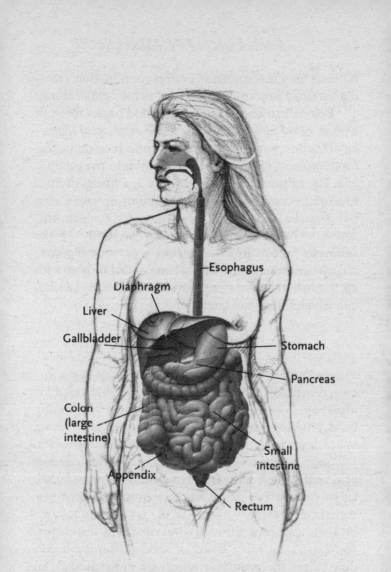

- Esophagus
- Diaphragm
- Liver
- Gallbladder
- Stomach
- Pancreas
- Colon (large intestine)
- Small intestine
- Appendix
- Rectum

The GI tract encompasses a lot more than just your stomach. To function smoothly, digestion requires the harmonious collaboration of all of these components.

sis. Each muscle contracts in perfect coordination, creating harmony in your digestive tract as food glides along.

Before it reaches the stomach, food passes through a point of no return called the *lower esophageal sphincter*. This one-way valve prevents stomach contents like food and acid from washing back up into the esophagus. The sphincter opens and shuts in a timed rhythm to work in concert with the movements of your digestive muscles. All of this takes incredible synchronization to keep digestion running smoothly. If the sphincter fails to function properly or your digestive muscles contract at the wrong time or out of sync with each other, digestive symptoms like heartburn can occur, which I'll explain later in this chapter.

Then You Digest

Although many women view their stomach as the enemy, it's actually a strong muscular organ that's vital for digestion. Your *stomach* serves as a great big mixing bowl, grinding down what you've just eaten and mixing in acidic juices until all that's left are tiny food particles.

Your stomach is also a great protector. Stomach acid helps kill off nasty invaders like food-borne bacteria or cold viruses that made their way onto your biscotti from a server's hands. While it's true that some invaders can pass through your stomach unscathed, you'd get a lot more bouts of food poisoning if you didn't have the protective effects of stomach acid. So think about this the next time you're about to curse your bulging stomach. (Besides, excess abdominal fat is *really* the culprit behind the belly bulge!)

After your stomach has done its job, food becomes a mushy liquid that is released slowly into the *small intestine*. If stretched straight out, your small intestine would measure an impressive 15 to 20 feet. To fit into your abdominal cavity, this length of tubing is folded over many times. It's composed of three main parts: the *duodenum* (at the top nearest the stomach), the *jejunum* (in the middle), and the *ileum* (at the end). When the liquid mush of food enters the duodenum, it gets mixed with juices from the *pancreas* that contain enzymes to help break down fats and protein. Your *liver* releases bile, which gets mixed into the mush and aids in the digestion of fats. Carbohydrates are broken down to simple sugars by specific digestive enzymes that are released from the lining of the small intestine.

In an intricate system of timed chemical reactions, fats, carbohydrates, and proteins are broken down into their simplest forms—that is, fatty acids for fats, glucose for carbohydrates, and amino acids for proteins. Your small intestine then extracts these vital nutrients, along with vitamins, minerals, and water, from your food. All of these elements get pulled through the cell wall of the small intestine to be absorbed into your bloodstream. The cell wall has an opening just large enough for these nutrients to squeeze through but small enough to keep out larger particles that may be toxic to your body. Again, your digestive tract finds ways to safeguard your health. Your body relies on all the nutrients for, among other things, providing energy and replenishing cells.

The passage of food through the small intestine usually takes about two to eight hours. Every particle must be tagged either as usable or as waste. As I mentioned, those usable nutrients that are small enough to pass through the intestinal wall can enter the bloodstream, but before they get far in the body, they must first pass through inspection by the liver. The liver serves as a filter, picking and choosing which particles it will allow to circulate through your body. Again, the goal here is to protect your body and prevent dangerous substances from getting to vital organs like your heart and brain. Besides acting like a filter, your liver makes and breaks down many substances, including cholesterol and hormones like testosterone and estrogen. It also regulates blood sugar levels and manufactures bile.

Any particles that don't pass your liver's inspection or that never get through the wall of the small intestine become waste products. This waste is shuffled off to the *colon* (also called the *large intestine* or *large bowel*) through the same synchronized contractions that moved food through your digestive tract from your esophagus downward.

Finally, You Excrete

The colon acts like a giant dehydrator, absorbing water from waste and turning it into a solid mass of stool. Your digestive muscles contract and squeeze stool into the rectum, where the stool remains until you're ready to sit down, relax, and push a bowel movement out through the anus. The control you have over your bowel movements results from two valves, or sphincters, in the anus that prevent stool from leaking out involuntarily. You trigger the opening of the outer of these two sphincters whenever you push out a stool.

A JOURNEY THROUGH THE FEMALE DIGESTIVE TRACT

When it comes to the actual machinery of the digestive system, women aren't built much differently from men. Both sexes have the same series of interconnected tubes that run the span from the esophagus through the colon. Women and men have an identical array of digestive organs such as stomach, liver, and gallbladder. Despite these similarities, the simple placement of a uterus between a woman's bladder and rectum can have vast consequences for gut function. This becomes obvious with pregnancy. The weight of a growing fetus can weaken the pelvic floor muscles that support the uterus, bladder, and rectum. As women age, these muscles can further weaken and cause a shift in the shape and location of the rectum, hindering bowel movements. The result is often pain, rectal prolapse, or constipation.

What's more, women are in general more petite than men. We have a smaller pelvis and a smaller abdominal cavity, which houses our digestive organs. We also tend to have a longer sigmoid (the lower portion of the colon) than men, which, when you add in our reproductive organs, means we have a lot more stuff squeezed into a much smaller space. This means our digestive organs don't have much give when they get filled with excess gas, air, or food or when our digestive muscles go into spasm. Thus, your digestive tract may be more sensitive to stress or dietary changes than a man's.

In fact, a wide range of studies have shown that women are more vulnerable to a variety of painful conditions, including abdominal pain of various kinds. Hormonal, biochemical, and anatomical differences all seem to contribute to sex differences in pain and may help explain why two-thirds of IBS sufferers are women.

I tell my patients to picture themselves alongside basketball star Michael Jordan. Both have the same digestive organs, yet Michael has far more room in his abdominal cavity for his intestines to stretch out. His GI tract has a lot more give than the average woman's, which is squeezed into a smaller body.

Female hormones, like estrogen and progesterone, can also have dramatic effects on the performance of our GI tract. The very hormones that allow us to create and nourish a new life can also disrupt the movement of food through our intestines. Certain female hormones can speed the process up, causing diarrhea, nausea, and abdominal pain. Other hormones can slow things down, causing constipation and bloating.

These female factors can send our finely mechanized digestive system into a tailspin. And they may account for some of the differences that gastroenterologists see between male and female patients. A review of ninety-five studies, published in the *Journal of Gender-Specific Medicine,* found significant differences between women and men when it comes to both the functions and malfunctions of our gut. What this means is that women may need a different diagnostic test or treatment to manage a particular problem.

Here's a top-to-bottom look at some of the key issues for women.

Esophagus

Unfortunately, the number of women suffering from chronic heartburn, known as gastroesophageal reflux disease (GERD), is on the rise. The condition now afflicts about three percent of women, up from one percent a few decades ago. Women now have about the same incidence of GERD as men. No one really knows why GERD has risen in women higher than ever before, but it could be due to the fact that more of us are overweight. The number of obese women has increased from 25 to 33 percent in the past decade, and packing extra fat around the abdomen seems to strain the lower esophageal sphincter, which can trigger heartburn.

The female hormone progesterone also plays a role in the development of GERD. During pregnancy, soaring progesterone levels cause a great slowdown in our digestive system. Food remains in the stomach for a longer time, which makes it more likely that it will wash back up. Taking oral contraceptives or hormone replacement therapy containing progesterone can also cause this slowdown. The good news is, these same female hormones may also protect us from certain diseases. One study found that breast-feeding lowers our risk of developing esophageal cancer later in life; the longer we breast-feed, the lower our risk. Additionally, women with a condition known as Barrett's esophagus have a lower risk of esophageal cancer than men with the same condition.

Stomach and Duodenum

Thanks again to estrogen and progesterone, food leaves a woman's stomach at a slower rate than it leaves a man's. As a result, we're more likely to experience cyclical bouts of nausea, bloating, belching, loss of appetite, abdominal pain, and fullness after eating, as our hormones ebb and flow during our menstrual cycle. Premenstrual syndrome can cause a decrease in the frequency of bowel movements or even constipation, which may also be directly related to a shift in hormone levels.

Certain medications that women are more likely to take can also cause stomach problems. For instance, long-term use of nonsteroidal anti-inflammatory drugs (NSAIDs) like ibuprofen (Motrin, Advil, and others) and naproxen sodium (Aleve) can increase the likelihood of an ulcer. That's because these medications can damage the lining of the stomach. Since women suffer more frequently from arthritis and other conditions that cause chronic pain, we tend to use these medications more than men.

Liver

Liver diseases present a special problem for women. Drinking excessive amounts of alcohol does more damage to our liver than to a man's—even if we pair up by weight and match each other drink for drink. We're also more likely than men to develop certain liver problems, although these are pretty rare. For instance, we have a higher risk of developing a type of autoimmune disease (in which the body attacks its own tissues) that can cause hepatitis, a serious liver disease that can sometimes turn deadly. Our risk is also higher for developing liver tumors and liver disease caused by the chronic use of certain medications, particularly oral contraceptives.

Estrogen may play some role in making our livers particularly vulnerable to disease. But my message here is not to cause you to panic or think that you're destined to develop a diseased liver. Rather, if your doctor does diagnose a liver problem, he or she should take your gender into account when choosing which diagnostic tests to perform and which treatments to recommend.

Gallbladder and Pancreas

As women, we have twice the risk of developing gall-stones as men. It's unfair but true. Estrogen and progesterone are partners in this crime. Estrogen increases the amount of cholesterol in bile, a digestive liquid made by your liver and emptied into your gallbladder. Progesterone slows the emptying of bile from the gallbladder, which gives the cholesterol time to harden into crystals, otherwise known as gallstones.

On the upside, estrogen and progesterone appear to protect against pancreatic disease, which could explain why men are three times more likely than women to develop pancreatic cancer, a particularly deadly form of cancer. Women who get pancreatic disease also have a slightly longer survival than men.

Intestines

Many women experience bouts of constipation or diarrhea associated with their menstrual cycle. For some women, constipation occurs a day or two after ovulation, when progesterone levels are at their highest. (Remember, progesterone slows the movement of food through your gut.) Others find that symptoms worsen premenstrually and during menstruation when certain hormones called prostaglandins are released. These ovarian hormones—the same ones that cause your uterus to contract during labor—can increase the movement, or motility, of your gut, which results in diarrhea.

Women make up two-thirds of the IBS sufferers in the United States, and whether our sex hormones play a role in our increased risk remains an unanswered question. Although this condition has no known cause, recent research has shown that people with IBS have an increased sensitivity in their gut that can trigger some very real symptoms. Sufferers often experience severe abdominal pain and bouts of constipation, diarrhea, or both.

Why are women in the United States particularly prone to IBS? It isn't all about having two X chromosomes. In different parts of the world, men and women have an equal incidence of IBS, and in India men with IBS outnumber women. Maybe it has something to do with the lifestyles American women lead and the stress we put on ourselves.

Female hormones, though, may also play some role. About one-quarter of IBS sufferers have decreased gut motility, which often results from elevated levels of the female hormone progesterone. Food takes longer to leave the stomach and weave its way through the intestines. So women with IBS are more likely to experience pain, bloating, nausea, and constipation. There are several medications available to treat symptoms of IBS, but medications that work in men often don't work in women—and vice versa. Two new therapies designed specifically for women are now available: alosetron (Lotronex) for diarrhea-predominant IBS and tegaserod (Zelnorm) for constipation-predominant IBS. These are discussed in more detail in Chapter 13.

Colon

I'll say this over and over again throughout the book: Colon cancer is the third-largest cancer killer of women. I can't say this enough because I want you to remember it and take action to get screened for this disease. (See Chapter 15.) *Today* show host Katie Couric has done an amazing job publicizing this disease, but many women still haven't gotten the message that colon cancer strikes women, too.

Certain "female" factors come into play in determining your colon cancer risk. If you've had uterine, ovarian, or breast cancer or have never had children, you have an increased risk. If you take hormone replacement therapy, you have a 35 percent lower risk of developing colon cancer, according to data from the Harvard Nurses' Health Study. (But this reduced risk disappears gradually once you go off the hormones.) Taking oral contraceptives for eight years or more can also reduce your colon cancer risk.

Reproductive Organs

I know I'm venturing beyond your digestive tract here, but your reproductive organs can sometimes play a role in your digestive symptoms. Endometriosis, a reproductive disorder that causes the uterine lining to grow beyond the uterus, can on occasion interfere with digestion if it involves the intestinal tract. Other conditions like pelvic inflammatory disease (caused by a uterine infection) or ectopic pregnancy (in which the embryo implants in the fallopian tube) can cause cramping or bloating, symptoms that may be mistaken for a digestive health problem.

In some cases the onset of persistent bloating, constipation, and pressure in the abdomen and pelvis can signal ovarian cancer. Just recently I saw a woman named Donna who had had IBS for years but suddenly noticed that her symptoms had changed. She was extremely bloated, a problem that had never bothered her before. By doing a CT scan, we quickly discovered that Donna had a large pelvic mass that was ovarian cancer. I don't want to scare you into thinking that every case of bloating means ovarian cancer. I just want you to trust your instincts. Donna knew that something different was going on. I want you to also trust your knowledge of your body. If your digestive symptoms deviate from their typical pattern, it's time to see your doctor.

IT'S NOT ALL IN YOUR HEAD— OR MAYBE IT IS

As I tell my patients nearly every day, there's a strong connection between the mind and the gut. The mind-body connection has been documented for other medical disorders like migraines, chronic back pain, and PMS. In recent years researchers have also found that certain gastrointestinal problems are exacerbated—and perhaps even triggered—by stress.

I've seen the mind-body connection at work in my own practice. Many of my patients who are students at the University of Virginia tell me they lose their appetites, experience a change in bowel habits, and develop stomach pains during final-exam week. Other patients, who work full time, tell me they get more bloated or constipated when trying to meet a huge job deadline. At this point we don't know if women are more likely than men to manifest stress in their digestive tract. What we do know is that women with IBS outnumber men by at least two to one and that this condition is often aggravated by stress, anxiety, and depression.

Nearly all of us have experienced the brain-gut connection. We've all had "butterflies" in the stomach before a big event like speaking in public or an important job interview. In some people it's just a little flutter, but others have diarrhea or even vomiting. We all react differently to varied levels of stress.

There's a real physiological explanation as to why your GI tract reacts so strongly to your emotional state. Your gut has its own separate nervous system, often called a minibrain, that sends messages back and forth to your brain. Your gut actually has more nerve cells than your brain's central nervous system. In fact, the number of nerve fibers that carry messages from your GI tract to your brain is nine times more than those that travel from your brain to your GI tract. If your GI tract sends out frequent warning signals to your brain, you're apt to be in trouble. In fact, having a

Sick to Her Stomach

"I've never had any real stomach problems, but I can tell you that I feel it in my guts when I'm stressed. Just the other day my son and daughter-in-law called to ask me if I could loan them a huge amount of money to buy the house of their dreams. My anxiety level shot through the roof as I imagined how I would manage my retirement on less money. Literally within a minute I was doubled over with cramps. I ran to the bathroom and had an explosive bowel movement. I'm a person who is normally on the constipated side, so I was pretty shocked to see the power that stress had over my body."

—**Rose**, 63, mother of three, grandmother of seven

malfunctioning digestive system can have a negative impact on the brain.

Your digestive system makes many of the same nerve chemicals that are manufactured in your brain. These chemicals, called *neurotransmitters,* are released in the gaps between nerve cells to help transmit nerve impulses from cell to cell. Serotonin, a feel-good neurotransmitter that gives you a feeling of calmness and tranquility, is pumped out in vast quantities by both your GI tract and your brain. People who are depressed often have low levels of serotonin and are treated with serotonin-boosting drugs to elevate their moods. Researchers at the Massachusetts Institute of Technology (MIT) have found that eating carbohydrate-rich food like pretzels, crackers, and cookies can boost serotonin levels in the brain. This may be one reason why certain depressed individuals self-medicate with food and develop binge eating disorders. What's more, many women with PMS experience a decline in serotonin just before their period, which brings on mood swings, depression, irritability, and carbohydrate cravings.

Serotonin may also play a role in how your digestive tract handles stress. In fact, a whopping 95 percent of the serotonin manufactured in your body is found in your GI tract. And research suggests that women may experience more GI disturbances in response to stress and anxiety than do men. Certain digestive problems like IBS are known to be exacerbated by emotional stress, and a major culprit may be serotonin. Women with diarrhea and IBS have been shown to have higher serotonin levels than women without IBS. IBS patients are also more likely to have concomitant depression and anxiety. Some women may experience an alleviation of pain symptoms associated with IBS after being treated with antidepressants.

TAKING TIME TO GET YOUR DIGESTIVE SYSTEM IN ORDER

I could expound for chapters on the physiological implications of living a harried lifestyle. I don't need to tell you that stress is no good for your GI tract. I also don't need to tell you that you need to put your health as a number-one priority. Still, as women, we face particular challenges when it comes to taking care of our health. We are the universal caregivers. Many of us must provide for the needs of our young children and our aging parents at the same time. The majority of us work full time outside the home, yet we haven't yet reached equality with men when it comes to sharing household responsibilities. What this all adds up to is a lack of time for ourselves.

You may be feeling the time crunch, even at this moment, as you catch a few minutes to read this book. But at least you're taking some precious time out to consider your health and your digestive problems. You're listening to the signals that your body is giving you about your digestive health. If you're suffering from constipation, diarrhea, bloating, or some other GI symptom on a regular basis, chances are you need to make some changes—whether it's in your diet, your exercise habits, or your stress levels. Or you may benefit from taking a medication to get your GI tract back on course.

As women, we have an added burden placed on us by our culture. Even in this day and age we are still expected to act with a certain femininity when it comes to our bodily functions. We're not given the freedom that men have to pass gas, belch, or unbutton our jeans in public. So too often we hold back and suffer through the consequences.

Some of us don't even feel comfortable eating a substantial meal in front of others, so we wait until we're alone at night and quickly raid the kitchen pantry, consuming most of our calories for the day. We're far more likely than men to skip a meal or go on a crash diet. These erratic eating habits can set us up for digestive distress like constipation, gas, and bloating. Many women find that these problems can last for months, even after they switch back to regular eating habits.

Sometimes we take our obsession with our weight to great extremes. We might read in a beauty magazine

THE MIGRAINE-NAUSEA CONNECTION

If you've ever suffered from a migraine, you know that the worst symptoms may not be the excruciating head pain but the accompanying nausea and vomiting. These GI disturbances are nearly universal to migraine sufferers. About 90 percent experience nausea, and one-third suffer from vomiting. Diarrhea strikes about 16 percent of patients. What's worse, these digestive disturbances often strike when migraines are more severe or prolonged.

No one knows exactly why migraines disrupt the GI tract. What is known is that vomiting stems from a strong stimulation to the vomiting center in the medulla. Nausea stems from a weaker stimulation in this area of the brain. Research suggests that cell receptors for the neurotransmitter dopamine may play a role in causing these symptoms and are also linked to the triggering of migraines. The activation of these receptors during the migraine slows the movement of food through the intestines, causing nausea and vomiting. In fact, some drugs, such as metoclopramide (Reglan), block the effects of dopamine, stopping nausea and speeding the movement of food through the GI tract. And they may help the migraine headache as well. What I find most interesting, however, is that this is one more piece of evidence showing the linkage between the gut and the brain.

that our favorite celebrity tried colonics to "lose weight quickly," then decide to give it a whirl ourselves. Some of us really abuse herbal laxatives and diuretics, and we're too ashamed to tell our doctors the real culprit of our abdominal pain or diarrhea.

I believe that the only way women are ever going to get over these embarrassments and concerns is by talking about them. That's why I spend a lot of time listening to my patients and trying to educate them about the physiological processes that are causing their symptoms. The good news is: Women pay more attention to their health than men. We're more likely to seek out a physician's care for our symptoms and are more likely to explore the reasons for our health problems. We're probably also more likely to take action to relieve our discomfort and improve our overall health.

Yet far too many of us still see our body as the "enemy" that burdens us with jiggly thighs and a mushy stomach. It took me a long time to learn to respect my body. Now I see my body as strong and capable of carrying me through my hectic days if I feed it the right fuel.

I have to admit that I don't always follow good eating habits. I often skip breakfast, and if I'm really busy at the clinic or doing endoscopies, I don't have lunch until three P.M., when I'll grab a bagel left over from a morning conference in the hospital. To a certain extent, I have an iron stomach and regular colon. Still, I always have a balanced dinner with my family. And in the summer, when my favorite fruits and vegetables are in season, I eat more healthily. As a result, I feel better and have a better-functioning GI tract.

JUST BETWEEN US: MY PERSONAL RX FOR YOUR DIGESTIVE WOES

Working as I do at a large hospital in a busy university town, I see women from many walks of life. Some have carefully chosen me after checking out my credentials, while others have no health insurance and haven't seen a primary care physician in years. I see women with digestive disorders that stem from years of alcohol or drug use or even physical abuse by their spouses. I see homemakers who can't be there for their children because they're so encumbered by stomach pain or constipation. I see professors with minor heartburn who ask me questions about the latest medication that just came on the market.

But regardless of whether my patient and I share the same zip code, fashion sense, or parenting problems, I always try to make a connection with her and meet her on some common ground. First and foremost I listen and take her problems seriously. I ask her to enter into a partnership with me to come up with a diagnostic plan and treatment regimen that is specific to her unique GI problem. This is not a one-sided relationship but rather a two-way free flow of conversation.

That's the kind of conversation I'd like to have with you. I'm asking you to put your trust in me. I in turn will put my trust in you to use this book wisely in conjunction with your own physician. I can't serve as a substitute for your doctor. Rather, my goal is to help you acquire the tools to understand your GI symptoms and to find someone you can trust with your digestive health.

This book is set up in three parts. Part I breaks new ground in describing GI concerns that are unique to women, including the role that our sex hormones play in our digestive health and how to manage our weight to combat digestive distress. Part II gives you an overall strategy for managing specific symptoms, including heartburn, gas, constipation, and diarrhea. It provides a wide range of self-treatment options and gives you guidelines for whether or when to see a doctor. Part III walks you through the process of finding the appropriate doctor and what to expect in terms of diagnostic tests and treatments for specific GI conditions.

Throughout the book I'll shed some light on the exciting new treatments that are available to combat your symptoms and reverse the course of your condition. Some of these breakthrough treatments like alosetron (Lotronex) and tegaserod (Zelnorm) for IBS have been designed specifically for use by women. You'll also see that getting properly diagnosed doesn't have to be a painful or embarrassing experience. High-tech diagnostic tools now help doctors peer into the GI tract without having to perform invasive exploratory surgeries. And I explore which new, less invasive tests are on the horizon. Hint: You may find that the colonoscopy experience changes dramatically within the next five years.

The goal of this book is to help you make an informed decision when it comes to looking for a doctor to deal with your digestive health concerns. You may also discover that you can treat many of your symptoms on your own simply by altering your diet or stepping up your activity level. I frequently recommend lifestyle approaches as the first course of action for my patients. Yes, prescription medications may be necessary, but most women would rather use them sparingly since every drug has its own set of side effects. As a doctor and a woman, I understand these concerns and prefer to take a comprehensive approach to treatment.

This book embodies my philosophy of patient care: Never send a patient home with just a medication prescription. My personal prescriptions usually include guidelines for exercise and an eating plan. If I think that stress, anxiety, or some other emotional problem is aggravating the symptoms, I might also write out a referral for professional counseling. Or if my patient is about to start an exercise plan from square one, I might recommend a personal trainer. If you suffer from digestive problems, you're entitled to more than a slip of paper to hand to a pharmacist. You need a full lifestyle approach that gets to the root of your symptoms.

I'll explore how taking certain steps to improve your overall health can also help improve your digestive health. We'll discuss complementary therapies like herbal remedies and progressive muscle relaxation. I refer to them as complementary—rather than alternative—therapies because I think these treatments can be a significant part of your overall medical program. Many women find they need both prescription medications and other therapies to restore their digestive health.

This book can serve as your road map to good GI health. If you're suffering from a digestive problem like constipation, gas, or abdominal pain, you probably need to make some changes in your life. It may be as easy as avoiding particular foods that aggravate the symptoms or increasing your intake of certain nutritious foods that your diet is lacking. Or you may have to probe deeper into your lifestyle habits and find better ways to manage stress, your weight, or lack of exercise.

As you try some of the self-help remedies that I

recommend, you'll find that you'll be rewarded for your efforts. Making some changes in your diet, exercise, and overall lifestyle will improve not only your digestive health but your overall health as well. In fact, the two are intimately connected. So grab the reins, and let's get started.

ARE YOUR SEX HORMONES TO BLAME?

I'M ABOUT TO VENTURE INTO UNCHARTED territory: I'm going to explore the role that sex hormones play in digestive function. The very same sex hormones that command the ebbs and flows of your menstrual cycle and enable you to sustain a pregnancy have an astonishing impact on your digestive tract. Understanding the connection between your female hormones and your GI tract is the first step toward understanding any digestive symptoms you may be experiencing.

MENSTRUATION

If you're in tune with your body, you may have noticed that your bowel movements are a little looser or firmer at certain times of the month. This is perfectly normal and probably results from fluctuating levels of the hormones estrogen and progesterone. Some women, however, can't help but notice their hormonal highs and lows because they become extremely bloated and

Periodic Symptoms

"I always know when my period's coming. I can predict it almost to the hour. I get horrible cramps combined with diarrhea almost immediately after eating. This happens about a day before my period starts and lasts for the first few days of menstrual bleeding. While I have my period, I feel queasy all the time, and I find I can't stomach anything more than a few crackers or a bowl of cereal. Even that can set off my cramps and diarrhea. When I was in college, my roommates knew that we had to eat at a dining hall table that was closest to the bathroom whenever I had my period. Sometimes I have only about thirty seconds to race there before I explode. Once my period ends, my symptoms vanish. I only have diarrhea once in a while the rest of the month—usually if I'm really stressed. What's strange and amazing, though, is that my symptoms have become much, much milder since my pregnancy and the birth of my daughter. I don't know what pregnancy did to my body to help cure this problem, but I'm certainly not worrying about it. I'm just thankful that I feel better."

—**Nicole B.,** 30, mother of a two-year-old, who has suffered from IBS for the past fifteen years

constipated during the last half of their menstrual cycle, from ovulation until their period begins.

When your period begins (day one of your cycle), your estrogen and progesterone levels are at generally their lowest levels. After your period ends, your hormone levels gradually rise, and the inner lining of your uterus, the endometrium, begins to grow and thicken in preparation for pregnancy. At the same time follicle-stimulating hormone (FSH), which is produced in a

MIDDLE-OF-THE-MONTH TWINGES

Some women can tell exactly when they're ovulating. They feel abdominal pain when the ovarian follicle ruptures and the egg is released. The pain can range from a mild sensation to severe pain that some women mistake for appendicitis. The pain is usually sudden, sharp, and localized to one side below the navel. This phenomenon is called *Mittelschmerz*, a German word that means "middle pain."

part of the brain known as the pituitary gland, is released, which triggers your ovaries to produce follicles (egg sacs). The follicles grow and ripen until luteinizing hormone (LH), another substance from the pituitary gland, is released, causing the largest follicle to burst and release an egg around day fourteen. This event is known as ovulation. What's interesting is that many women whose digestive problems are tied to their menstrual cycle often find that their symptoms get better, or are at least less noticeable, during these first fourteen days of their cycle, which is called the follicular phase.

The last fourteen days of the menstrual cycle, called the luteal phase, or premenstrual period, is when women are most likely to feel digestive twinges. Estrogen and progesterone levels are at their highest, which sets the stage for reflux, bloating, and constipation. Progesterone is thought to decrease the movement of food through the digestive tract, according to a number of research studies. It can delay stomach emptying, which can cause heartburn (also known as reflux) as the acid and food sitting in the stomach can backwash up into your esophagus. Rising progesterone levels can result in bloating and constipation as food moves more slowly through the intestines. It can also aggravate hemorrhoids. Estrogen may also play a role in this process, but the research is too scant to know for certain.

After ovulation, the ruptured follicle becomes the corpus luteum, a clump of yellow tissue that churns out progesterone. Acting in harmony, estrogen and progesterone activate the tissue lining in the uterus to prepare a thick carpet of blood vessels where, if pregnancy occurs, a fertilized egg can attach and develop. If an egg is fertilized, this blood-vessel blanket will supply nutrients for the developing placenta. Gastrointestinal symptoms can get worse as estrogen and progesterone levels soar to nourish the pregnancy.

If pregnancy doesn't occur, estrogen and progesterone levels plunge, and the endometrial lining is shed during menstruation. Blood vessels are shorn off as the lining is shed, which causes the release of prostaglandins, chemicals that clot the blood to prevent hemorrhaging. These very same chemicals also interact with the digestive tract—increasing the movement of food through the system. As a result, you may experience looser stools or even diarrhea during the first few days of your period. (High levels of prostaglandins are released during labor, which is why some women in labor experience acute vomiting and/or diarrhea.)

I've outlined the possible digestive disturbances you may experience due to cyclical hormonal changes. But I can tell you that every woman is different. Some of my patients tell me that the only time they're free of digestive distress is during the ten days in the middle of their

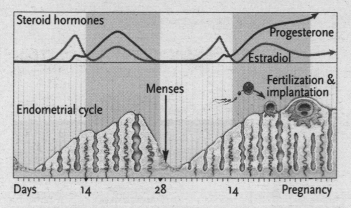

The female hormones released during a menstrual cycle impact the GI tract. This is why some women experience bloating, constipation, cramps, and other digestive symptoms during their period.

cycle. Others say they notice absolutely no change in their symptoms during the course of their cycle.

What is known is that 30 to 50 percent of all women report having some change in their bowel habits during the course of their menstrual cycle. Researchers believe that hormonal fluctuations may be the cause. Most women find that they can live with the monthly symptoms if they make a few dietary adjustments. You may, however, need to see a doctor if you find that any monthly gastrointestinal symptoms are interfering with your life.

Premenstrual Syndrome (PMS): Your GI Action Plan

An estimated 80 percent of women in their reproductive years experience some emotional or physical symptoms

MENSTRUAL PHASE	TYPICAL NUMBER OF DAYS	HORMONAL ACTIONS	DIGESTIVE CHANGES
Follicular (Proliferative) Phase	Days 1 to 6: beginning of menstruation to end of blood flow	Estrogen and progesterone start out at their lowest levels. FSH levels rise to stimulate the maturity of follicles. The ovaries start producing estrogen and levels rise, while progesterone remains low. Prostaglandins are released, which speeds the motility of the GI tract.	Diarrhea and looser bowel movements occur, sometimes accompanied by cramping. IBS sufferers may develop symptoms during this time, probably due to a sudden drop in hormone levels.
	Days 7 to 13: The endometrium thickens to prepare for the egg implantation.	Estrogen levels continue to rise.	This may be the best time of the month, when digestive symptoms are least likely to occur.
Ovulation	Day 14:	LH surges. The largest follicle bursts and releases the egg into the fallopian tube. Estrogen levels are at a peak.	Stomach pain may arise around time of ovulation, which could be due to the ovary releasing the egg—not a GI problem.

MENSTRUAL PHASE	TYPICAL NUMBER OF DAYS	HORMONAL ACTIONS	DIGESTIVE CHANGES
Luteal (Secretory) Phase, also known as the Premenstrual Phase	Days 15 to 28:	The ruptured follicle develops into the corpus luteum, which produces progesterone. Progesterone and estrogen stimulate a blanket of blood vessels to prepare for egg implantation.	Progesterone levels reach their peak, triggering constipation, reflux, and bloating in some women. Women may experience PMS symptoms like mood swings, depression, and headaches.
	If fertilization occurs:	The fertilized egg attaches to the blanket of blood vessels, which supplies nutrients for the developing placenta. The corpus luteum continues to produce estrogen and progesterone.	Digestive problems like nausea, bloating, and constipation may become worse as hormone levels soar.
	If fertilization does not occur:	The corpus luteum deteriorates. Estrogen and progesterone levels drop. The blood-vessel lining sloughs off, and menstruation begins. Prostaglandins are released to stem blood flow.	Women usually notice a change in bowel habits during their periods. Some get looser stools or diarrhea due to the release of prostaglandins.

in the days leading up to their periods. Along with weight gain, headache, depression, and irritability, PMS can also cause gastrointestinal disturbances like abdominal bloating, constipation, and diarrhea. Research suggests that changing your diet and exercise habits during the two weeks before your period may help to reduce gastrointestinal problems and other symptoms associated with PMS.

What to Eat:
Unrefined Carbohydrates.   Eating carbohydrates in moderation can help ward off the mood swings, depression, and irritability that come with PMS. Your body uses glucose—a basic sugar that your body makes from all the carbohydrates you consume—to manufacture serotonin, a brain chemical that improves your mood. Women with PMS often have low levels of serotonin, and research suggests that this may fuel cravings for pretzels, brownies, and other carbohydrate-rich foods. All too often we give in to our cravings in an attempt to take the edge off of PMS moodiness.

I'm not going to tell you to fight these cravings, but I do recommend that you feed them with low-fat, nutritious carbohydrates like whole-grain bread, high-fiber cereal, brown rice, fruits, and vegetables. They'll increase your serotonin levels as much as starchy snack foods will, but their high-fiber content will also help you avoid constipation. What's more, they'll help keep your blood sugar levels stable, so you won't get the sugar highs and lows that can exacerbate mood swings associated with PMS. And you'll wind up eating fewer calo-

DO YOU HAVE ENDOMETRIOSIS?

GI problems that get worse when you have your period may be caused by endometriosis, a painful, chronic disease that affects more than five million women in the United States. It occurs when the endometrium grows outside the uterus and wraps itself around other pelvic organs like the ovaries, fallopian tubes, and bowel. It may also grow in the cavity between the vagina and rectum and on the cervix, bladder, and vulva.

This misplaced tissue responds to the menstrual cycle in the same way the uterine lining does. Each month it builds up, breaks downs, and sheds during menstruation. But the blood and tissue shed from endometrial growths have no way of leaving the body. This results in internal bleeding, inflammation, and the formation of scar tissue and adhesions, which can lead to abdominal pain, bowel problems, and infertility.

You may have endometriosis if you have:

- painful bowel movements during your period
- diarrhea, constipation, or nausea that gets worse during your period
- very painful periods
- pain during sex
- infertility
- painful urination

If you suspect you have endometriosis, you should seek help from your gynecologist. After a pelvic exam, your doctor may begin treatment, though the condition can be definitively diagnosed only via a laparoscopy. This procedure involves making a small incision (usually near the belly button), through which a flexible lighted tube called a laparoscope is inserted. Your doctor can see any endometrial lesions through the laparoscope. Treatment de-

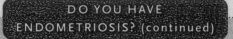

DO YOU HAVE
ENDOMETRIOSIS? (continued)

pends on the degree of your symptoms and can range from simple observation to treatment with hormones (progesterone pill
or injections or oral contraceptives) to a hysterectomy in women
who are finished with childbearing.

For more information on endometriosis, contact:

Endometriosis Association
8585 North 76th Place
Milwaukee, WI 53223 U.S.A.
tel. (414) 355-2200
fax (414) 355-6065

ries, helping you avoid weight gain during this time of
the month.

Some of my patients have told me that they've found
relief from their mood swings and depression from an
over-the-counter complex-carbohydrate powdered
drink called PMS Escape. They've found that their carbohydrate cravings disappear when they have this
drink, and that it helps them avoid weight gain during
this time of the month. Still, you can probably save
money and get the same result by switching from white
bread to whole-wheat bread, from sugar cereal to oatmeal, and from pretzels to apple slices and celery sticks
spread with peanut butter.

Lower Your Intake of Saturated Fat. When you have PMS,
lowering your intake of fatty cuts of beef and whole-
milk dairy products may help reduce abdominal bloat-

ing. A 2000 study reported that women who followed a low-fat vegetarian diet for two menstrual cycles experienced less bloating and a shorter duration of premenstrual symptoms than those who ate a typical American fast-food diet. A handful of studies have also found that women who eat one or two servings a day of fish rich in omega-3 fatty acids (dark-fleshed fish like salmon, tuna, and mackerel) experience less PMS discomfort.

Less Salt? Moderating your salt intake probably won't hurt you, but will it help reduce fluid retention? I suppose it probably can reduce swelling in the arms and legs in women who are salt sensitive, but I don't think it has much impact on abdominal bloat. All the research I've seen points the other way—that reducing salt intake won't help abdominal bloating. The best advice I can give is to try cutting back on salt if you are bloated in your abdomen or your extremities to see if it works for you.

What to Drink: To help reduce bloating, drink plenty of water. Avoid sugary soft drinks, caffeinated beverages, and alcohol.

Supplements to Consider:

Calcium. Research has found that supplemental calcium can dramatically reduce PMS symptoms. In one study, women who took 1200 milligrams of calcium a day for three months had a 50 percent reduction in the severity of their PMS symptoms. One caveat: Calcium supplements can be very constipating, so if you suffer from premenstrual constipation, I wouldn't recommend taking them. Instead, you can get your calcium from foods like low-fat dairy products, dark green vegetables, nuts, grains, beans, and canned salmon and sardines (which include bones). On the other hand, if you experience premenstrual diarrhea, a calcium supplement may help alleviate this symptom.

Vitamin B_6.   Some clinical evidence suggests that vitamin B_6 may be beneficial in reducing PMS symptoms, including depression. You can take 50 to 100 milligrams a day; start with a lower dose, and increase if the lower dose doesn't have much effect. I wouldn't go beyond 100 milligrams, however, since high doses of B_6 (500 milligrams or more daily over a long period) can lead to nerve damage, causing instability and numbness in the feet and hands. Note: If you take 50 milligrams or more of vitamin B_6 for a prolonged time and stop suddenly, you might develop what's known as rebound deficiency. Taper off the supplements slowly, and increase your intake of vitamin B_6 foods like lean cuts of beef (top round, sirloin, eye round), omega-3-rich fish, poultry, whole grains, dried fortified cereals, soybeans, avocados, baked potatoes with skins, watermelon, plantains, bananas, and peanuts.

Vitamin B_1.   One study found that taking B_1 (thiamine) relieved menstrual pain. Thiamine is found in almost all foods, but the best source is pork. Stick with the lean cuts. Other good sources are vitamin B–fortified cereals, oatmeal, and sunflower seeds.

Oral Contraceptives to Combat PMS?

If you aren't trying to get pregnant, oral contraceptives may be one way to help alleviate gastrointestinal symptoms by keeping your hormone levels fairly stabilized throughout the month. Oral contraceptives are extremely effective at preventing pregnancy and may also have other benefits like a reduced incidence of ovarian cancer and less painful periods. You should use a type of pill that delivers the same dose of hormones every day (except for the placebo days) rather than a formulation that delivers varying doses of hormones.

My colleague Dr. Kathie Hullfish, an obstetrician-gynecologist at the University of Virginia Hospital, recommends first trying a very-low-dose pill that contains 20 micrograms of estrogen, such as Loestrin 1/20 or Alesse. (Progesterone levels don't vary much from pill to pill.) Compared to other oral contraceptives (which typically have 30 to 50 micrograms of estrogen per pill), these low-dose pills are potentially less likely to cause problems with bloating and constipation. They do, though, have a downside: They're more likely to cause spotting and breakthrough bleeding.

Two new contraceptive options, the contraceptive patch and the vaginal ring, may prove to be gentler on the digestive tract. The patch is worn on the skin, so the hormones are absorbed into the blood without passing through the liver. The vaginal ring is worn in the cervix, so once again hormones bypass the digestive tract. These devices, though, haven't been around long enough for researchers to see if they can indeed ease

Pregnancy Woes

"When I'm pregnant, I have every digestive malady known to man. I get up in the middle of the night from heartburn, and one antacid often doesn't do the trick. I have to take three or four. With my first two pregnancies, I was constipated all the time. And of course, I'm always nauseous for the first three months from morning sickness. What always amazes me is how quickly my stomach troubles clear up after labor. Maybe it's nature's way of helping me care for my newborn baby."

—Judy C., 36, mother of three and pregnant with her fourth

bloating, constipation, and other digestive symptoms that are tied to the menstrual cycle. We'll have to wait and see over the next few years as more and more women try these products, which came onto the market during the last year.

There really is no one-size-fits-all approach to hormonal contraceptives. Many women find that switching to this form of birth control really provides the solution to their symptoms. Others find that these contraceptives have no effect on their symptoms, and a small number find their symptoms get worse. Unfortunately, I can't tell you which particular contraceptive might work best for you. I can only say that if you are debilitated by GI problems every month around the time of your period, it's worth trying the pill, patch, or ring. You might have to try different formulations of hormones to see which one, if any, provides relief.

If you decide to try a new contraceptive, stay on it for

two to three months to see if you notice any improvement in your symptoms. (You may feel worse during the first few weeks as your body adjusts to the hormones.)

PREGNANCY

An astonishing 90 percent of women develop gastrointestinal complaints during pregnancy. Everything about pregnancy sets you up for digestive problems. First of all, pregnancy creates the "big squeeze." As your expanding uterus and developing fetus take up room in your abdominal cavity, all your other organs get squeezed upward into a smaller and smaller space. As a result, you're more likely to suffer from heartburn and indigestion.

Some women find that certain foods or smells make them queasy; others have to eat small amounts of food throughout the day to avoid nausea, indigestion, and heartburn. Altered bowel functioning may cause bloating and constipation—or have the opposite effect. The good news is that all of these symptoms are common and normal during pregnancy, and most pregnant women don't need to see a gastroenterologist for treatment.

Morning Sickness

Pregnancy bathes your body in hormones. During the first few weeks, rising levels of estrogen and the pregnancy hormone beta-HCG trigger changes that can cause nausea and cause your stomach to empty more slowly than usual. This combination sets the stage for morning sickness—although the 70 percent of pregnant

MY QUICK CURES FOR MORNING SICKNESS

DO . . .

- Keep a box of crackers by your bed, and nibble a few in the morning before getting up. Nausea and vomiting frequently strike on an empty stomach.
- Eat smaller meals more frequently throughout the day. Symptoms can get worse if your stomach is too full or too empty.
- Have a dose of ginger. Steep a piece of fresh ginger in some boiling water to make ginger tea. Several studies have found that ginger root is an effective remedy for nausea.
- Try acupressure: Acupuncture and acupressure devices that stimulate the acupuncture point P6 (which is found just above your wrist) have been shown to decrease the nausea of pregnancy. Drugstores and health food stores carry wristbands (one product is called Sea Bands) embedded with a small plastic bead that will press on this point when you wear them.
- Get plenty of rest. Most of us need at least eight hours of sleep a night, and many pregnant women need even more. Catch a catnap in the afternoon, or go to bed an hour earlier.
- If the nausea and vomiting continue, ask your doctor if you can take antacids, which are generally considered safe for pregnant women. Some prescription medications like metoclopramide (Reglan) may be safe to take when you're pregnant as long as you get your doctor's okay.

DON'T . . .

- Drink too much water with meals. A combination of food and excess fluid can fill your stomach to capacity, triggering nausea and worsening heartburn.
- Eat greasy or fried foods. These can be harder on your system because they empty more slowly from your stomach, and— with your enlarging uterus pressing against your stomach— having food in your stomach for too long can set you up for heartburn and make you feel queasy.

Note: In some cases nausea and vomiting may be severe enough to warrant medical intervention. If your distress is severe and is causing dehydration or keeping you from gaining enough weight during your pregnancy, talk with your doctor.

women who experience these symptoms know that they can occur at any time of day.

Morning sickness does run in families, so if your mother and sister suffered from it, you're more likely to experience it as well. It is also linked to a heightened sense of smell and taste during pregnancy. You may have strong aversions to certain foods, which can trigger nausea and vomiting.

The good news is, morning sickness does seem to serve a purpose. Women who experience nausea and vomiting have decreased rates of miscarriage and preterm labor. In severe cases, morning sickness may require a woman to be hospitalized due to severe dehydration caused by excessive vomiting. But this condition, called hyperemesis gravidarum, is rare, only occurring in about one percent of pregnancies.

Heartburn

This condition is perhaps even more common than morning sickness, afflicting as many as 80 percent of pregnant women. Once again the squeezing of the organs and the delayed emptying of the stomach are to blame. Heartburn occurs when a small amount of the acid and food churning around in your stomach washes back up into your esophagus. Normally, the one-way "valve" called the lower esophageal sphincter (LES) closes off your esophagus from your stomach and opens only when you swallow to let food enter your stomach. This valve, though, sometimes opens at inappropriate times, especially as LES pressure decreases throughout pregnancy. (Pressure reaches a nadir immediately before delivery, when estrogen and progesterone levels peak.)

Heartburn most commonly strikes during the third trimester (28 to 40 weeks), though plenty of patients come to see me in their first or second trimester complaining of symptoms. Many women feel the classic signs of a burning pain in their sternum or chest area and food and acid backwash in the back of their throat. Some have less common symptoms like throat clearing, hoarseness in their voice, or a chronic cough. No matter how heartburn manifests itself, most pregnant women just have to live through it or seek relief through over-the-counter antacids, which are generally safe to take if you have your doctor's approval. Over-the-counter acid-blockers (like Zantac, Pepcid, Tagamet, and Axid) are usually safe, but again, speak to your doctor before you take them. (See Chapter 4 for additional tips on

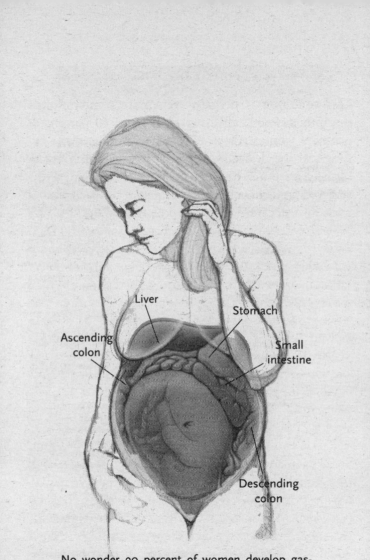

Liver

Ascending colon

Stomach

Small intestine

Descending colon

No wonder 90 percent of women develop gastrointestinal complaints during pregnancy! As the fetus grows, the uterus pushes against your internal organs, resulting in heartburn, indigestion, and other discomforts.

	DRUG NAME	SAFETY IN PREGNANCY AND BREAST-FEEDING	COMMENTS
For Peptic Ulcer Disease and Heartburn	**Antacids** calcium, magnesium, and aluminum antacids	safe	no controlled trials, but widely used and believed to be safe
	sodium bicarbonate	unknown	avoid in pregnancy because of potential for fluid overload in mother and fetus
	H₂ blockers cimetidine (Tagamet)	probably safe	no association with birth defects; excreted into breast milk
	famotidine (Pepcid)	probably safe	no evidence of adverse effects; less excretion in breast milk than cimetidine and ranitidine
	nizatidine (Axid)	unknown	no studies in humans; birth defects seen in rabbits
	ranitidine (Zantac)	probably safe	no association with birth defects; excreted into breast milk

	DRUG NAME	SAFETY IN PREGNANCY AND BREAST-FEEDING	COMMENTS
For Peptic Ulcer Disease and Heartburn (continued)	**PPIs** esomeprazole (Nexium)	probably safe	no adequate studies in women; excretion into breast milk has not been studied
	lansoprazole (Prevacid)	probably safe	no adequate studies in women; excretion into breast milk has not been studied
	omeprazole (Prilosec)	unknown	no adequate studies in women; excretied into breast milk
	rabeprazole (Aciphex)	probably safe	no adequate studies in women; excretion into breast milk has not been studied
	pantoprazole (Protonix)	probably safe	no adequate studies in women; excretion into breast milk has not been studied
	Prokinetics metoclopramide (Reglan)	unknown	effects of long-term use in pregnancy unknown; excreted into breast milk

	DRUG NAME	SAFETY IN PREGNANCY AND BREAST-FEEDING	COMMENTS
For Peptic Ulcer Disease and Heartburn (continued)	Other misoprostol (Cytotec)	contraindicated	can induce abortion; may possibly cause birth defects; excretion into breast milk unknown but potential cause of severe diarrhea in nursing infants
	sucralfate (Carafate)	safe	no association with birth defects; breast-feeding likely safe due to minimal excretion into breast milk
For Diarrhea	loperamide (Imodium)	probably safe	probably safe for short-term use
	diphenoxylate (Lomotil, Lonox)	unknown	should be used only when clearly needed during pregnancy; excreted into breast milk, but probably safe for breast-feeding
For Constipation	castor oil	unknown	may cause premature contractions

	DRUG NAME	SAFETY IN PREGNANCY AND BREAST-FEEDING	COMMENTS
For Constipation (continued)	hyperosmotic agents, lactulose (Kristalose, Chronulac)	probably safe	approximarely 3% absorbed; should be used only if clearly needed during pregnancy; excretion into breast milk has not been studied
	fiber (Metamucil, Citrucel)	safe	not absorbed by the body; preferred treatment for constipation
	mineral oil	unknown	chronic use may lead to decreased absorption of fat-soluble vitamins, which can cause malnutrition in the fetus
	saline laxatives (milk of magnesia, Fleet's Phospho-Soda)	unknown	may cause volume overload or electrolyte disturbances
For Irritable Bowel Syndrome	**Constipation-dominant**		
	tegaserod (Zelnorm)	probably safe	should be used only when clearly needed during pregnancy; unknown excretion into breast milk

	DRUG NAME	SAFETY IN PREGNANCY AND BREAST-FEEDING	COMMENTS
For Irritable Bowel Syndrome (continued)	**Diarrhea-dominant** alosetron (Lotronex)	probably safe	should be used only when clearly needed during pregnancy; unknown excretion into breast milk
	Antispasmodics dicyclomine (Bentyl)	probably safe	should be used only when clearly needed during pregnancy; excreted into breast milk and should not be used during breast feeding
	hyoscyamine (Levsin, Anaspaz)	unknown	should be used only when clearly needed during pregnancy; may be excreted into breast milk
For Inflammatory Bowel Disease	**5-ASAs** sulfasalazine (Azulfidine)	probably safe	widely used and considered safe, but should supplement diet with folate; excreted in breast milk and one case report of bloody diarrhea in breast-fed infant
	mesalamine (Asacol, Canasa, Colazal, Pentasa, Rowasa)	use caution	considered safe; excreted in breast milk; may cause diarrhea in breast-fed infant

	DRUG NAME	SAFETY IN PREGNANCY AND BREAST-FEEDING	COMMENTS
For Inflammatory Bowel Disease (continued)	olsalazine (Dipentum)	safe	excreted in breast milk; be on guard for diarrhea in breast-fed infant
	Steroids corticosteroids (prednisone, prednisolone)	probably safe	extensive experience has found them to be safe
	budesonide (Entocort EC)	unknown, use with caution	should be used only when clearly needed during pregnancy; excreted into breast milk
	Immunomodulators azathioprine (Imuran)	unknown, use with caution	use with caution only when clearly needed during pregnancy; may cause growth retardation in fetus and premature delivery
	6-mercaptopurine (Purinethol)	unknown, use with caution	use with caution only when clearly needed during pregnancy; excretion into breast milk has not been studied, but probably should not be used during breast-feeding

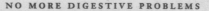

**DIGESTIVE MEDICATIONS DURING PREGNANCY
AND NURSING: WHAT'S SAFE, WHAT'S NOT
(CONTINUED)**

	DRUG NAME	SAFETY IN PREGNANCY AND BREAST-FEEDING	COMMENTS
For Inflammatory Bowel Disease (continued)	cyclosporine (Neoral)	unknown, use with caution	should be used only when clearly needed during pregnancy; excreted into breast milk and should not be used during breast-feeding
	infliximab (Remicade)	unknown, use with caution	should be used only when clearly needed during pregnancy, no studies in pregnant women; unknown excretion into breast milk
	methotrexate	contraindicated	may harm fetus

relieving heartburn.) The good news is that although heartburn is common during pregnancy, it's rarely serious. Esophageal damage from pregnancy-induced reflux doesn't occur very often. What's more, in 98 percent of women who had symptoms during pregnancy, heartburn disappears almost immediately after birth.

Constipation

As your body expands and your baby grows at an ever-quickening pace, you may not think of pregnancy as the great body slowdown. But that's exactly what it is: High levels of the hormone progesterone cause your GI tract muscles to relax, causing food to move through it more slowly. This can bring on constipation. Taking a calcium or iron supplement or a prenatal vitamin that contains iron can add to your troubles.

As a general rule, if you go more than three days without a bowel movement, you're setting yourself up for constipation. To stay regular, increase your intake of fiber-rich foods like dried prunes or figs, vegetables, legumes, bran cereals, and whole-grain breads. Drink several glasses of water a day to increase the fluid content of your stool. And keep yourself moving by walking, swimming, or other moderate exercise. Exercise speeds digestion and helps food move through your intestines at a quicker rate. *Note: Don't take any herbal remedies for constipation or over-the-counter laxatives when you're pregnant, without your doctor's consent. Many of these can be harmful to the fetus.*

Hemorrhoids

The pressure of the fetus in the uterus, worsening constipation, and hormonal changes can all cause your hemorrhoidal veins to enlarge. These veins are located around your anus and tend to dilate and swell due to an increase in blood volume during pregnancy. Excess straining or constipation can make swelling worse, causing irritation, itchiness, and bleeding. You may get hemorrhoids for the first time during pregnancy, or you may find that pregnancy makes existing hemorrhoids more severe. All too frequently hemorrhoids remain after childbirth and become a chronic condition. On some occasions these veins—placed under severe pressure during delivery—may even fall down (prolapse) through the anus and protrude outside the body. When this happens, the vein may become irritated and painful and require removal by your doctor.

Like other GI problems that occur during pregnancy, the best way to deal with hemorrhoids is to avoid getting them in the first place by preventing constipation. You should also avoid sitting in one position for a long period of time. Over-the-counter treatments like Preparation H can be safely used during pregnancy and can help provide relief. But make sure to get your doctor's okay before using them.

MENOPAUSE

Kristy came to me several years ago complaining of severe rectal pain and told me she was always constipated. "I spend hours every day glued to my toilet seat straining and straining," she complained. "I've missed important meetings at work, and I think my husband is losing patience. We missed the first act of an opera the other night because of my date with the bathroom." The fifty-five-year-old woman, who had remarried only a few months earlier, told me her honeymoon with her new husband was definitely over.

I examined Kristy by performing a rectal exam and

discovered that she had a rectocele, or small hernia between the vagina and the rectum. It is a type of pelvic
floor dysfunction, or a weakening of the pelvic floor muscles, tissues, and nerves, that often occurs from previous
pregnancies, aging, and menopausal changes. Kristy had
two children with her first husband, and ever since her
second child was born fifteen years ago, she had had occasional trouble with urinary incontinence—when she
laughed too hard or sneezed repeatedly. Kristy was
amazed to find out that her constipation was actually related to her pelvic floor muscles. I gave her instructions
for treating her constipation with the standard remedies
like stool softeners, milk of magnesia, and an occasional
enema when her constipation was at its worst. But I also
taught Kristy how to squeeze and tighten her pelvic floor
muscles (using what are called Kegel exercises; see the box
on page 72) to help prevent constipation and avoid urinary incontinence. She promised to do them for a few
minutes every day.

After listening to Kristy's misery over her lost honeymoon, I decided to refer her to a psychologist that I work
with. Kristy talked to the psychologist about the stress of
her marriage and the difficulties her teenagers were hav
ing adjusting to her new husband. She noticed that her
constipation got worse when she was depressed or on
edge. "I just needed to talk through some of my family
problems," she later told me, "and I realized that I was
beating up my body—straining and straining and straining—to try to get some control over my life. I would force
my body to do what I wanted it to, even if I couldn't force
my family to get along." Having this self-realization,

A WORD ABOUT HRT

The medical community now recognizes menopause for what it is: a natural life transition. Not all women need to be "treated" with hormone replacement therapy (HRT), contrary to what some doctors believed years ago. HRT can play a beneficial role if you suffer from hot flashes, mood swings, or vaginal dryness, but it isn't risk free. That was certainly made very clear after researchers decided to halt a large-scale clinical trial, called the Women's Health Initiative, ten years before it was slated to end. Preliminary results showed that women who took a combination of estrogen and progesterone for more than five years had a 26 percent increase in breast cancer, a 41 percent increase in strokes, and a 29 percent increase in heart attacks compared to women who did not take hormones. These health risks outweighed the benefits of a 37 percent reduced risk of colorectal cancer and a 34 percent lower rate of hip fractures. The general consensus among medical experts is that HRT certainly shouldn't be given routinely to women entering menopause, although it can still be useful on a short-term basis to alleviate hot flashes, mood swings, and other menopausal symptoms. When deciding whether to take HRT, you need to consider your own health history and talk with your doctor about your personal risks and benefits.

I have to admit that I feel conflicted about the results of this and other HRT research. I think they have given women the wrong message: that they shouldn't take hormones, no matter what. The truth is, HRT may be necessary if menopausal symptoms are destroying the quality of your life. The therapy may also be beneficial if you have a strong history of colon cancer in your family—say, a mother and sister who

had colon cancer. Ditto if you have a family history of osteoporosis or a bone scan showing significant bone loss. So I'm
not just taking an easy way out by saying talk to your doctor. I
really do think you need to consider your own personal health
issues and your own risk of developing certain diseases—not
the overall risk of the general female population that was rep-
resented in this research.

Kristy no longer spent hours straining in the bathroom or
allowed herself to get stressed when she couldn't have a
bowel movement. Learning that she could have some
positive influence over her body with the exercises and
the treatments enabled Kristy to relax, which helped her
deal with her condition—and her life.

Menopause can have profound effects on gastrointestinal function. For some women, these effects can be
positive. For instance, women who take iron supplements or medications for uterine fibroids and conse-
quently experience constipation and bloating often find
that these symptoms clear up when they enter menopause and no longer need to take these medications. (Fibroids, benign tumors that can cause heavy periods,
usually shrink and disappear on their own after menopause, so treatment is no longer necessary.) Case in
point: About 60 percent of women with IBS who had
hysterectomies to remove large fibroids experienced an
improvement in their symptoms after undergoing the
procedure, according to a study from the University
Hospital of South Manchester in Great Britain. This may
be because these women were finally able to abandon
their fibroid-shrinking medications.

Some women, however, do experience gastrointestinal problems when they reach menopause. Symptoms often appear well before complete cessation of menstruation, during the period known as perimenopause. They are thought to be a result of the wide swings in levels of estrogen and progesterone that can continue throughout the decade or so before a woman's last period. With the onset of menopause itself, hormones stabilize at their lowest levels since puberty. Researchers at Stanford University found that perimenopausal and postmenopausal women have a high prevalence of bowel-related problems (diarrhea, constipation, abdominal pain, gas/flatulence) compared to premenopausal women. In a study of 228 women, the researchers found that 14 percent of premenopausal women reported having bowel problems compared to 36 percent of perimenopausal women and 38 percent of postmenopausal women. Perimenopausal women seemed to have the most severe symptoms.

I wish I had a simple explanation for why these symptoms strike at the onset of menopause. The truth is, we don't really know for sure. Declining levels of estrogen and progesterone should help alleviate digestive disturbances that are linked to the menstrual cycle. And yes, many women do find that they feel better when they reach menopause. But some women may find that the hormonal decline actually exacerbates symptoms.

Here's what we do know: Postmenopausal women are more likely to suffer from constipation. The decline in estrogen can cause extensive vaginal dryness, and dry tissues tend to be weaker and offer less support. Thus, your rectum has less-supportive tissues and muscles surrounding it. Stool may be difficult to pass if your pelvic floor muscles are weak, and this can cause constipation. Another possible explanation: Aging causes cells lining your intestinal tract to secrete less of the mucus that lubricates your stool. As a result, stools are harder and drier, which makes them more difficult to pass. All this straining can lead to other problems in the rectal area like rectal prolapse (in which part of the rectum protrudes through the anus) or a rectocele (a small hernia between the rectum and vagina), the problem that brought Kristy to my office.

Weight gain can also play a major role in GI problems that occur in your fifties. The average woman (and man, for that matter) gradually gains about 25 to 30 pounds between age twenty and fifty, which greatly increases the likelihood of getting GI problems like gastroesophageal reflux disease (GERD) and gallbladder disease (more on weight issues in the next chapter).

Pelvic floor dysfunction can factor in as well, especially in lower-GI problems that occur in middle age. Nerves and muscles in the pelvic floor are normally stretched during vaginal childbirth, and for most women these muscles spring back without causing problems. Some women, though, may develop a permanent weakness in their pelvic floor muscles if they had difficult vaginal labors with prolonged pushing. Others find that their muscles got weaker with each pregnancy. Pelvic floor dysfunction—as the condition is called—commonly causes urinary incontinence since the muscles that surrounded and supported the bladder are weakened.

Pelvic floor muscles also support the tissue layer between the intestines and rectum. Without this support, you may experience an array of digestive ills from constipation to hemorrhoids to fecal incontinence, all of which become more common after menopause.

ANATOMY OF YOUR PELVIC ORGANS

When medical professionals talk about "pelvic organs," they mean much more than just the reproductive organs. Yes, your ovaries, uterus, fallopian tubes, and vagina lie in the space between your pelvic bones. But so do your rectum, anus, bladder, and urethra. All of these can be affected if you develop weakness in your pelvic support muscles.

The urethra (a short, narrow tube) and bladder lie in front of the vagina. The bladder receives and stores urine from your kidneys and expels it through the urethra. The uterus is at the top of the vagina. Behind the uterus is a space within the pelvic cavity called the cul-de-sac. This space contains some of the small intestine. Along the back of this space is the rectum, which continues down the back of the vagina and ends at the anus. The pelvic organs are held in place by three types of support:

1. Layers of connecting tissue called endopelvic fascia

2. Thickened parts of the fascia called ligaments

3. A paired group of muscles that lies on either side and around the openings of the urethra, vagina, and rectum

If any of these tissues weaken, stretch, or fail to provide support, various problems can result. For instance, the bladder can drop from its normal place and push into the vagina, creating a type of hernia known as a cystocele. You may leak urine if you cough, sneeze, or lift something heavy, or you may have trouble emptying your bladder. A rectocele is another type of hernia in which the rectum

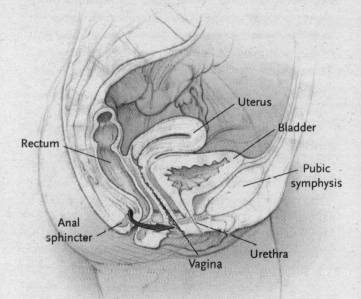

The pelvic floor muscles provide crucial support for the GI tract, bladder, and uterus. If any of these tissues weaken or sag, incontinence or difficulty in having a bowel movement can result. The arrow represents the puborectalis muscle.

STRENGTHEN YOUR PELVIC
FLOOR MUSCLES: DO KEGELS

I strongly recommend Kegel exercises to almost every woman who comes to see me. Kegels (which get their name from Dr. Arnold Kegel) are also referred to as pelvic floor squeezes, perineal exercises, or tightening exercises. They strengthen the pubococcygeus (PC) muscle, one of the main muscles of the pelvic floor that supports your urethra, vagina, uterus, and rectum. Women who strain excessively and have chronic constipation often have weak pelvic floor muscles, as do women who suffer from urinary incontinence. You can treat some forms of pelvic floor dysfunction, and perhaps even prevent it, by doing these exercises. Here's a step-by-step guide for doing Kegels.

1. **Find the right muscles:** More than one-third of women start out squeezing the wrong muscles. Try this helpful tool for finding your PC muscle. Imagine sitting on a chair. On the chair is a marble. Pick up the marble with your vaginal muscles *only* and hold it for a moment. You should feel a small lifting motion as you contract the muscle. You can also find this muscle by placing a finger in your vagina and squeezing around it. When you feel tightening around your finger, you're using the correct muscle. (This is the same muscle that starts and stops the flow of urine, but you shouldn't do Kegels when urinating because this may prevent your bladder from emptying completely, which can promote urinary tract infections.)

2. **Start slowly:** Start by doing Kegel contractions for one to three minutes at a time, twice a day. At first you may not be able to squeeze for longer than a second or two. As your muscles strengthen, you should be able to squeeze for a

count of four and then eventually to a count of ten. Try to keep all your other muscles relaxed as you squeeze the muscle right around your vagina. Do not bear down or squeeze the thigh, back, or abdominal muscles. You should feel a small lifting motion as you contract the muscle. Practice the exercises as you go about your day (though not while urinating). Do fifteen contractions three times a day. You'll also work your muscle more if you do the exercises with your knees apart.

Your pelvic muscles may be sore for the first few days, but that should improve with time, just as with any other exercise. If you need assistance learning this technique, your health care provider may be able to refer you for pelvic floor physical therapy.

3. **Fit them in anytime, anywhere:** Since no one knows when you're doing Kegels, you can do them whenever you feel like it. Do them while standing in line at the bank, while sitting in your car at a red light, or while watching TV. Some women even claim that doing Kegels during intercourse creates a tightness in their vagina that enhances their and their partner's sexual pleasure!

pushes against weakened tissues in the back wall of the vagina. A rectocele may cause constipation by interfering with the rectal muscle contractions. Both of these conditions cause a bulging into the vagina and can be the result of aging, surgery, or pregnancy with vaginal delivery.

Celebrating yourself as a woman is a vital part of staying healthy. I don't want you to see menstruation, pregnancy, and menopause as impediments to your gastrointestinal health. They are natural life phases, not weaknesses. I know they can alter the way your body handles food, and yes, you may experience GI disturbances as a result. But this doesn't mean you're doomed to feel lousy the rest of your life. Rather, it means you need to tune in to your body. Listen to its signals, and make some small adjustments in your lifestyle to keep your digestive system running smoothly. Maybe you need to drink extra water or eat a little more fiber if you're constipated during your period. Perhaps you should eat smaller, more frequent meals during the course of your pregnancy.

In addition to hormones, a host of lifestyle factors, like eating habits, activity levels, and stress levels, can all play a role in digestive disturbances. First, though, you need to think about your weight and what damage you can do trying to achieve the "ideal" weight that every woman envisions for herself. Weight issues come up all the time in my practice. I see overweight women who have heartburn, constipation, or gallbladder disease related to their obesity, and I see emaciated women with eating disorders who have constipation and chronic abdominal pain. I also see women of average weight who seem to be on a new diet every month and don't realize that their chronic dieting can lead to chronic digestive distress. As you'll see in the next chapter, when it comes to gastrointestinal health, weight is definitely a weighty issue.

A WEIGHTY PROBLEM FOR
DIGESTIVE HEALTH

I HAVE YET TO MEET A WOMAN who is completely satisfied with her weight. You may weigh yourself religiously once a day. Or you may eagerly buy any magazine that promises to help you "shed ten pounds in two weeks!" You may just stare in the mirror cursing the bumpy cellulite on the backs of your thighs. Even when a patient comes to my clinic for reflux or constipation, we almost always touch on some aspect of her weight. In most cases we discuss ways that weight affects her digestive tract and really her overall health. For most of my patients (and most Americans), weight issues center on being overweight and ways we can try to lose weight.

I also, though, see patients who are underweight and desperately trying to gain pounds. These women usually suffer from some form of malnourishment due to a particular GI disorder. Some women have celiac sprue, a disorder resulting from an intolerance to wheat and grain products that can cause a decreased absorption of food from the upper GI tract. Others have inflammatory bowel disease, which can prevent the absorption of certain nutrients because of damage to the intestines. Many of us may think that needing to gain weight would be a great problem to have, but in reality underweight patients may struggle as much as overweight patients to reach a healthy weight.

We have become a society of chronic dieters. Just look at the raging popularity of the Atkins diet, Sugar Busters, and the latest Palm Beach Diet. Millions of Americans try these high-protein, low-carbohydrate diets, and yes, many do lose weight on them. But the minute they return to their normal eating habits, they gain it back. And in the process they often wreak havoc on their digestive systems, which I'll talk about a little later.

With all of us dieting, you'd think we'd be thinner as a population. Yet we're not. Americans are heavier than we've ever been. More than 50 percent of us are overweight, and one-third of us are obese. A 2003 study published in the *New England Journal of Medicine* found that although dieters did lose more weight after spending six months on a high-protein, low-carbohydrate diet—they lost an average of fifteen pounds, compared to a six-pound weight loss for those on a reduced-fat, standard-carbohydrate diet—they didn't keep it off. Neither group of dieters in the study was able to successfully maintain the weight loss after one year. What's more, researchers point out that high-protein diets may pose long-term risks such as clogged arteries (from the high saturated fat and cholesterol content), decreased bone mass, and an exacerbation of kidney problems in those with renal disease.

Even clothing designers have recognized that women in this country are getting larger. Plus-size designers have seen skyrocketing profits. And traditional clothing designers have been cutting their sizes larger and larger because they know women are reluctant to buy clothes in a larger size. For instance, today's size 10 really is about the same cut as a size 12 or 14 from the 1980s.

While women indulge in their favorite foods, many of us also feel an enormous sense of guilt that we don't look like the actresses and supermodels that grace the pages of our favorite magazines. Yes, we may realize (somewhere in the rational part of our minds) that these airbrushed, cellulite-free bodies would be impossible for us to attain even if we followed Atkins for the rest of our lives. And yet we still beat ourselves up about the shape of our own bodies.

I admit that I fall into this trap myself. My weight falls into a healthy range, yet whenever I get a compliment about my appearance, my first response is "Oh, but I need to lose a few pounds." I simply can't accept the fact that my body looks fine even with the small protruding tummy left over from my pregnancies. I probably have the same hang-ups that plague most women, and eventually I'll have to just come to terms with my body's flaws.

Some women, however, carry this recognition to an extreme and become obsessed with making their bodies perfect—which usually means excessively thin. They may turn to starvation diets or constant, high-intensity exercise to get as reed-thin as Courteney Cox Arquette on the TV show *Friends*. Eating disorders are on the rise in this country, especially among teens. Many American girls begin dieting as early as age nine and continue to see food as the enemy throughout their teenage years.

Entire books have been written about our love-hate relationship with food, and I can only touch on this subject briefly in this chapter. What I'm leading up to, however, is how your eating habits and weight issues affect the functioning of your digestive tract. Dieting can have a negative impact on how well your body digests food and can lead to constipation, bloating, and other symptoms. Some herbal weight-loss products can cause diarrhea. If you're overweight, you have a higher risk of developing reflux, gallbladder disease, and liver problems. Being unnaturally underweight due to an eating disorder can cause a host of digestive problems, including constipation, bloating, diarrhea, and reflux.

A few months ago Hope, a forty-five-year-old woman struggling with her weight, came to my clinic for some "answers" to her weight problems. Since the birth of her two sons in her late twenties, Hope has been desperately trying to shed the extra forty pounds she gained during her pregnancies. She tried the grapefruit diet, downed Slim Fast shakes, and even managed to lose twenty-one pounds in three months on the Atkins diet—though she says she was always constipated from forgoing her morning bowl of bran cereal. Unfortunately, Hope gained back the weight she'd lost and then some.

Hope's obesity recently began taking a toll on her digestive tract. She had severe attacks of abdominal pain and was diagnosed with gallstones. She had surgery to have her gallbladder removed and was told by her surgeon that the combination of her excess weight and crash-dieting habits probably led to the gallstones in the first place. I don't need to tell you how frustrated Hope was to hear this. She was at the point of throwing in the towel when she came to see me. She posed this question to me: "What's the best way to reach and maintain a healthy weight so I don't have digestive problems in the future?"

That's the billion-dollar question, and it's one that I will answer in this chapter—though as you'll see, I don't give a single-sentence solution or quick-fix approach. I'll explore healthy lifestyle approaches that will help you achieve the weight you desire. Researchers are finding that those who have the most success with maintaining a healthy weight often have to make several attempts at losing weight before they succeed for life. You yourself may have to experiment a little before you find the eating and activity plans that work best for you. The changes you make will have to be ones that you can stick to *for the rest of your life,* whether you need to lose weight or overcome an eating disorder.

Making a commitment to permanent change will have vast rewards. Reaching and maintaining a healthy weight can help you sidestep a wide range of health ills such as diabetes, heart disease, and breast cancer. It can also help improve your digestive function. For instance, eating smaller portions at mealtimes can help you avoid heartburn. Replacing high-fat snacks with fruits and vegetables can help prevent constipation and gallbladder disease. What's more, your weight, independent of your diet, can determine whether you have a healthy digestive tract—especially if you're at either extreme of the weight spectrum.

THE OBESITY EPIDEMIC

Our nation is in a crisis when it comes to obesity. During the 1970s only 14 percent of Americans were obese, compared to 33 percent of Americans who are obese today. At any time about 45 percent of women in this country are actively seeking to lose weight. Why are we losing the weight war?

The issue is complex, but it mostly involves a lot of mixed messages. We've become a lot more savvy about nutrition as more magazines and newspapers cover the latest nutritional research findings. While I applaud these efforts to educate the public, I think a lot of us have wound up confused. In the early 1990s heart disease researcher Dean Ornish published a best-selling book that touted the virtues of a fat-free, high-carbohydrate diet for losing weight and reversing heart disease. We all believed that we could eat more carbohydrates and lose weight, as long as we avoided fat. We piled on the pasta and consumed endless amounts of fat-free cookies and cakes. And guess what? We gained weight.

Striking out against the fat-free movement, researchers at Harvard University told us it was actually the *kind* of fat we were eating—not the *amount*—that led to health ills. They cautioned us to stay away from the saturated fats found in meat, eggs, and whole-milk dairy products and told us to embrace olive oil and other monounsaturated fats.

For about a decade nutrition researchers have

been debating about the best type of eating plan for weight loss. We've seen the resurgence of the Atkins high-protein diet plan, which advocates eating as much fat and protein as you want as long as you abstain from nearly all carbohydrates. Atkins dieters have lost weight by gorging on steak, cheddar cheese, and pork rinds, and Dr. Atkins's diet books have sold more than ten million copies. Diet books touting food-combination eating plans (eat carbohydrates and proteins but not together) have also surged in popularity. Some weight-loss gurus have even designed diets for your specific blood type or personality.

With all the brouhaha over these popular diets, we're definitely getting mixed messages about what we need to do to lose weight. What's more, the most popular weight-loss methods are often far from the healthiest. The Atkins diet is severely lacking in fruits and vegetables—and the vitamins and fiber they contain. Herbal remedies for weight loss are also flying off the shelves, despite the fact that they can be downright dangerous. Some women have suffered strokes or even sudden death after taking weight-loss supplements containing ephedra.

Clearly, our nation has gotten itself into a mess when it comes to weight control. As we search for the magic bullet diet or potion that will melt away pounds, however, we continue to eat more and more calories. Many restaurants have increased portion sizes over the last ten years and actually serve meals on larger plates to accommodate the extra food. Supersize fries and shakes have become a way for fast-food chains to lure in customers.

And let's face it: Many of us have abandoned regular mealtimes and instead eat constantly—snacking our way through the day. (I'm amazed at the amount of food passed around at my children's swim meets!) As a result, we've lost our ability to know when we're hungry and when we're full. Then we wonder why our weight is creeping up when we never actually sit down for a meal. Nutritionists call this Pinocchio dieting, where we trick ourselves into thinking that calories don't count if we don't keep track of the portions we're eating.

The truth is, it doesn't take much overeating to gain weight. Eating just 50 more calories a day than your body burns will cause you to gain five pounds a year. That doesn't leave a lot of leeway for indulging in treats.

That's why exercise is so important. Boosting your calorie burn by 300 calories a day (the equivalent of forty-five minutes of brisk walking or an hour-long leisurely stroll) will help tip the scales in your favor. You'll have more wiggle room to have a dessert you enjoy without tipping the calorie balance to the weight-gain side. With all the complicated nutritional messages being bandied about, the most important one that rings true is this: If you eat more calories than your body burns throughout the day, you will gain weight. If you eat fewer calories than your body burns, you'll lose weight.

IS BEING HEAVY IN YOUR GENES?

You may think you're doomed to be overweight because obesity is in your genes. If your grandmother and mother were overweight, you're bound to be overweight as well, right? Well, yes and no. Genetic patterns

THE HUNGER GENE

Recent research suggests that the digestive system helps control whether a person tends to overeat and gain weight. We've known for years that there are receptors in your stomach and small intestine that sense when you've eaten a large meal and then send signals to your brain that the feeling of hunger has been satiated and that you should stop eating. When your stomach is empty and your body needs food, these same receptors send out a feed-me message to the brain. New findings, however, show that sometimes these messages get mixed up or are never sent. The brain never gets the message of satiety and keeps processing hunger messages.

The culprit may lie in a stomach hormone called ghrelin, which makes people hungry, slows metabolism, and decreases the body's ability to burn fat. Your stomach releases ghrelin in peak amounts before meals and cuts off production of the hormone toward the end of a meal. Studies have shown that people who are injected with ghrelin have huge appetites and eat 30 percent more food than they normally would. Those who have excess levels of ghrelin in their bloodstream appear to have a higher likelihood of becoming obese.

This hormone may be foiling dieters: According to a 2002 study published in the *New England Journal of Medicine*, dieters who lost weight and kept it off made more ghrelin than they did before dieting—as if their bodies were attempting to regain the lost fat. The study also found that people who had a stomach-reduction surgery called gastric bypass to lose weight wound up producing very little ghrelin, which could explain why they have a large appetite reduction after surgery.

This exciting piece of research made national headlines,

THE HUNGER GENE (continued)

but I'm reserving judgment on how big a role ghrelin plays until more studies are done. This particular study included only twenty-eight people, and experts say that ghrelin may not be involved in most cases of obesity. Still, I think it's intriguing that the gastrointestinal tract may hold one key to managing obesity.

for obesity do run in families. In studies of obese children, one or both parents were obese in 72 percent of cases. Having two obese parents gives a child a ten times greater risk of becoming obese as an adult. What's more, there are a variety of genetic syndromes that can trigger obesity, like polycystic ovarian syndrome, a hormone imbalance occurring in women that prevents ovulation and leads to excess abdominal fat.

But obesity genes only partly explain why our nation is overweight. They certainly don't account for the recent rise in obesity. The proportion of obese Americans has increased by more than 50 percent during the past two decades, yet it takes thousands of years for our genes to change. Our bodies, however, are genetically programmed to conserve fat in the good times in order to prepare us for the lean times like war or famine. Fortunately, most Americans haven't experienced these lean times, so our bodies continue to conserve fat while waiting for the war to break out.

For the most part, people who become obese have a chronic energy imbalance: They take in more calories than their body uses. Why this occurs may be due to certain genes that control whether they feel hungry or full and whether their body uses food for energy or fat storage.

Clearly, though, a mixture of genes and environment plays a role in most cases of obesity. Unfortunately, once obesity sets in, it tends to be lifelong unless adjustments are made in food-intake or activity levels. Yes, taking off weight does take work, but not as much as you might think. It's far more effective to make small changes—like cutting out your predinner snack or taking a daily one-mile stroll—that you'll stick with forever than it is to go on a drastic diet.

WHAT'S YOUR WEIGHT RISK?

Whenever I see a patient for the first time, I measure her weight and height, and then I calculate what is called a body mass index (BMI). This calculation, which is a ratio of height to weight, gives me a pretty clear indication if she's underweight, normal weight, overweight (up to thirty pounds above her ideal weight range), or obese (thirty pounds or more above her ideal weight range). Use the chart on page 86 to find your own BMI.

These calculations are based on obesity research linking weight to an increased risk of health problems like heart disease and diabetes. But I personally think that if you're at the upper limit of your appropriate weight range, you're already a little on the heavy side. I've seen many patients with digestive problems linked to their weight who are at the upper end of normal, and sometimes losing just ten pounds can make all the difference.

BMIs also don't tell the whole story with regard to weight. In recent years researchers have been focusing on

BODY MASS INDEX CHART

HEIGHT (FEET AND INCHES)

	5'0"	5'1"	5'2"	5'3"	5'4"	5'5"	5'6"	5'7"	5'8"	5'9"	5'10"	5'11"	6'0"	6'1"	6'2"	6'3"	6'4"
100	20	19	18	18	17	17	16	16	15	15	14	14	14	13	13	12	12
105	21	20	19	19	18	17	17	16	16	16	15	15	14	14	13	13	13
110	21	21	20	19	19	18	18	17	17	16	16	15	15	15	14	14	13
115	22	22	21	20	20	19	19	18	17	17	17	16	16	15	15	14	14
120	23	23	22	21	21	20	19	19	18	18	17	17	16	16	15	15	15
125	24	24	23	22	21	21	20	20	19	18	18	17	17	16	16	16	15
130	25	25	24	23	22	22	21	20	20	19	19	18	18	17	17	16	16
135	26	26	25	24	23	22	22	21	21	20	19	19	18	18	17	17	16
140	27	26	26	25	24	23	23	22	21	21	20	20	19	18	18	17	17
145	28	27	27	26	25	24	23	23	22	21	21	20	20	19	19	18	18
150	29	28	27	27	26	25	24	23	23	22	22	21	20	20	19	19	18
155	30	29	28	27	27	26	25	24	24	23	22	22	21	20	20	19	19
160	31	30	29	28	27	27	26	25	24	24	23	22	22	21	21	20	19
165	32	31	30	29	28	27	27	26	25	24	24	23	22	22	21	21	20
170	33	32	31	30	29	28	27	27	26	25	24	24	23	22	22	21	21
175	34	33	32	31	30	29	28	27	27	26	25	24	24	23	22	22	21
180	35	34	33	32	31	30	29	28	27	27	26	25	24	24	23	22	22
185	36	35	34	33	32	31	30	29	28	27	27	26	25	24	24	23	23
190	37	36	35	34	33	32	31	30	29	28	27	26	26	25	24	24	23
195	38	37	36	35	33	32	31	31	30	29	28	27	26	26	25	24	24
200	39	38	37	35	34	33	32	31	30	30	29	28	27	26	26	25	24
205	40	39	37	36	35	34	33	32	31	30	29	29	28	27	26	26	25
210	41	40	38	37	36	35	34	33	32	31	30	29	28	28	27	26	26
215	42	41	39	38	37	36	35	34	33	32	31	30	29	28	28	27	26
220	43	42	40	39	38	37	36	34	33	32	32	31	30	29	28	27	27
225	44	43	41	40	39	37	36	35	34	33	32	31	31	30	29	28	27
230	45	43	42	41	39	38	37	36	35	34	33	32	31	30	30	29	28
235	46	44	43	42	40	39	38	37	36	35	34	33	32	31	30	29	29
240	47	45	44	43	41	40	39	38	36	35	34	33	33	32	31	30	29
245	48	46	45	43	42	41	40	38	37	36	35	34	33	32	31	31	30
250	49	47	46	44	43	42	40	39	38	37	36	35	34	33	32	31	30

☐ Underweight   ▧ Weight Appropriate   ▨ Overweight   ▩ Obese

HEALTH RISKS OF BEING OVERWEIGHT

Your body mass index helps determine your risk of developing obesity-related diseases. In 1998 the National Heart, Lung, and Blood Institute issued a groundbreaking report on the health hazards of being overweight. The report summarized the latest research. Here are some of the key findings:

- **Hypertension:** Your risk of high blood pressure increases with every excess pound you carry. If you have a BMI of 30 or greater, you have a 32 percent risk of developing high blood pressure; women with a BMI under 30 have a 17 percent risk.

- **High Cholesterol:** Higher body weight is directly associated with high cholesterol levels, especially if you carry more fat around your abdomen (compared to your hips).

- **Diabetes:** Gaining just eleven pounds or more after age eighteen increases your risk of developing Type 2 diabetes. Your risk of diabetes increases by 25 percent for every one-unit increase in your BMI above 22.

- **Heart Disease:** Moderately overweight women (with a BMI of 25 to 29) have twice the risk of developing heart disease, and obese women (with a BMI of 30 or greater) have three times the risk compared to women who aren't overweight.

- **Stroke:** If your BMI is greater than 27, you have a 75 percent higher risk of suffering a stroke; if it's greater than 32, you have a 137 percent higher risk compared to slender women.

- **Osteoarthritis:** For every two- to three-pound increase in weight, an overweight woman's risk of developing

HEALTH RISKS OF BEING OVERWEIGHT (continued)

osteoarthritis increases by 9 to 13 percent (about one BMI unit), according to a study that tracked sets of middle-aged female twins in which one had developed arthritis. By the same token, a decrease in weight of two BMI units or more decreases the odds of developing osteoarthritis by 50 percent.

- **Cancer:** If you have a BMI of 30 or more, you have twice the risk of developing colon cancer as a woman with a BMI of less than 21. If you tend to have more fat around your abdomen than your hips, you have a higher risk of developing colon polyps, which can be precursors to cancer. Being obese also increases your risk of breast cancer. Researchers have found that gaining just twenty pounds from age eighteen to midlife doubles your risk of breast cancer.

- **Premature Death:** Mild obesity (a BMI of 25 to 29) doubles your risk of dying in the next ten years, and severe obesity (a BMI of 40 or over) can cut five to twenty years from your life span. More than 300,000 Americans die each year as a direct result of their obesity.

where your weight is distributed, whether it's on your hips and thighs (pear shaped) or around your abdomen (apple shaped). Apple-shaped women are at greater risk of developing heart disease and diabetes than pear-shaped women. The National Institutes of Health address this problem with a simple statement that the health risks of being overweight increase further for a woman if her waist size is greater than thirty-five inches.

For men, the risks increase if their waist is greater than forty inches.

We're all aware that excess body fat means a greater risk of heart disease and diabetes, but patients are sometimes surprised when I tell them it also increases their risk of digestive disorders. The three most common problems linked to excess weight are gallbladder disease, GERD, and fatty liver disease.

Gallbladder Disease

Being overweight dramatically increases your odds of developing gallstones. According to 1995 data from the National Health and Nutrition Examination Survey (NHANES) III, obese women have a 25 percent risk of developing gallstones compared to normal-weight women, who have a 9 percent risk. The most common type of gallstones form when excess amounts of cholesterol empty into your gallbladder from your liver. Your gallbladder serves as a holding tank for this cholesterol, which can harden into crystallized lumps or gallstones. The more you weigh, the more cholesterol your body produces, which increases your risk of gallstones.

Losing weight can help reduce your risk of gallstones, but you need to avoid losing weight too quickly. Obese individuals who lose more than two pounds a week have a 25 percent chance of developing gallstones within four months of dieting. Those who lose five pounds or more a week have a 70 percent chance. Losing weight too quickly causes your liver to mobilize cholesterol, which eventually gets emptied into your gallbladder. I recommend losing no more than one or two pounds per week. You can also help lower your risk of gallbladder disease by avoiding foods high in cholesterol and saturated fat (such as red meat, fried foods, full-fat cheeses, and cream sauces), which can raise your cholesterol levels.

GERD

Obesity can also increase your risk of developing gastroesophageal reflux disease (GERD). Carrying extra weight in your abdomen can increase pressure on your lower esophageal sphincter valve, the one-way valve that separates your esophagus from your stomach. With this extra pressure, the valve opens more frequently, causing food and acid to backwash from the stomach into the esophagus, resulting in heartburn and other reflux symptoms. What's more, studies suggest that obese individuals who have diabetes have delayed stomach emptying, which means that food remains in the stomach for longer periods of time. The longer food remains in your stomach, the more likely it will wash back up into your esophagus.

A recent study published in the *Journal of the American Medical Association* found that the link between obesity and GERD is particularly strong in women. Those with a BMI over 35 were more than six times as likely to have GERD as women with a BMI below 25. The research suggests that estrogen may play a role in GERD since it occurs more frequently in premenopausal women and in postmenopausal women who take estrogen.

Weight loss can reverse reflux symptoms and completely cure GERD in some overweight people. I know that it's far easier to control GERD by taking antacids and prescription medications, but I can tell you from my patients' experiences that losing weight is far more effective over the long haul—not to mention the fact that you'll lower your risk of other chronic diseases that can be far more serious than GERD.

Fatty Liver Disease

If you're apple-shaped (you carry more fat around your stomach than on your hips) and overweight, you're far more likely to carry fat around your vital digestive organs like your pancreas and liver. Fatty infiltration of the pancreas doesn't cause specific gastrointestinal disturbances in most people. Those who are severely obese may lose some pancreas function, but this may not cause any problems since the pancreas usually churns out more digestive enzymes than we need to digest food.

Fatty infiltration of the liver, however, can be far more serious. Like the pancreas, the liver can function pretty normally with a certain amount of fat contained within it—up to a certain point. The condition called nonalcoholic fatty liver disease strikes 10 to 24 percent of the general population, but the incidence increases to as high as 74 percent in obese individuals. Being obese in combination with having diabetes increases this risk even further. One study found that nearly 100 percent of obese diabetics had at least mild fatty liver

IS YOUR MEDICATION TO BLAME FOR WEIGHT GAIN?

If you recently started a new medication and found the scale inching upward, the drug may be to blame. Some prescription medications are notorious for causing weight gain. For instance, many women put on ten to fifteen pounds after they begin taking the tricyclic antidepressant amitriptyline (Elavil). The drug rosiglitazone maleate (Avandia), used to treat Type 2 (adult-onset) diabetes, can increase appetite, leading to a larger consumption of calories. This creates a vicious cycle of weight gain and a need for a higher dose of the medication.

If you think you're gaining weight from your medication, I urge you to speak to your doctor to see if you can take an alternative medication not associated with weight gain. Metformin hydrochloride (Glucophage) is a diabetes drug that's associated with a small degree of weight loss rather than weight gain. Antidepressants such as buproprion (Wellbutrin, Zyban), sertraline (Zoloft), and fluoxetine (Prozac) cause little, if any, weight gain.

disease. Occasionally, a fatty liver can become inflamed, which can lead to more serious liver disease.

Like liver problems caused by excess alcohol consumption, nonalcoholic fatty liver disease can lead to scarring and progress to cirrhosis and eventually liver failure. One study of obese diabetics found that 19 percent of them had full-blown cirrhosis. The frightening part is, you may not experience any symptoms until your liver is severely damaged. (Some of my patients, though, do complain of fatigue or malaise and a sensation of fullness on the right side of their upper abdomen.) Because fatty liver disease can be a hidden condition, I do standard blood tests to measure liver function in most of my obese patients. This condition is the most common cause of abnormal liver test results, and I find it very frequently in obese patients. Once there is scarring or cirrhosis, the damage may not be reversible, so it is vital to lose weight before the condition progresses.

Colon Cancer

Many studies have shown a relationship between obesity and colon cancer. Obese women who are diagnosed with colon cancer have a much worse prognosis compared to thin women who are diagnosed, according to a new study from the Dana-Farber Cancer Institute in Boston. Harvard University researchers found that twice as many women with a BMI of greater than 29 developed colon cancer that had spread than did women with a BMI of less than 21. Being overweight increases blood levels of certain hormones and proteins, such as estrogen and insulin, which can feed the growth of tumors. Other research has linked obesity to cancers of the esophagus, gallbladder, and pancreas.

OVERCOMING PSYCHOLOGICAL IMPEDIMENTS TO WEIGHT LOSS

I strongly oppose fad weight-loss diets. Yes, you can lose weight on the "grapefruit" or "cabbage soup" diet or by loading up on red meat while avoiding bread. But these diets are often just gimmicks. They work only as long as you're on them, and the pounds come flying back on the minute you're off them.

If you really want to lose weight permanently, you need a plan—one that you can follow for the rest of your life. Theresa Anderson, R.D., a nutritionist who works with the Women's GI Clinic, draws up eating plans for many of my overweight patients. Her philosophy is that barriers to weight loss are in large part psychological. "People generally know the basics of healthy eating," she says. "They know they're supposed to eat ample amounts of fruits and vegetables and to eat pretzels, chips, and candy bars only in moderation. They know that whole-wheat bread is better than white and that high-fiber bran cereal is better than sugar cereal.

DID YOU KNOW?

More than twice as many children are overweight today as twenty-five years ago, some 13 percent of girls and 15 percent of boys ages six to eleven. What's more, overweight children are twice as likely to become overweight adults. Losing weight yourself can help your child. Children under ten who have a weight problem and who have a least one overweight parent have a 60 percent chance of being overweight as adults—more than double the risk of their overweight peers who have thin parents, according to one study. Bottom line: Adopting healthy eating and activity habits can help both you and your family achieve a healthy weight.

They know they're supposed to exercise—or at least walk around the block or do a few laps at the mall."

Janice thought she had the perfect excuse for being overweight. She had no time to prepare and eat nutritious meals. Janice taught full time and had two school-age children who were involved in after-school sports and academic activities. "I'm constantly on the go and always eat on the run," she says. "For dinner, the kids and I usually stop in a fast-food restaurant and get takeout for my husband." Janice came to our clinic because she had GERD that was related to her obesity. I told her she could help relieve her symptoms if she lost twenty or thirty pounds, and I referred her to Anderson for nutrition counseling.

After listening to Janice's hectic schedule, Anderson told her that she had to get rid of her excuses. "I explained to Janice that adding structure in her life, which included regular meals at regular times, would actually add more time to her day," she said. "I had her go home and make dinner menus on three-by-five index cards with her husband and kids. They put their favorite foods on the cards, like meatloaf, grilled chicken and rice, meatballs, and spaghetti. They worked together and came up with four weeks of meals that they shuffled and rotated every week. I told her to go shopping once a week to buy what she needed for these meals and to post a menu on the wall."

Janice found that her husband and kids enjoyed having a hand in planning the meals as well as the family time they now had every night around the dinner table. They also found they were eating much more healthily. As the weeks went on, Janice discovered that she had the time and energy to begin her fitness plan. After six months Janice returned to Anderson for a follow-up appointment—ten pounds lighter.

Like Janice, says Anderson, many women often say they don't have time to live a healthy lifestyle. In the superstressed, time-crunch world we live in, who has a free moment to cut up vegetables for a salad? It's far easier to grab a candy bar on the run or microwave a burrito. But the issues often run deeper than a lack of time. Some women feel a loss of control over their lives and use food to gain comfort and an anchor in the rough waters. Others use food to quell boredom and simply can't pass up the jar of M&M's on a co-worker's desk or the half-eaten cupcake left on their child's plate.

Before Anderson even gets into eating preferences, she works with women on building a foundation. "I have them identify bricks that they feel are crumbling," she says. "Do they have support from their spouse? Are they overloaded at work? Do they live their life from moment to moment instead of planning out their day and their week?" She contends that once these roadblocks are surmounted, women often lose weight naturally because they can focus on switching to healthy food choices and more organized meal planning instead of using food as an antidote to their emotional problems. She also encourages them to find alternate pleasures to replace food, like a soothing bubble bath or a night out at the movies. (Note: These techniques work for emotional eaters and may not be appropriate for morbidly obese individuals who need calorie-restricted meal plans.)

MAKING THE
EXERCISE CONNECTION

I am a huge advocate of exercise, both because it helps maintain the proper function of your digestive tract and because of its weight-loss benefits. That's why I talk about making the exercise connection throughout this book, whenever I think it can help improve a GI condition. I also don't think you can lose weight and successfully keep it off without increasing your activity level. This is purely a matter of science. If you reduce your body weight, your body requires fewer calories to maintain that new, lower weight. So you have to be really careful to keep a lower food intake even after you've lost weight if you don't want to gain it back. If you exercise, however, you'll be giving your metabolism a boost, making it easier to keep off lost pounds.

Getting active isn't only about joining a gym or having formal workouts in sweats. In fact, making minor adjustments to your activity level may be more effective than "exercise" if you have a hard time sticking to your fitness commitment. One study found that people who made minor lifestyle adjustments, like climbing stairs instead of taking elevators, opening the garage door themselves, and getting up to change TV channels instead of using the remote, had more long-term success with weight loss than those who initiated an exercise program for the first time in their lives. That's because people find it too tempting to skip exercise days or quit altogether, whereas those who make minor activity adjustments see these changes as a permanent part of their lifestyle.

I recently attended a symposium given by former surgeon general David Satcher, where he emphasized the need for doctors to promote fitness to their patients in order to combat the obesity epidemic. After I saw the glaring statistics on the rise of obesity in this country just in the past decade alone, I took his words to heart.

I regularly counsel my patients to exercise—even if they aren't overweight, but especially if they are. I recommend all kinds of exercise programs, from finding a walking buddy (to keep you motivated) to swimming or water aerobics (for patients with arthritis or other musculoskeletal ailments). I actually write out a "prescription" for exercise using my prescription pad. I'll say "Walk for 15 minutes, 3 days a week" or "Take 2 water aerobics classes and swim 5 laps each week." I might also write a prescription for a patient to get evaluated at the cardiac fitness center at our hospital if she has heart disease, or I'll write a prescription for her to visit a medically supervised gym in our area. This gym is staffed with a doctor and a nurse as well as personal trainers and is designed for those who are obese or have heart disease or other ailments that prevent them from exercising on their own. These kinds of gyms are sprouting up throughout the country. Many of my patients tell me they love Jazzercise, and my secretary Susan can vouch for its effectiveness. She danced away dozens of pounds by going to class several times a week.

Just as with eating, there are psychological barriers to exercise. I can't tell you how often I've heard "I can't afford to join a gym" or "I can't find any time to exercise." My first answer is "You can't afford not to exercise if you want to avoid the health risks and health expenses associated with obesity-related diseases." I may not be a digestive health role model when it comes to my eating habits, but I do find time to exercise. Three nights a week I run on my elliptical trainer for twenty to thirty minutes. During the summer my kids and I play badminton in the backyard at night and hit the community pool.

After I turned forty, when I put on those few extra pounds, I realized that the best way for me to keep my weight in check was to try hard to exercise. I tell my patients, "I work full time—sometimes twelve-hour days—and have two young kids. If I can find time to exercise, then you can, too."

FINDING A SENSIBLE EATING PLAN THAT'S RIGHT FOR YOU

I don't want to call this a weight-loss plan because I don't want you to become focused on the number on your scale. I think the reason so many of us fail to lose excess weight and keep it off is because we use weight, rather than a healthy lifestyle, as the endpoint. We exercise for weight loss, and we eat for weight loss. Once we reach our weight goal, we go back to our old habits.

Overweight patients who come to my Women's GI Clinic are counseled to think healthy and live healthy and to consider weight loss to be an added bonus. When we talk about weight loss, we emphasize slow loss—no more than one or two pounds a week. This is the safest and most effective way to lose weight and will minimize gastrointestinal problems, like gallstones, that can come with rapid weight loss.

So how can you take off weight in a safe and effective way? The answer lies in healthy eating and finding a plan that you can stick with for life. Some general guidelines issued in the U.S. Department of Agriculture (USDA) 2000 Dietary Guidelines for Americans are:

- Get no more than 30 percent of your total calories from fat. Choose a diet low in saturated fat and cholesterol and moderate in total fat.
- Choose a variety of grains daily, especially whole grains.
- Choose a variety of fruits and vegetables daily.
- Choose beverages and foods to moderate your intake of sugars.
- Choose and prepare foods with less salt.
- If you drink alcoholic beverages, do so in moderation.

The USDA also recommends following its Food Guide Pyramid, which was issued nearly fifteen years ago. Nutritionists and physicians, myself included, agree that this model is outdated. It suggests that you get most of your calories from cereals, starches, and other grains and recommends consuming red meat on a daily basis. Except for the brief mention about limiting saturated fats, it lumps all fats and oils together, not distinguishing between heart-healthy monounsaturated fats and fish oils and heart-damaging fats like trans fatty acids (found in margarine and baked goods with partially hydrogenated oils).

For this reason I generally don't recommend the USDA Food Guide Pyramid. Instead, I recommend following an alternative like the Mediterranean Diet Pyramid (shown below). This pyramid was established by researchers from Harvard School of Public Health and other universities in conjunction with Oldways

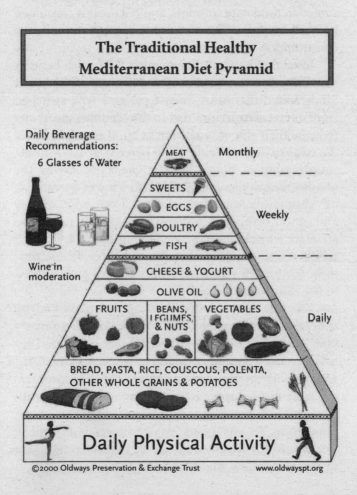

The Traditional Healthy Mediterranean Diet Pyramid

Daily Beverage Recommendations:
6 Glasses of Water

MEAT — Monthly

SWEETS
EGGS
POULTRY — Weekly
FISH

Wine in moderation

CHEESE & YOGURT

OLIVE OIL

FRUITS | BEANS, LEGUMES, & NUTS | VEGETABLES — Daily

BREAD, PASTA, RICE, COUSCOUS, POLENTA, OTHER WHOLE GRAINS & POTATOES

Daily Physical Activity

©2000 Oldways Preservation & Exchange Trust   www.oldwayspt.org

Preservation and Exchange Trust. It is based on the typical diets found in Greece, southern Italy, and Crete, which use olive oil and nuts as primary sources of fat and are rich in high-fiber carbohydrates (fruits, vegetables, whole-grain cereals, legumes). Fish and chicken are consumed in moderate amounts, and red meat is consumed in small amounts. The diet also encourages a moderate consumption of red wine.

Several clinical studies support the health benefits of the Mediterranean diet. The 1994 Lyon Diet Heart Study found that heart disease patients who switched from a typical American diet to the Mediterranean diet reduced their risk of heart attacks by 73 percent and reduced their risk of dying by 70 percent. A 2003 observation study of 22,000 healthy Greeks following the Mediterranean diet found they had a lower overall risk of death and a lower risk of dying from heart disease and cancer compared to their Greek counterparts who ate more American-style fare. This study found that no single nutrient or food contributed to this disease protection; rather, a synergistic effect among nutrients led to less disease and death.

You may have noticed that daily physical activity appears on this pyramid, and I think this is an important point. Any eating plan should incorporate an active lifestyle, whether it's biking to work, walking to do your errands, or playing tag with your kids. Incorporating these dietary approaches with an increased activity level will help you lose weight the natural way—without dieting. Yes, weight loss will be slower, but it will be steady, and the weight will stay off permanently if you continue to follow your new lifestyle.

I realize that you may not want to eat Mediterranean every day, and you may definitely explore other alternatives. The same developers of the Mediterranean pyramid also developed Asian, Latin, and Vegetarian pyramids. You can find details on all of these at the Oldways Preservation and Exchange Trust website: www.oldwayspt.org. I'm not trying to force a particular diet program on you. I think these pyramids provide good general guidelines for healthy eating. Use them to adapt your meals, whether you're making Mexican, Chinese, or Italian fare.

A LITTLE MIND OVER MATTER

Everyone knows that eating involves much more than the simple act of putting food in our mouths. If we all had the willpower to close our mouths tightly whenever a doughnut or chocolate bar came in sight, we wouldn't need diet books or weight-loss elixirs. Getting a handle on emotions that may trigger eating (stress, anger, sadness, boredom, happiness) will help you go a long way toward losing weight. Here's how to get into a healthy eating mind-set:

1. **Find your hunger:** The ability to recognize true hunger, and to know when you're eating for other reasons, is the key to controlling your weight. With food available all the time, many of us have forgotten what it's like to feel hungry. On the flip side, we've also ignored the signals of feeling full. What is true hunger? Technically, it can't be defined, but researchers have found that many healthy people

BEWARE THE FAT-FREE POTATO CHIP!

If you're trying to cut calories without giving up your favorite foods, fat-free potato chips, made with the fake fat olestra, may seem like a great option. Fat-free chips like Frito-Lay's Wow! and Utz's Yes! contain just 70 calories and 0 grams of fat per serving, compared to 150 calories and 10 grams of fat in regular potato chips. Olestra, approved by the Food and Drug Administration several years ago for use in savory snack foods like potato chips, cheese puffs, crackers, and popcorn, is basically made of table sugar and vegetable oil. Since molecules in olestra are much larger than those in ordinary fats, it is not digested or absorbed by the body. Thus, it adds rich taste and smooth texture to food without adding calories.

The trouble is, olestra can have some nasty gastrointestinal side effects. Since it adds nondigestible bulk to the diet, it can cause side effects like bloating, cramping, loose stools, and flatulence in some people who eat as little as the 10 grams of chips contained in a serving-size bag. A small percentage even experience anal leakage of stool after eating the chips. Evidence suggests that these side effects are more common in people with chronic inflammatory bowel disease like Crohn's or ulcerative colitis.

Another potential problem with olestra: Fat-soluble vitamins like A, D, E, and K seem to attach themselves to this large fatty acid molecule and are carried out with it instead of being absorbed by the body. The FDA requires foods containing olestra to have vitamins A, D, E, and K added.

Still, some experts are concerned that other fat-soluble nutrients, like certain cancer-preventive carotenoids, are also being flushed out with olestra. One study from Holland found that people who ate just 3 grams of olestra daily for a month (an amount contained in only six potato chips) had 40 percent less lycopene in their blood compared to controls who didn't eat any olestra. Lycopene, a carotenoid found in tomatoes, has been linked to lower rates of prostate cancer and possibly other cancers.

I believe that the jury is still out on whether olestra is truly safe to eat on a regular basis. If you decide to replace fattier snacks with snack foods that contain olestra, eat them in moderate amounts and reduce your intake if you experience digestive disturbances.

who feel hungry report having a growling stomach and an achy stomach emptiness. Hunger can also cause headaches, dizziness, weakness, fatigue, and a loss of concentration, due to low blood sugar levels.

Feeling a little hungry before a meal is a good thing. Hunger should rise slightly before you eat and should decline after you've consumed a meal. The trick is to space out your eating so you don't eat too soon or feel too ravenous when you do eat.

2. **Identify your eating style:** How often and how you eat ultimately determine how much you eat. To determine how often you eat, count the number of times a day you put food in your mouth. If the answer is "too many to count," you're probably a mindless snacker. You could probably lose weight simply by controlling the number of times a day you eat. Think three meals a day plus one or two snacks—a total of four to five times.

How you eat is a bit more complicated. You need to identify your eating styles: when you eat, how fast you eat, whether you eat while doing other activities like watching TV, your attitude about when to stop eating, and problem foods. For instance, do you eat when you're hungry or when you're stressed, tired, or down in the dumps? Sometimes just being aware of why you're eating can help you find nonfood ways to comfort yourself. Exercising is a much healthier way to de-stress than downing a box of cookies. Eating too quickly can also derail you. About twenty minutes pass between the time you begin eating and the time your brain gets the signal that you're full. If you consume your meal faster than that, you might overeat before getting the satiety signal.

You need to be conscious of habits you picked up as a child. Do you always feel compelled to leave a clean plate because your mom told you not to waste food? You may have certain "trigger" foods that you can't consume just in small amounts. Perhaps you can't resist gooey chocolate chip cookies like those your mom made you whenever you had a bad day at school or a bag of greasy potato chips of a kind that was never allowed in the house.

3. **Cut yourself some slack:** Did you "cheat" and have a doughnut during your coffee break at work? That doesn't mean you've ruined your eating plan for the day and might as well go on an all-out binge. The key is to aim for balanced eating. You don't have to get your quota of fruits and vegetables, starches, and

low-fat protein at every meal. In fact, you'll probably overeat on some occasions and undereat on others. Your body can compensate when you veer away from healthy behaviors—as long as you don't veer away too much. Yes, you should try to eat healthy foods throughout the day and dole out moderate-size portions that leave you full but not stuffed. But you also need to build in flexibility that allows you to have a piece of cake at your child's birthday party or a strawberry daiquiri on your night out.

4. **Think of food as empowerment:** Certain foods contain substances that can help ward off disease. Eating fish rich in omega-3 fatty acids (salmon, tuna, mackerel) can help prevent depression, arthritis, and cardiovascular disease. Fruits and vegetables contain beneficial substances called phytochemicals; some, such as lycopene found in tomatoes, can help prevent cancer. The greater the variety of colors you eat, the wider the variety of phytochemicals you'll get. You can also use food to gain sustained energy by eating a combination of protein, carbohydrates, and fat in every meal. Food can indeed be a powerful medicine if you eat a balanced diet.

SHOULD YOU CONSIDER MEDICAL INTERVENTION FOR WEIGHT LOSS?

For most people, diet and exercise should be the first course of action when initiating a weight-loss program. Cutting your calorie intake by 500 a day, burning off that amount through exercise, or doing a combination of

LIQUID FASTS AND OTHER DIET FADS

Whenever I read about a new weight-loss fad that will magically melt away pounds with minimal effort, I always think, "If only." If only we could lose weight with a tea or tonic that will boost our metabolism or cleanse our system of toxins. If only life were that easy—we would all be thin.

The trouble is, permanent weight loss does require permanent lifestyle changes, and the quick-fix approach is often harmful to your health and your digestive tract. I already mentioned that losing weight rapidly increases your risk for gallstones. The type of product you use can increase your risk of other problems as well. For instance, liquid fasts, which are all the rage at health spas throughout the country, are touted for ridding the body of dangerous toxic substances and for quick weight loss. Women down thirteen beverages (one an hour) a day containing psyllium (a natural laxative), chlorophyll, and plant juices—and that's it. Some say they lose seven or eight pounds after five days on the 200-calorie-a-day liquid diet.

Surviving on so few calories puts your body into starvation mode. Not only does metabolism drop, but blood pressure, body temperature, pulse, and breathing rate fall. You can lose muscle and can become constipated. Some women get light-headed and suffer from abdominal pains due to a lack of calories. A healthy thirty-five-year-old woman sheds about four and a half pounds of water in a day or two, which she'll immediately gain back once she goes off the diet. Some fasters even put on more weight than they started with, after they begin eating again. What's more, there's absolutely no medical evidence that fasting rids your body of "toxins."

Sometimes the weight-loss elixirs themselves are harmful. Weight-loss teas and tablets containing the herb ma huang (or ephedra) have been linked to seizures, strokes, and sixty deaths, according to the FDA. Herbal weight-loss teas that contain natural laxatives like senna, aloe, rhubarb root, buckthorn, cascara, and castor oil can also cause major gastrointestinal problems in healthy women who take them. Used for centuries to treat constipation, these herbal teas, when taken in excessive amounts, can cause diarrhea, vomiting, nausea, stomach cramps, chronic constipation, fainting, and perhaps even death, according to the FDA. Since these herbal products aren't regulated for safety or effectiveness, your best bet is to stay away from them altogether. "All-natural" definitely isn't synonymous with "safe."

the two will lead to a weight loss of one or two pounds a week. But, if you are moderately obese (a BMI over 30) or have a BMI over 27 and medical complications of obesity, you may benefit from a medical therapy for weight loss. Several options are available, although none are without side effects and risks. You need to talk to your doctor about which method is right for you. Make sure you understand how much weight loss you can expect to achieve and the possible side effects and lifestyle changes you'll need to make to sustain the weight loss.

Weight-Loss Medications

These medications have been on the market for decades but continue to come under fire for their health risks. Amphetamine-type appetite suppressants were found to be highly addictive and to cause dangerous cardiac side effects. Other drugs, which altered the amount of serotonin in the brain, caused circulatory problems. A few years ago the FDA pulled the diet drug dexfenfluramine (Redux) after it was linked to heart valve problems in some women who used the drug. Phentermine (which was used with fenfluramine in a combination called phen-fen) was also implicated in possible heart problems. The product's manufacturer now recommends using it for no longer than three months.

Two newer weight-loss medications appear to be useful in helping severely overweight people lose enough weight to get themselves out of the danger zone. Sibutramine (Meridia) acts like an appetite suppressant, working to balance two brain chemicals, serotonin and norepinephrine, while also increasing metabolism. It can be used safely for one year, nine months longer than phentermine. Like phentermine, though, it can cause blood pressure to rise and shouldn't be taken with certain antidepressants. Other side effects may include dry mouth or drowsiness.

The other new drug, orlistat (Xenical), works directly in the digestive tract. The pill is taken with meals and is released in the small intestine, where it inactivates a digestive enzyme called lipase. Without this enzyme, fat cannot be digested and absorbed. Fat passes through the body undigested—sometimes in a rushed fashion. Users commonly experience diarrhea as a result. Other side effects include oily and foul-smelling stools, flatulence, incontinence, and malabsorption of fat-soluble vitamins. All patients on orlistat should take a vitamin supplement containing the fat-soluble vitamins A, D, E, and K. This supplement should be taken at least two hours before or two hours after the dose of orlistat.

The average woman who takes one of these medications loses five to ten percent of her initial body weight. These drugs aren't appropriate for you if you want to drop ten or fifteen pounds—they're recommended only for those who are extremely overweight. More important, these drugs aren't a cure-all on their own. They need to be part of a weight-loss program that includes a reduced-calorie diet and appropriate physical activity. Your doctor should help you fit these medications into an overall weight-loss program or should refer you for weight-loss counseling.

Surgical Options

Surgery to lose weight is a drastic option, but I can tell you it's a popular one, and it can be extremely effective for appropriate candidates: those whose obesity seriously threatens their health and who cannot lose weight any other way. It may be life-saving for patients who have repeatedly failed to respond to regular diet, exercise, and medical therapies and who have significant complications from obesity like diabetes, liver disease, and arthritis. Known as *gastric bypass* or *stomach stapling* or by the medical term *bariatric surgery,* weight-loss surgery came into the national spotlight when pop singer Carnie Wilson underwent the procedure, which was broadcast live on the Internet. Weatherman Al Roker's experience, which he talked about repeatedly on the *Today* show, also increased awareness.

More than 63,000 gastric bypass procedures were

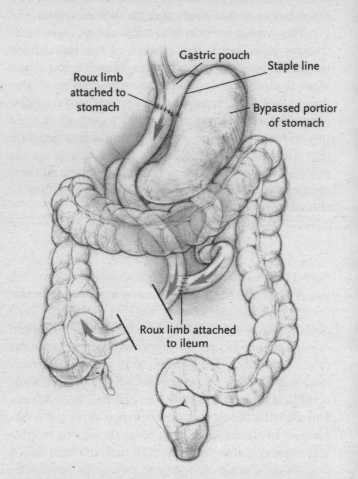

Gastric pouch

Staple line

Roux limb attached to stomach

Bypassed portion of stomach

Roux limb attached to ileum

The most popular form of gastric bypass surgery, Roux-en-Y, involves stapling the stomach to create a pouch the size of a small egg. This pouch is then sewn to the lower portion of the small intestine, creating a shorter surface area for absorption. The surgery is irreversible.

performed in the United States in 2002, three times the number from five years ago. At the University of Virginia Hospital (UVA), about a hundred women opt to undergo the surgery every year. This number is continuing to rise, and we have a nine-month waiting list for the procedure. Even so, only a small percentage of the women who come see us actually qualify as candidates for this radical surgery. The vast majority are turned away with the explanation that it is not for the overweight individual who wants to lose thirty or forty pounds in a quick-fix way. "This is really a last resort only for women who have exhausted all medically supervised weight-loss programs," stresses Anna Miller, R.N., the nurse at UVA who works with Bruce Schirmer, M.D., the bariatric surgeon who does this procedure.

According to a National Institutes of Health consensus panel of experts, a weight-loss-surgery candidate should suffer from "clinically severe obesity" with a BMI of 40 or higher. Those with a BMI of 35 or above may also qualify if they have severe health problems caused by obesity, like uncontrolled diabetes, high blood pressure, or high cholesterol.

Several types of gastric bypass surgery are available, all of which are intended to shrink the stomach from a capacity of 48 to 64 ounces (6 to 8 cups) to just one or two ounces. The most popular surgery, called Roux-en-Y, involves stapling off the upper portion of the stomach to create a small pouch. It is irreversible. The pouch, which becomes the new stomach, is about the size of a thumb initially, but eventually stretches to the size of a small egg. (In contrast, the stomach of an average-weight woman can stretch to about the size of a football.) The surgeon then connects this new stomach to the upper portion of the small intestine, bypassing much of the surface area through which calories and vital nutrients are absorbed.

After the operation patients slowly introduce tiny amounts of solid food, sometimes one teaspoonful at a time, to see how much they can tolerate. Some discover they can't digest meat, fats, dairy products, or sugar and may have vomiting or diarrhea whenever they eat these

Sutures or staple

Adjustable band

A new technique in weight-loss surgery involves the placement of an adjustable band to section off the stomach. The stomach is not bypassed, but the creation of a small pouch requires you to eat less in one sitting.

foods. What's more, instead of taking in several thousand calories a day, they can eat only about 1,000 calories a day without getting sick. Because of this, excess body fat melts away.

Patients lose an average of 65 to 70 percent of their excess weight (20 to 35 percent of their initial body weight) during the first year. So a 300-pound woman trying to reach a healthy weight of 140 would lose about 115 pounds. Weight tends to stabilize after the first year, and some patients gain back some of the weight. Research suggests that the average patient is able to keep off half of the excess weight that she started with.

It's important to realize that gastric bypass won't make you stick-thin if you're obese. It will, though, take off a lot of excess weight, which will give you energy to exercise and help reverse health conditions related to obesity. Studies show that it results in a greater weight loss and more improvement in health problems like diabetes, sleep apnea, and gastroesophageal reflux disease than conventional diet and exercise programs.

But these benefits come at a price. You'll never be able to enjoy food in the same way again. All-you-can-eat buffets are out. Ice cream sundaes are out. Supersize fries are out. In fact, carbonated beverages, caffeine, and alcohol are all discouraged. And there's a total ban on sweets and starchy snack foods. Trouble is, the surgery won't banish your desire for these foods, but it will make you feel sick after you have them. If you overindulge or eat sugar, you're likely to experience the dumping syndrome, an extremely unpleasant reaction that includes nausea, sweating, fainting, and diarrhea. Think back to your last bout of food poisoning, and you'll get the picture. To avoid vomiting after a meal, you won't be able to eat anything more than about half a Lean Cuisine meal in a single sitting. And you'll have to eat it slowly and chew it thoroughly over about thirty minutes.

You should also realize that weight-loss surgeries, like other surgeries, pose a small but real risk of serious side effects. These include chronic malnutrition, osteoporosis, infections, and intestinal leaks. Some patients need repeat surgery to get rid of scar tissue and adhesions, which can cause severe abdominal pain. And one patient in every two hundred who has the surgery will die from the procedure. These complication rates are reduced if you use a surgeon who is very experienced in the procedure—one who has done at least seventy-five bypasses. Your surgeon should be a member of the American Society for Bariatric Surgery. Log on to www.asbs.org for a referral to a surgeon in your area.

A newer procedure that uses an adjustable band to section off the stomach is considered to be a kinder, gentler form of weight-loss surgery. It's easier to perform and has a lower rate of complications than the Roux-en-Y. And it's reversible. It also doesn't cause the dumping syndrome, so patients can still eat sweets in moderation. It is, though, less effective for weight loss than traditional gastric bypass surgery. In FDA clinical trials, patients initially lost an average of 36 percent of their excess weight— about half the amount that gastric bypass patients lose. If you're considering weight-loss surgery, talk to your doctor about the various options to see which is best for you.

Before I refer any of my morbidly obese patients for surgery, I refer them to a clinical psychologist, Dr. J. Kim Penberthy, who spends a good deal of time with them discussing the risks and implications of the surgery. She asks patients what they expect from the surgery, to make sure their expectations are realistic (i.e., they won't become stick-thin and can't eat anything they want afterward).

Dr. Penberthy insists that surgical candidates completely alter their eating habits before surgery. She has them keep a food diary and teaches them to eat four to six small meals a day that are low in fat and sugar, the diet they will have to follow after the surgery. She also prepares them for a drastic body change. "Many of these women have been extremely overweight for decades," says Penberthy. "They may not remember what it's like to get sexual attention from men they pass on the street. A significant number of women who get this surgery were sexually abused in the past and gained weight as a protective cloak to keep away men. I help them to become mentally prepared to deal with this."

EATING DISORDERS AND GI PROBLEMS

Jill, a twenty-year-old who has been underweight her entire life, came to see me about five years ago. She literally had to be dragged into the clinic by her mother, who had called me several times before convincing Jill to come in to see me. She told me that her daughter had not faced up to the fact that she had an eating disorder. Jill was going to a local university, and her mother didn't realize how serious her daughter's condition had become until Jill had come home for winter break. She was extremely thin and was having severe abdominal pains and bloating after every meal, and often she didn't even eat at mealtime.

When I saw Jill in my office, she looked a little on the thin side in her baggy jeans and oversize sweatshirt. But when I saw her sitting in a flimsy gown in my examination room, I had to keep myself from gasping out loud. Jill was profoundly emaciated. She looked skeletal, and at five foot six, she weighed only ninety-two pounds.

When I questioned Jill about her eating habits, I found out she was eating no more than 7 grams of fat per day and less than 1,000 calories. She counted every single calorie and fat gram and refused to go over her daily quota. She was a classic anorexic. Jill told me that she simply could not tolerate fat. "If I eat a turkey sandwich with mayonnaise spread on the bread," she explained, "I get really bad cramps and bloating."

I knew Jill's GI symptoms were related to her eating disorder, but I wanted to gain her trust by ruling out other conditions. I ran some blood tests, which showed she did not have a fat-malabsorption disorder; Jill could tolerate a lot more fat than she was actually eating. I also ordered some other tests to see if her anorexia had damaged her body. When I got the results, I met with Jill again and told her I had some troubling news. "Your stomach cramps are the least of your problems," I said. "They are indicative of the amount of weight that you've lost." I wasn't really certain as to what was causing Jill's abdominal pain. She probably had some slow-motility problems due to the reduced amount of food she was eating. Some studies have shown that anorexia can cause a prolonged transit of food through the intestines. Researchers have also found that motility problems improve once the patient gains weight.

I explained to Jill that her abdominal pains weren't life-threatening; rather, they were a symptom of a much bigger problem: her anorexia. I told her I was more concerned by the results from her other medical tests. She

GASTROINTESTINAL COMPLICATIONS OF EATING DISORDERS

Side Effects of Starvation (Anorexia)	Side Effects of Bingeing and Purging (Bulimia)
Delayed stomach emptying; could lead to reflux	Bloody vomit
	Bloody diarrhea
Bloating	Inflammation or ulcers in the cheeks, tongue, or lips (stomatitis)
Early satiety during meal	
Constipation	Reflux
Diarrhea	Swelling in the neck near the ear (parotid gland enlargement)
Reduced taste	
Abdominal pain of unclear origin	Constipation
	Diarrhea
	Esophageal tears
	Expansion of the stomach (gastric dilation)
	Abdominal pain of unclear origin
	Low muscle tone in the colon (atonic)

Source: D. Blake Woodside, M.D., "Eating Disorders," *Clinical Perspectives in Gastroenterology* (November–December 2001), 333–39.

Hunger Pangs

"When I first got married about fifteen years ago, I became anorexic and only allowed myself to consume about 700 calories a day. I think I was punishing myself because I felt so guilty for moving far away from my family when I got married. My sister had died in a terrible house fire a year before, and I was pitching in to help raise her two little boys. When I moved away, I felt like I was abandoning my nephews. I don't even know if I was consciously aware that I had an eating disorder even though I was skin and bones. I'm five foot seven, and I thought that an acceptable weight for me was 107 pounds. Once I reached this weight, though, I found myself suffering from severe stomach pains. One day I was doubled over in pain that kept coming in waves. My husband thought I was having an appendicitis attack and rushed me to the emergency room. Although I came in for abdominal pain, all my medical tests were normal. My doctor approached me about my eating habits and made me realize that I was extremely underweight and that I was probably having 'hunger pangs' and that I needed to get more nourishment. What ultimately convinced me to eat? I wasn't menstruating because I was so thin, and my doctor told me I would have trouble getting pregnant. I was told how much weight I needed to gain in order to get pregnant and have a healthy baby. I wanted a child so much that I entered an outpatient eating disorders program and eventually gained fifteen pounds."

—Jackie D., 39, mother of four

had a DEXA bone scan (an X-ray test that measures bone density), which showed that she had severe bone loss and was heading toward osteoporosis. Her bones looked like those of a seventy-five-year-old woman. Her body lacked bone-building nutrients like vitamin

D, magnesium, and calcium, which she should have been getting in her diet.

Jill also had an essential fatty acid deficiency, which is caused by malnutrition and not taking in enough or the right kinds of fat. She and I looked in the mirror at her thinning hair, dry skin, and brittle nails. "Those are all caused by a lack of fat in your diet," I stressed. "You will look so much better if you give your body the food it needs to stay healthy." I explained that fat is an essential part of our diet and plays a vital role in the body—like providing the structure for brain tissue, hair, nails, and cells. Fat also provides the insulating sheath that surrounds our nerves and helps the brain transmit messages to the rest of our body. We talked about the fact that her near-complete avoidance of fat could be extremely detrimental.

But I knew that my pleas and her medical test results weren't enough to get Jill to start eating again. I knew her mother had to be a partner with me in convincing Jill to get professional counseling. "This eating disorder could kill her," I warned. Jill's mother convinced her to enter an eating-disorder program at the University of Virginia. Jill decided to take a semester off school so she could receive treatment. "I don't want to die," Jill told me. "I just want to feel better and have a normal life."

Now, five years later, Jill is still battling her anorexia, but she's much healthier. She managed to get her weight up to within a few pounds of her minimum healthy weight. And she earned her university degree. She is continuing her therapy sessions and recognizes that she has a disease that needs to be managed for the rest of her life. But she fights the good fight because her will to survive is stronger than her will to keep her weight down.

All too frequently young women come into my office with gastrointestinal complaints when the root of their problem lies not in their digestive tract but in their brain. Eating disorders like anorexia and bulimia are considered to be serious psychiatric illnesses. Both of these conditions disrupt the normal functioning of the gastrointestinal tract and may cause severe gastrointestinal symptoms.

More than 90 percent of people with eating disorders are women, probably because of the value that our society places on a woman's being thin. Anorexia affects about one percent of women in their teens and twenties, and these women have twelve times the risk of dying (from starvation or suicide) as women their age who don't have an eating disorder. Anorexia is defined as being in the 15th percentile or lower for the average weight for a person's height. The condition is usually accompanied by an intense fear of gaining weight and a distorted body image or refusal to acknowledge low weight. Most anorexics stop menstruating because of their low percentage of body fat.

The second major eating disorder, bulimia, affects about four percent of women in their teens and twenties. Bulimics frequently binge on large amounts of food in a short time and then purge their food by vomiting, taking laxatives, or engaging in vigorous exercise. Like anorexics, they're preoccupied with their weight and shape.

You may be surprised to learn that gastroenterologists are frequently the first health care providers to diagnose eating disorders. Many young women with eating disorders present with stomach pain or heart-burn as the first indication of a problem. Unless the doctor asks targeted questions, he or she won't know that the bulimic patient, who is most likely of normal weight, is bingeing and purging. And anorexics, who look malnourished, aren't usually forthcoming about their eating habits and usually deny that they have a problem. But when a bulimic has bloody vomit or diarrhea or an anorexic has severe cramps or heartburn, she may come to my office—without realizing that her eating disorder is the root cause of her GI distress.

A few years ago *binge eating disorder* was identified as a third type of eating disorder by the *Diagnostic and Statistical Manual of Mental Disorders,* the official publication of the American Psychiatric Association. Binge eaters have recurrent, sometimes daily, bouts of uncontrollable eating, during which they eat an unusually large amount of food over a short period of time. The person usually feels out of control while bingeing. Unlike bulimics, binge eaters don't engage in purging behaviors like vomiting, laxative use, or excessive exercise. As a result of their excess food intake, binge eaters are usually severely overweight. They carry the same increased risk of digestive disorders that plague overweight people who don't have binge eating disorder: gallstones, GERD, and fatty liver disease. Binge eaters, however, may have additional complications resulting from their massive food intake at a given time. They may become constipated and bloated, or they may suffer from severe indigestion that brings on vomiting or abdominal pain.

More recently, another eating disorder has begun to receive national attention. It's called *orthorexia,* and it hasn't yet been recognized as an "official" eating disorder. Still, nutrition professionals are encountering this disorder more and more in their practices. Orthorexia is literally an obsession with correct eating. A person with the condition takes "healthy eating" to such an extreme that it causes a nutrition imbalance and ill health. The planning and preparation of special foods becomes an end in itself. The orthorectic's inner thoughts become dominated by efforts to resist temptation on a rigid, self-imposed eating plan. Choices become narrow and limiting, and the orthorectic frequently becomes malnourished due to a lack of fat and protein. She may lose significant amounts of weight and take on the appearance of an anorexic.

Whenever I encounter a patient with an eating disorder, I'm honest and direct. I explain that her gastrointestinal symptoms are valid but that her treatment will center on management of her eating disorder. Yes, I can prescribe medications to ease the pain of an esophageal ulcer brought on by self-induced vomiting. But I can't keep the esophagus from being damaged again unless a patient stops vomiting.

I'm also a strong believer in professional counseling for patients with eating disorders. Patients need to address the way they feel about themselves and accept that their bodies will change as they get to a healthier weight. Fixing a compulsion with food usually requires a psychologist's intervention and counseling from a nutritionist. Both of these professionals should work together to heal the patient. Antidepressants and antianxiety medications can also be helpful for treating these disorders.

EATING DISORDER ORGANIZATIONS

American Anorexia/Bulimia Association
tel. (212) 575-6200

Anorexia Nervosa and Related Eating Disorders
tel. (541) 344-1144; www.anred.com
ANRED provides information related to recovery from and prevention of eating disorders.

Eating Disorders Awareness and Prevention
tel. (206) 382-3587; members.aol.com/edapinc
EDAP works with prevention and outreach; it sponsors National Eating Disorders Week.

National Association of Anorexia Nervosa and Associated Disorders
tel. (847) 831-3438; www.anad.org
ANAD works to prevent eating disorders through education, referrals, hotlines, national and local training, free support groups, and research.

Overeaters Anonymous
tel. (505) 891 2664; www.overeatersanonymous.org
OA is a 12-step self-help organization with support groups for individuals with eating disorders.

O-Anon
tel. (206) 382-3587
O-Anon is a 12-step organization with support groups for relatives or friends of individuals with eating disorders.

If you have an eating disorder, you are the one who is responsible for seeking out treatment for your condition on your own time. No one can force you to receive treatment, and the only effective treatment is voluntary. What you need to realize, though, is that you may be damaging your body permanently in pursuit of your "ideal" body. Anorexia can lead to heart problems, hormonal problems, skin disorders, and osteoporosis. Bulimia can cause heart damage, kidney failure, and tooth decay. The longer you have an eating disorder, the more likely your medical problems will persist after you're successfully treated.

Unfortunately, I don't have the space to launch into the various treatments for eating disorders. (Entire books have been written just on that topic.) You can, however, get more information on treatment from the resources on page 125.

I cannot emphasize enough what an important role weight plays in your digestive tract function. If you aren't at a healthy weight, chances are you don't have a healthy GI tract. Achieving a healthy weight and healthy body image will make you feel better about yourself. You'll have a healthier outlook and will probably take better care of yourself by fueling your body with high-quality, nutritious foods. And your digestive system will reward you in the long run by naturally working the way it should.

Part II

MANAGING YOUR SYMPTOMS

CAN YOU SPELL
INDIGESTION?

On TV AND IN MAGAZINES YOU hear a lot of medical lingo like "esophageal reflux" and "dyspepsia" to describe symptoms that you may know only as indigestion. Indigestion can mean a wide range of symptoms, from heartburn to stomach pain to nausea. And not surprisingly, it is our most common gastrointestinal complaint. On one occasion or another we've all had a meal that doesn't sit quite right. Indigestion, though, means different things to different people. One woman might describe her indigestion as a burning sensation that moves upward from her upper abdomen to her chest. Another woman might say she feels bloated and uncomfortably full after eating a large meal. Someone else might find that heartburn symptoms plague her throughout the night. Indigestion often—though not always—occurs after eating a meal. It's really an all-encompassing term that includes one or more of the following symptoms:

- heartburn (a burning feeling or discomfort in the stomach that moves up into the chest)
- reflux (a feeling of "hot water" in the back of the throat)
- upset stomach
- nausea
- bloated feeling
- abdominal pain, burning, squeezing, fullness, tightness

Although these symptoms usually resolve on their own, they can also indicate a serious medical condition, such as heart disease, that warrants treatment. So while I don't want you to jump to any alarming conclusions, I don't think you should ignore warning signs. I discuss the distinguishing differences between heartburn and heart disease on pages 150–152. Also in this chapter (and all the other chapters in Part II), I include a section called "When to See the Doctor," where I list the red flag symptoms that need to be immediately checked out by your doctor. This section is a *must read*.

THE AMAZING ABILITIES
OF YOUR STOMACH

I have been practicing gastroenterology for over ten years now, yet I'm still fascinated by the way the stomach functions. Ever wonder why your stomach rumbles when your meal is delivered to you in a restaurant? The very act of seeing and smelling food initiates the digestive process. You begin to salivate, and your stomach starts churning, increasing its production of acid and digestive enzymes to prepare for the delectables heading its way.

With a capacity about the size of a football, the stomach contains a chemical soup of stomach acid and the digestive enzymes lipase and pepsinogen. The acid produced by the stomach serves to activate these enzymes and kill off bacteria and viruses in your food. At any given time, the stomach holds about 25 percent of the total volume of food and liquid in the digestive tract. That's an incredible amount, considering its size compared to the rest of the digestive tract.

More food for thought: Each day your gastrointestinal tract moves about 2.5 gallons of fluid from the beverages you drink, the food you eat, and the juices released from the stomach and other digestive organs. The small intestines absorb about 2 gallons of this fluid into your bloodstream, some of which makes its way into your bladder to be expelled as urine. The colon absorbs 90 percent of the half-gallon that's left. Barely 3 ounces of fluid reach the rectum and get expelled from your body in the stool you pass. Your body has a pretty efficient system for not wasting water!

With all the machinations that have to occur to keep your GI tract running smoothly, it's a wonder we don't all suffer from digestive problems 24/7. But there is beauty in the way we were designed. All of our digestive organs work in synchronicity, even the wavelike motions of digestive muscles as they contract to push food down the esophagus, through the stomach, and into the intestines. There is beauty in the design of the plumbing that connects your esophagus to your stomach. The lower esophageal sphincter (LES) neatly opens when food needs to pass through into your stomach, then quickly closes shut so food can't wash back up.

And there is beauty in your stomach—yes, your stomach—and the way it stretches and expands to accommodate the food you've just eaten. The average woman can hold 4 to 6 cups of food in her stomach, while those who are overweight can hold up to 7 or 8 cups. When your stomach stretches to its capacity, special stretch receptor cells in the stomach send a message to your brain that you're full. If you have a habit of eating a lot of food at one time during the day, your stomach capacity may be greater, and it may take you longer to feel full during a meal. On the flip side, if you spread your calories evenly throughout the day, your stomach capacity may be smaller.

You may be surprised to learn that you can shrink your stomach capacity. The less you eat during meals, the less your stomach expects to get. In a study published in the *American Journal of Clinical Nutrition*, obese individuals who were put on a reduced-calorie diet for four weeks felt the sensation of fullness at a 36 percent smaller stomach capacity than obese nondieters. Thus, your stomach may be the key to successful weight loss. Feed it less, and it will expect less. It will activate the "full" signal *before* you've overeaten.

WHAT DOES YOUR INDIGESTION MEAN?

Whenever I see a patient who complains of heartburn or other symptoms of indigestion, I have to consider any number of gastrointestinal conditions including gastroesophageal reflux disease (GERD), ulcers, gastritis (inflammation of the stomach lining), and gallbladder disease. Specific symptoms and experiences can help me pinpoint one cause over another. For instance, if you're plagued by heartburn and acid regurgitation, you probably have GERD. If you have pain that bores into your midsection right under your rib cage, you might have an ulcer. This pain gets either better or worse with food and is usually short lived. I would suspect an ulcer even more if you told me you're taking a nonsteroidal anti-inflammatory drug (such as Advil, Nuprin, Motrin, Aleve, or aspirin) on a regular basis to relieve chronic pain caused by arthritis or premenstrual symptoms, headaches, or some other condition. These drugs can erode the stomach lining over time.

If you're diabetic and you have heartburn or reflux, you might have a condition called *gastroparesis,* a motility disorder of the stomach that causes a delayed emptying of food and often occurs with diabetes. Gallbladder disease could be a possibility if you have nausea and pain in the upper-right-hand side of your abdomen that begins shortly after a meal and lasts for several hours. Of course, you could have all the symptoms of indigestion without any clinical finding on an X-ray or via an endoscopy. In this case, you might have "nonulcer dyspepsia," a diagnosis given when all other conditions have been ruled out. It is similar to irritable bowel syndrome, except that it affects the upper part of your digestive tract rather than the lower portion.

That's all I'm going to say about these gastrointestinal medical conditions in this chapter. If your symptoms are only occasional and relatively mild, you may not have any of these illnesses. They may simply result from something you ate, some medication you're taking, or some other lifestyle factor. In this case, *you* can be your most effective healer—and I don't mean by reaching automatically for one of dozens of over-the-counter remedies that promise you instant relief.

Living in America, we're all on a search for quick fixes for our health problems. We live in a land of e-mails, cell phones, and beeping Palm Pilots that have our lives scheduled down to the minute. Who has time to be sick? If we could, we'd take a pill to cure all our aches and pains rather than take the time to change our lifestyle.

Unfortunately, medications aren't always the best answer when it comes to digestive health problems. Many drugs cause unwanted side effects, and nearly all treat the symptoms without actually fixing the underlying cause of the problem. For this reason, I'm a big believer in starting your "fix" with lifestyle modification—that is, making a change in the way you eat, exercise, and live your life overall. You can still try an over-the-counter remedy to relieve your symptoms, but by altering your lifestyle, you'll help prevent the underlying condition in the first place. This is especially true for indigestion.

As I was writing this chapter, a new patient, Joanne, came to see me because she was suffering from severe heartburn. She also complained about her breath. She told me she always had a bad taste in her mouth and was concerned that others would notice her breath. "I pop Altoids like crazy," she said. I told Joanne that halitosis, or bad breath, is a common problem that goes hand in hand with reflux. I asked her if she noticed that her heartburn had become more severe since she started taking the mints, and she raised her eyebrows in surprise and told me that her heartburn had gotten worse over the past few weeks. "Altoids contain peppermint," I explained, "and peppermint relaxes the sphincter valve at the bottom of your esophagus that opens and closes to keep food from backwashing from your stomach into your esophagus. Eating peppermint can cause this valve to open more frequently than necessary, which can result in heartburn." Joanne immediately opened her purse, grabbed two packets of Altoids, and threw them away in my trash can.

Joanne and I then went through a list of other foods that could be heartburn offenders. She told me she drank about six cups of coffee a day and ate a chocolate bar as a midafternoon snack. I told her she would need to cut back on the coffee and chocolate since these foods, like peppermint, relax the LES muscle. On our next visit a month later Joanne told me that her heartburn symptoms now bothered her only once every two weeks, instead of every day. Her symptoms became much more tolerable and, to her, definitely less worrisome. She was able to manage her infrequent bouts of heartburn with antacids. Joanne was particularly surprised that her bad breath improved *after* she stopped taking the breath mints. She still has a mint or two occasionally after, say, eating pizza with garlic and onions, but she no longer keeps Altoids with her at all times.

WHAT CAUSES INDIGESTION?

There's no one simple cause for all cases of indigestion. That's because symptoms can arise from various malfunctions in the digestive tract. Here are some of the biggest culprits.

Harmful Stomach Acid

Most people believe that "too much stomach acid" is the cause of indigestion. Truth is, most indigestion occurs because of where the acid is located rather than how much acid is produced. If stomach acid winds up in your esophagus because of a malfunction in your LES, you can get a nasty case of heartburn. Your stomach has special features that protect it against the ravaging effects of stomach acid—such as a mucus layer and tight connections between stomach cells that keep acid from seeping in. Your esophagus doesn't have these same features. This means that every time acid splashes up through your esophageal sphincter, it can sear and burn the esophageal lining, causing pain.

Certain foods can promote acid backwash (heartburn) or give you a feeling of indigestion. Gassy foods like carbonated sodas, beans, and cruciferous vegetables (broccoli, cauliflower, brussels sprouts) can make you belch and feel bloated. Acidic foods like citrus fruit, coffee, and tomatoes put more acid in your stomach. And alcohol, chocolate, and mints can cause a relaxation in the LES, causing acid to backwash more easily.

In certain cases, the stomach can produce too much acid, which can set the stage for an ulcer. This usually occurs from an infection with the bacteria *Helicobacter pylori*. These bacteria cause gastritis, or an irritation of the lining of the stomach, and increase the production of stomach acid. This increased acid can also damage the more fragile lining of the duodenum (the first part of the small intestine), causing ulcers to form there. (See Chapter 10 for more on ulcers.) The more acid you have churning around in your stomach, the worse the pain.

Some people have the opposite problem: They produce too little stomach acid. Although this won't lead to heartburn, it can cause bloating, gas, or diarrhea. What's more, low acid can prevent the proper absorption of vital nutrients such as iron, zinc, and B-complex vitamins. (Folic acid is a B vitamin necessary in early pregnancy for the prevention of birth defects.)

The most common cause of low acid is long-term infection with *H. pylori*. I know I seem to be contradicting myself, but the latest research shows that people who have a chronic *H. pylori* infection that goes undiagnosed for years eventually wind up with lower levels of stomach acid. Over time *H. pylori* causes changes in the lining of the stomach that result in decreased acid production. This chronic infection is probably the cause of decreased acid production in the elderly population. When we lack enough stomach acid, bacteria from our food can multiply in the stomach and small intestine. This can alter the motility of the digestive tract, resulting in the bloating and gas. What's more, chronic bacterial overgrowth can damage the lining of the small intestine, making it less able to digest and absorb nutrients. This undigested food makes its way to the colon, where it is fermented by colon bacteria, causing even more gas and bloating as well as diarrhea.

Motility Problems

The motions or motility of the stomach can cause indigestion, especially if motility is too slow, which delays the emptying of food from the stomach. The main function of stomach motility is to churn and grind food into smaller and smaller particles. When the particles are tiny enough, this liquid mixture of acid and particles is then allowed to pass in measured amounts into the small intestine. If the stomach empties too slowly (a common complication of diabetes), you may feel full after eating just a small amount of food, which can feel like bloating or indigestion. Plus, you have a greater chance of experiencing reflux and heartburn because food remains in your stomach for a longer period of time. Delayed stomach emptying can also be caused by diet. High-fat foods take longer for the stomach to digest, so they empty from the stomach more slowly. This is why you get the "I can't believe I ate the whole thing" feeling after eating a piece of stuffed pizza or a chocolate-cream-filled doughnut.

Heightened Sensitivity

You may be very sensitive to the inner workings of your GI tract, which causes you to feel pain or indigestion from the normal passage of food. A heightened sensitivity in the colon is often caused by IBS. If you have indigestion symptoms with no apparent cause, you may have nonulcer dyspepsia, a condition I discuss in Chapter 10.

Dietary Habits

If you suddenly fill your stomach beyond its capacity, you could be asking for trouble. Remember that one-way valve that keeps food from backwashing into your esophagus? Well, it tends to relax and let food splash back up if you eat too much. As your stomach stretches to accommodate the extra food, it can push up against this sphincter, causing it to relax and open. What's more, your stomach will need to produce more acid to digest all that food, which can make heartburn hurt even more. Overindulging in heartburn-promoting foods can exacerbate indigestion.

PREVENTING INDIGESTION

If you've been experiencing any of the symptoms on pages 129–130, your first course of action should be to do everything you can to prevent the symptoms from happening in the first place.

Eat Smaller, More Frequent Meals

Eating smaller, more frequent meals can help prevent indigestion. Try eating four to six small meals a day instead of three large ones, to avoid overloading your digestive system with too much food at one time. Eating smaller meals provides the added benefit of shrinking your stomach capacity so you'll feel less hungry and be less likely to overeat in the future.

Eat Slooooowly

Try not to eat on the run. Take a few minutes to sit down and really taste and savor your food. Eating too quickly can cause you to swallow air, leaving you with bloating and indigestion. When you sit down for a meal, cut the food into small pieces and chew it thoroughly. You'll enjoy it more, and your body will, too.

Watch What You Eat

Certain foods increase the acid in the stomach or slow digestion, causing symptoms. Some foods can relax the LES, which can cause food and acid to backwash into your esophagus, causing heartburn. You may want to cut back or avoid the following:

- Fatty foods: High-fat foods like cheese, fried foods, and butter take longer for your stomach to digest, so they sit in your stomach and cause you to feel fuller longer.
- Gassy foods: Carbonated sodas contain gas that can cause bloating, belching, and that too-full feeling. So too can foods that increase the production of gas by colon bacteria, such as high-fiber foods, green leafy vegetables, and beans.
- Acidic foods: Some foods that are naturally acidic may cause stomach upset by altering the pressure on the LES, causing it to open at inappropriate times. These foods include citrus fruits, tomatoes, orange and tomato juice, colas, coffee, tea, and beer.

- Heartburn offenders: Eating chocolate, peppermint, or onions can relax your LES.

Fill Your Shopping Cart Wisely

Stock up on nonacidic fruits (such as apples, pears, and bananas) to substitute for more acidic fruits like oranges and tomatoes. Go for low-fat, low-calorie, high-fiber foods (which will help you lose excess weight). Keep some antacid products (available without a prescription) in your medicine cabinet for occasional relief from heartburn.

Moderate Your Alcohol Intake

Alcohol can increase stomach acid, aggravating heartburn. It also is broken down into a chemical that gets into your bloodstream and causes your esophageal sphincter to relax. I'm not going to tell you to avoid alcohol altogether. I myself enjoy a glass of wine occasionally and recognize that it helps protect against heart disease. You should, though, determine how much you can tolerate without getting severe heartburn and try not to exceed that amount. Also, make sure you don't imbibe on an empty stomach. Food slows the absorption of alcohol into your bloodstream, so you'll be less likely to get heartburn, nausea, and a hangover the next day.

Don't Smoke

You already know this is a dangerous habit. Smoking is responsible for the deaths of tens of thousands of women each year from lung cancer, emphysema, and heart disease. In addition, the nicotine found in to-bacco can make heartburn worse by decreasing the ability of the LES to work properly. One report found that heartburn was 50 percent more likely to occur after a woman smoked a cigarette than before she smoked. Smoking also changes the composition of saliva, which normally contains acid-neutralizing chemicals called bicarbonates. Smokers' saliva contains smaller amounts of these bicarbonates, so the ability of saliva to neutral-ize stomach acid before it backwashes is diminished. Of course, I realize it's difficult to quit, but a variety of re-sources are available that can help ease the break. Nic-otine patches and gum can help you wean yourself off nicotine. Support groups like the American Lung Association's Freedom from Smoking group can help you deal with the emotional aspects of quitting; log on to www.lungusa.org for more information.

Lose Weight and/or Take the Pressure off Your Waist

Too much pressure on your stomach can cause reflux. To help ease the pressure, maintain a healthy weight or, if you're overweight, lose excess weight. You should also loosen your belt and avoid wearing tight jeans and skirts. If you know you're going out for a big business lunch, for example, choose the suit with the looser-fitting skirt. Also, avoid bending over right after eating.

If you have a stretching routine, do it before meals rather than after.

Avoid Eating Before Bedtime

Try to avoid eating within two or three hours of bedtime. If you lie down on a full stomach, the food and acid don't have the pull of gravity to prevent them from washing back up. If you must lie down, lie on your left side, since this appears to keep heartburn at bay.

MEDICATIONS AND DIETARY SUPPLEMENTS THAT LEAD TO INDIGESTION

Several years ago I developed arthritis in my wrist from doing endoscopies, a medical procedure that requires a lot of repetitive wrist motions. I took over-the-counter ibuprofen (Advil) every day to reduce the pain, and it worked. Trouble was, I developed a new pain, one in my stomach. I would walk around all day with my fist clenched in my belly to ease my pain. I didn't even realize I was doing it until the nurses pointed it out to me. I finally switched to a prescription anti-inflammatory pain reliever called rofecoxib (Vioxx), which doesn't cause stomach upset. I didn't realize just how bad my indigestion was until it was gone. Many drugs can cause chronic heartburn or stomach upset, so I urge you to make a list of any prescription and nonprescription medications you may be taking as well as any dietary supplements (herbal products, vitamins, nutritional supplements) and discuss this list with your doctor.

Nonsteroidal Anti-inflammatory Drugs (NSAIDs)

These drugs, which include aspirin, ibuprofen (Advil, Motrin, Nuprin), and naproxen sodium (Aleve, Naprosyn), can irritate the stomach lining and decrease its ability to protect against damage from harmful acid. As a result, the stomach lining can erode, causing stomach upset, heartburn, and eventually an ulcer. Read your medication labels: Even cold and flu remedies contain aspirin (salicylates) or ibuprofen. If you're taking an NSAID for arthritis or other chronic pain condition and have stomach upset, talk to your doctor about switching to one of the newer anti-inflammatory COX-2 inhibitor drugs—such as rofecoxib (Vioxx) or celecoxib (Celebrex)—that may cause fewer gastrointestinal side effects.

Bisphosphonate Drugs

These prescription medications, such as alendronate sodium (Fosamax), are extremely effective for the treatment and prevention of osteoporosis in women with bone loss. The trouble is, the pill is fairly large and sticky and sometimes gets lodged in the esophagus. As the pill dissolves, it can cause corrosion in the esophagus that, in rare instances, can lead to an ulcer. This causes *extreme* pain for up to a week until the ulcer heals. Women who take these medications must take the pill with 6 to 8 ounces of water and shouldn't lie down for at least thirty minutes to help the pill reach the stomach more quickly and reduce the potential for irritation of the esophagus.

Other Medications

Potassium supplements, antibiotics—such as doxycycline (Doryx), tetracycline (Achromycin V, Sumycin), ciprofloxacin (Cipro), clindamycin (Cleocin)—sustained release iron supplements, NSAIDs, and vitamin C and vitamin A supplements can all cause "pill esophagitis." These pills, like alendronate, are sticky and may dissolve in the esophagus, causing a large esophageal ulcer if they become stuck. A female physician friend of mine was taking doxycycline for an infection and ended up with terrible esophagitis. She had pain every time she swallowed that lasted for over a week. She had a hard time eating and drinking and lost several pounds before her symptoms subsided.

Herbs Linked to Indigestion

Herbal products, home remedies, and other dietary supplements (vitamins and minerals) can also cause indigestion. These products aren't regulated by the FDA, so the exact incidence of digestive side effects isn't known. (Supplement manufacturers don't want to publicize this information, and who could blame them?) Although research is lacking, certain products have been shown in studies to be associated with digestive ills. Garlic pills may cause stomach burning and nausea. Ginkgo, feverfew, and chaste tree berry may cause gastrointestinal disturbances like gas, bloating, diarrhea, or constipation. Saw palmetto may cause stomach upset.

MEDICATIONS COMMONLY ASSOCIATED WITH INDIGESTION

The *Physicians' Desk Reference* lists literally hundreds of medications that have "dyspepsia, stomach upset" as a significant side effect. Here are some of the more common ones. If you're worried that your medication might be causing indigestion, talk to your doctor or pharmacist.

- acarbose (Precose)
- alendronate (Fosamax)
- codeine
- corticosteroids (Prednisone)
- iron pills
- metformin (Glucophage)
- nonsteroidal anti-inflammatory drugs: ibuprofen (Advil, Motrin, Nuprin), naproxen sodium (Aleve)
- oral antibiotics such as erythromycin
- orlistat (Xenical)
- potassium supplements
- theophylline (Theo-Dur)

RELIEVE INDIGESTION WITH . . .

Antacids

These drugstore remedies to reduce stomach acid can help relieve heartburn or stomach upset. They quickly neutralize the excess stomach acid that is produced when you've kicked back a few drinks or eaten a hefty dinner at your favorite restaurant. Over-the-counter antacids like

Alka-Seltzer, Maalox, Mylanta, Pepto-Bismol, Rolaids, Riopan, and Tums use a combination of magnesium, calcium, and aluminum to neutralize acid. They're pretty benign and have few side effects. Some people, though, who take antacids containing magnesium may experience diarrhea. Those who take antacids containing aluminum or calcium may experience constipation.

As the commercials say, an antacid can bring you the quickest form of relief (within minutes), but this relief is usually short-lived. It won't prevent heartburn from happening in the first place, and it probably won't help you sleep through the night if you have a bad case of indigestion.

Taking an antacid to relieve an occasional bout of indigestion is fine, but I would avoid taking it on a daily basis. Antacids containing calcium can stimulate the release of gastrin (a stomach enzyme), which causes the secretion of acid—a phenomenon known as acid rebound. Whether acid rebound actually causes any adverse effects, like the production of more stomach acid over time, isn't known. To be on the safe side, don't take an antacid continuously for more than two weeks. (If you have kidney problems, you should check with your doctor before taking any antacid, since these drugs can cause toxic levels of minerals in the blood if the kidneys are impaired.)

Acid-Blockers

Over-the-counter acid-blockers such as Zantac, Pepcid, Tagamet, and Axid come in half the dose of the prescription strength. (Pepcid is now also available over the counter in full prescription strength.) They take longer to work than antacids because they must be absorbed into your bloodstream to become effective. But they bring longer-lasting relief, from four to eight hours. As this book was going to press, another acid-blocker, Prilosec (omeprazole) also became available over the counter in full prescription strength. Prilosec is a more potent acid-blocker that lasts for twenty-four hours so it may provide longer-lasting relief of heartburn symptoms. Prilosec is indicated for frequent heartburn symptoms; if your symptoms continue despite this medicine, you need to see your doctor.

To prevent heartburn and indigestion, I recommend taking an over-the-counter acid-blocker an hour *before* going out for a big dinner or drink fest. You might also want to keep an antacid on hand in case you experience symptoms afterward and need immediate relief. One product, Pepcid Complete, which contains both an antacid and an acid-blocker in the same tablet, may be more convenient.

Alternative Remedies

If you prefer to find relief the more natural way, you can try an herbal product. Some studies suggest that herbal remedies that contain peppermint oil, chamomile, or ginger can relieve indigestion. In general, I'm not a big fan of herbal remedies because of the lack of scientific research confirming their effectiveness and because of the lack of safety regulations for these products. However, the following herbs are fairly benign and may bring relief from indigestion.

Peppermint can be very helpful in relieving stomach pain and nausea, with one caveat: It can relax the LES sphincter. So if you have heartburn, drinking peppermint in tea form probably isn't a good idea. Instead, you may want to try an enteric-coated peppermint pill, recommends Paul Lebovitz, M.D., a gastroenterologist who often uses alternative medicine in his practice at the Allegheny General Hospital in Pittsburgh. Such a pill prevents heartburn by passing through the stomach before it is digested. Dr. Lebovitz finds that two products, Pepogest by Nature's Way and Peppermint Plus by Enzymatic Therapy, work particularly well in his patients.

Chamomile is thought to cause a relaxation effect on the gastrointestinal tract. It's been used for centuries in Europe to relieve gastrointestinal complaints, but few studies have been done to see whether it really works. You can purchase chamomile teas and extracts in any health food store. One caveat: Since chamomile is part of the ragweed family, you shouldn't drink chamomile tea if you're allergic to ragweed.

Ginger works similarly to chamomile and has been studied extensively for the treatment of nausea during pregnancy. It has recently been found to be helpful for the treatment of other symptoms of indigestion. You can purchase ginger capsules, ginger teas, and crystallized ginger in health food stores. You can also buy pure gingerroot in the supermarket. If you buy crystallized or pure ginger, slice off a thin piece and place it on your tongue for several minutes. You can chew and swallow it, or suck the juice out and spit out the rest.

Fennel is used in several cultures to prevent gas and upset stomach. Chewing the seeds after a meal freshens the breath and releases a compound called terpenoid anethole. This compound may relieve gas pain and upset stomach by inhibiting spasms in the GI muscles and increasing stomach motility. Whole seeds may be chewed or used in tea. To make a tea, boil 2 to 3 grams of crushed seeds in one cup of water for 10 to 15 minutes. Cool, strain, and drink up to three cups per day.

HEARTBURN OR HEART ATTACK?

A few months ago a fifty-four-year-old African-American woman, Rhonda, came to the clinic complaining of chest pain. Rhonda's family doctor was concerned that her heartburn and chest pain were caused by reflux. Rhonda did have heartburn and occasional regurgitation of hot liquid into her mouth. Her symptoms were usually worse after big meals. But she also told me she had pain that radiated from her chest up to her neck and down her left arm that occasionally woke her when she slept. She had a strong family history of heart disease. I noted that Rhonda was obese and diabetic, two significant risk factors for heart disease, and decided I couldn't simply write off her heartburn as GERD. I referred her to a cardiologist at the University of Virginia Hospital, who discovered that her chest pain was really angina that was caused by several blocked coronary arteries. After opening these blockages with stents, Rhonda still had some heartburn symptoms, but they were mild and could be relieved by diet modifications.

When it comes to heart disease, women have been given the short end of the stick. For too long doctors neglected to take women's heart disease symptoms seriously. Many women still aren't aware of the fact that heart disease is the number-one killer of women in the United States. Sometimes the symptoms of heartburn can mimic those of a heart attack and vice versa. I don't want to scare you into thinking that every case of heartburn warrants a visit to the emergency room. I do, though, think you need to be aware of the warning signs that can help you distinguish the minor from the serious.

Distinguishing between chest pain caused by a heart attack and chest pain caused by heartburn and indigestion can be tricky even for the most skilled gastroenterologists and cardiologists. In the majority of cases heartburn (defined as a burning pain behind the sternum) and regurgitation (the backwash of gastric contents into your mouth) indicate an attack of acid reflux. If pain occurs after meals and gets worse when you lie down, heartburn is the more likely cause.

Heart pain is generally just that—pain or aching in the midchest. This pain is more common after physical exertion and tends to produce a pressure sensation in the middle left part of the chest that sometimes radiates to the neck and to one or both arms. Other possible signals of a heart attack include light-headedness, fainting, sweating, nausea, or shortness of breath.

Still, you can't count on these hallmark differences. Many people experiencing a heart attack describe the pain as a "burning" discomfort. Up to 50 percent of patients with heart disease have symptoms that mimic heartburn. On the flip side, a significant number of people with chest pain who get evaluated by a cardiologist actually have indigestion. Bottom line: You shouldn't diagnose yourself. If you have severe chest pain, which can be indicative of heart disease, seek immediate medical attention.

WHEN TO SEE THE DOCTOR

If your indigestion symptoms are accompanied by any of the following symptoms, call your doctor *immediately.* They are warning signs for more serious conditions:

- difficulty swallowing
- blood in the stool
- vomiting blood
- unexplained weight loss
- chest pain
- choking, chronic cough

The Two-Week Rule

If you have indigestion *without* any of the above symptoms, follow my two-week rule. Try making the lifestyle changes that I suggested starting on page 139. If after two weeks, you find your indigestion is still bothering you on a regular basis and causing major discomfort, make an appointment with your doctor. Before you go in for a visit, keep a symptom journal for a week. Every time you feel discomfort, write down what you're feeling. Bring your journal to your next appointment. Use specific adjectives to describe your pain, like *burning, stabbing, crampy, nauseating, sharp, dull.* Ask yourself these questions: Is the indigestion constant or intermittent? What makes it better, and what makes it worse? When are the symptoms most likely to occur? How long do they last? By the same token, note when you feel symptom free. Do you feel your best after breakfast or right before dinner? Record your answers in your journal. These are the types of questions your doctor will ask you, so he or she can determine the cause of your symptoms. Being prepared and knowing what your doctor will ask at your visit will help ensure you get a correct diagnosis.

GAS AND BLOATING

LISA S. CAME TO SEE ME FOR THE first time as I was writing this chapter. She told me her symptoms were more annoying than painful. As an attorney at a highbrow law firm, she felt extremely embarrassed when she burped repeatedly in the middle of an afternoon meeting. She was afraid her clients would think she was unprofessional and uncouth. I listened to Lisa's abdomen with my stethoscope and heard air rumbling in her upper GI tract. I told her I thought her symptoms were caused by air swallowing. This phenomenon—which most of us aren't even aware of—can cause excess air in the GI tract that has to be expelled through burping, or else it may travel into the intestines and cause abdominal bloat and flatulence.

Lisa probably gulped large amounts of air when she was stressed. She was also a fast eater, which added to the problem. I told her she needed to cut out the chewing gum and carbonated drinks, which can increase air in the GI tract. I also told her she needed to

Stress and Gas

"I'm a fast-paced person. I work ten-hour days at my engineering firm, and the day is packed with stressful meetings, deadlines, and phone calls. I brown-bag my lunch and wolf it down in ten minutes at my desk because I usually don't have time to go out. I love the work, but I notice that when I'm superstressed, I get extremely gassy after lunch. It's like a pressure pushing down on my diaphragm that becomes more intense until I belch and belch and belch. Sometimes I even wake up in the morning feeling bloated, and when I sit up, I burp repeatedly—even though I haven't eaten in ten hours. My husband looks at me strangely whenever I have a belching episode, but it's the only thing that makes me feel better."

—**Dawn F.**, 28, an engineer who has suffered from gas symptoms for the past five years

slow down her eating, taking thirty minutes to consume her lunch instead of ten. I suspected that the reason she woke up feeling gassy was that she was taking her stress to bed. I suggested she engage in ten minutes of meditation or relaxation exercises just before she went to sleep.

As I was polishing the final draft of this chapter, Lisa came to see me for a follow-up appointment. She told me she tried some of the changes I suggested and found that her symptoms occurred far less frequently. "I take a few bites of my lunch, put it aside, and read a magazine or take a phone call before I continue to eat. This forces me to eat less quickly," she said. She completely cut out the diet soft drinks and instead drank bottled water. She also bought a relaxation tape that she listened to with her husband every night before bed. "We find it a nice way to unwind together," she said. "He's a doctor, so he understands the importance of reducing stress, and I find it a nice way to end the day."

Gas and bloating can be very vague symptoms. Unlike constipation and diarrhea, gastroenterologists can't medically define them in black-and-white terms. Thus we rely on our patients' descriptions of symptoms to make a diagnosis. Medical tests may or may not show evidence of excess gas in the intestines, and feeling bloated is often just that: a feeling. Even if your body isn't actually making excess gas, you can be bothered by the normal amounts of gas passing through your intestines.

I've had patients try to prove to me visually that they were bloated. One woman took a home video of herself every day to show how her abdomen expanded on days she was feeling bloated. She lifted up her shirt and wrapped a tape measure around her belly to show me how the measurements changed from her "bloat" to her "no-bloat" days.

The truth is, I don't need the visual image of a rounded belly to convince me that a person is feeling bloated. Bloating and gassiness are very real symptoms, regardless of the source of the discomfort.

I was tempted to call this chapter "Gas and Bloating: The Woman's Problem" because these symptoms are so predominantly associated with women. Although gas and bloating may strike at the same time, they are really two separate gastrointestinal problems. They can be treated in similar ways but may be caused by different things. For this reason, I discuss gas separately from bloating. I do, however, give one set of recommendations for reducing both gas and bloating, since both can be alleviated by the same measures.

As women, we politely say we're feeling "gassy" instead of describing our true symptoms: excessive belching and flatulence. Can't you just see your mother frowning right now? It's important for you to know that everyone passes gas. Women need to fart just as much as men do. And yes, we're going to pass gas at inappropriate times, like during intercourse or in the middle of an important business meeting. Belching and flatulence are normal. To convince my patients of this, I keep a copy of *The Gas We Pass—The Story of Farts* by Shinta Cho in my waiting room. It looks like a children's cartoon book, but it carries a strong message that it's okay to pass gas. In fact, it's normal and healthy for your digestive tract.

WHAT CAUSES GAS?

Gas gets into your body in two ways: Either you swallow it, or your body makes it from the foods you eat. The average woman passes about 700 milliliters of gas a day—which could fill two soda cans—and passes flatus about ten times per day. You may have noticed that some farts are smellier than others; this has everything to do with the type of gas passed. Your flatus is composed of varying amounts of five gases: nitrogen, oxygen, carbon dioxide, hydrogen, and methane, plus trace amounts of other gases. Sulfur, one of the gases found in only trace amounts, is what gives gas its unappealing odor—the kind that makes you want to exit a crowded elevator *tout de suite.* Certain sulfur compounds in garlic can make your farts smellier.

Researchers have found that activated charcoal can eliminate the smell of sulfur so that farts are odor free. One company, UltraTech Products in Houston, has decided to take advantage of this research finding and now markets Flatulence Filters, a foam seat cushion coated with activated charcoal that traps about 90 percent of odor-causing sulfur gas.

During those times when you fire off a rapid succession of farts (I know I'm being blunt and unladylike here), you're probably releasing gas with high amounts of hydrogen and carbon dioxide and low amounts of nitrogen. Carbon dioxide and hydrogen in the flatus are thought to be produced from the fermentation of food particles by bacteria in the colon. For instance, fruits and vegetables (particularly legumes) often contain high amounts of sugars called oligosaccharides that can't be digested by enzymes in the small intestine but are fermented by bacteria in the colon; this causes the production of hydrogen. Hydrogen production also increases after eating flour made from wheat, oats, potatoes, or corn. Production of this gas is also increased in lactose-intolerant people who eat a lot of lactose-rich dairy products in one sitting. Carbon dioxide is produced from eating high-fat foods when stomach acid gets neutralized from breaking down the triglycerides in fats.

Those who swallow excessive amounts of air due to stress or eating too rapidly often have a problem with belching or flatus. The nitrogen in air is usually the culprit behind these symptoms. Gas expert Michael Levitt,

M.D., a gastroenterologist at the Minneapolis Veterans Affairs Medical Center and a colleague of mine, saw a patient who farted an average of 170 times a day. After collecting all his rectal gas and finding that it was mainly nitrogen, Dr. Levitt concluded that his patient was an air-gulper.

Excess gas can be released from the body in one of two ways: belching or farting.

Belching

Gas that occurs in the upper GI tract leads to belching. Most of this gas comes from swallowing air when you're stressed or nervous, eating or drinking too quickly, drinking carbonated beverages, chewing gum, or smoking. People with sleep apnea or reflux may also swallow excessive amounts of air.

Burping or belching is the way most swallowed air leaves the stomach. The remaining gas moves into the small intestine, where it is partially absorbed. A small amount travels into the large intestine, where it is released through the rectum. An occasional belch after meals is perfectly normal, but belching frequently may mean that you're swallowing too much air.

Flatulence

Air or gas that you pass through your rectum is called flatus. Again, I want to reiterate that it's normal to pass gas and that the average woman farts about ten times per day. Sometimes excess flatulence can be caused by an inability to digest certain foods properly, like the milk sugar lactose (in those who are lactose intolerant). Starting a high-fiber diet can also cause excess flatulence at first, since your body may not have enough bacteria to digest the extra fiber. Your body does adjust, and within a few weeks of beginning a high-fiber diet, excess flatulence should improve.

WHY AM I SO BLOATED?

I suspect that most men don't ponder this question on a regular basis—and not many men own up to feeling bloated. Either they aren't bothered by bloating, or they just don't like to talk about it. I think it's safe to say, though, that far more women are annoyed by abdominal bloat than men. In fact, statistics show that 10 to 25 percent of people have regular bouts of bloating and that twice as many women suffer from bloating than men. One study conducted by researchers at the University of North Carolina found that bloating affected 19 percent of women but only 10 percent of men.

Bloating and abdominal distension really are about the *perception* of increased gas. Most of the time they're not actually caused by an increase in gas, which has been confirmed in research studies. People who suffer from irritable bowel syndrome, especially women, often experience abdominal bloating. Studies have shown that most don't actually produce excess gas but may, instead, be more sensitive to the sensation of gas passing through their intestines. Some IBS sufferers may also have difficulty passing gas through their lower GI tract. Gas may collect there, causing abdominal pain and bloating.

Bloating can be caused by a variety of reasons, from the obvious to the surprising. You may be all too familiar with the bloating brought on by your period or by gassy foods, but have you ever considered that stress, a cough syrup, or a crash diet could be causing your bloating? Once you figure out what's causing it, you'll probably be able to manage your symptoms and even eliminate them altogether.

HORMONAL HAVOC

A rise in the sex hormones estrogen and progesterone during the latter half of your cycle can cause premenstrual bloat. (Bloating is one of the first signs of pregnancy, also due to a rise in these two hormones.) Medical experts aren't certain how hormonal changes cause bloating, but one reason may be that progesterone slows down the movement of food through the intestines, which can lead to that too-full feeling. Once hormone levels decline at the onset of menstruation, bloating usually disappears.

Try the following measures to avoid premenstrual bloat:

- **Get moving.** Doing thirty minutes of steady activity at least three or four days a week throughout the month—or at least during the week before you get your period—helps speed the movement of food through your digestive tract, counteracting the effects of estrogen and progesterone.
- **Stick to a regular sleep schedule.** Go to bed and rise at the same time each day. Disrupting your

DOES BLOATING CAUSE WEIGHT GAIN?

You may have a hard time believing this, but it's true: Abdominal bloating doesn't result in significant weight gain. You might put on half a pound to a pound—due to water retention—if you're bloated, but any weight gain beyond that isn't caused by bloating. Excess gas weighs almost nothing. You're not crazy, though, if you find you can't button your jeans when you're bloated. Bloating definitely causes your waistline to expand, making your clothes feel tighter. In fact, a 1994 study of more than a hundred Canadian women found that bloating can cause a person's waistline to expand by more than two inches.

Now here's the unanswered question: Does excess gas in the intestines actually cause the abdomen to expand like a balloon? Or do people tend to push their abdomen out when they feel gassy and uncomfortable, which causes it to look larger than normal? My colleagues have been debating this question for decades and have come to no resolution. My answer to them is: Does it really matter? We women know that we have trouble buttoning up when we're bloated, and we feel and look thinner when we're not. Enough said.

sleep pattern activates a gland that slows the movement of water through the intestines, which can lead to water retention.

• **Avoid salt and starchy carbohydrates.** PMS may make you crave pretzels, chips, and chocolate chip cookies, but salty and starchy foods increase water retention, which can lead to bloating. When I have the PMS munchies, I eat celery and carrot sticks dipped in salsa. Some of my patients find that eating unsalted peanuts or soy nuts dipped in chocolate (available in whole-food supermarkets) can help feed their cravings without the bloating. To avoid weight gain, stick with a serving-size portion—just enough nuts to cover the palm of your hand.

- **Watch out for oral contraceptives.** They can cause bloating, but the problem usually can be alleviated by switching to a different formulation—probably one with a lower dose of estrogen, as I discussed in Chapter 2.

- **Watch out for hormone replacement therapy (HRT).** In a 2001 study published in the *Journal of Women's Health and Gender-Based Medicine,* 15 percent of women who took HRT stopped taking the drugs due to side effects they were experiencing. Bloating was the number-two reason women cited for discontinuing HRT. It bothered 18 percent of those who quit, compared to just 3 percent of women who decided to stay on HRT. Other symptoms like breast tenderness, bleeding, and spotting affected women in both groups about the same. Of course, HRT has other potential problems, which I discussed in Chapter 2, so if you're suffering from menopausal symptoms, you need to consider your own health profile when making a decision about whether to take hormones.

You may find that bloating becomes a problem around the time of perimenopause, the years leading up to menopause when your periods begin to change in frequency and duration. The hormonal fluctuations that occur during this time can cause abdominal bloat.

THE FEMININITY FACTOR

Being polite and "feminine" sometimes has its drawbacks—especially when it comes to gas and bloating. Little boys smirk when they fart in class. Little girls get shunned. My eight-year-old daughter told me that kids in her class were making fun of a little girl who passed gas in the middle of art class. When I asked her why, she said, "It smelled so bad! None of us wanted to play with her after that because we thought she was gross." My eleven-year-old son, on the other hand, tells me that boys in his class have contests to see who can "make the loudest fart." When I asked him if girls participated in this game, he just rolled his eyes, implying, "No way, Mom."

Unfortunately, we can't change the way society thinks. Farting and belching are still considered uncouth or impolite. And no one wants to be a social outcast. Still, if you don't pass gas when your body gives you the signal, you might wind up feeling bloated later. Most of us learn to pass gas discreetly without feeling too embarrassed. But for some women this is a real problem that requires professional intervention. I've seen patients who won't pass gas in public under any circumstances. They hold it in and often aren't even aware that they have a problem. Many come to me complaining of severe appendicitis-like pains in their abdomen that wax and wane throughout the day and are usually tied to mealtimes.

When I ask them if they regularly pass gas, they give me a funny look and tell me that they feel comfortable doing that only when they have a bowel movement. Some women I've seen won't even pass gas in a public bathroom. Darlene, a forty-five-year-old woman who recently came to see me because of chronic abdominal pain, had this problem. On her first visit she told me, "I would be incredibly embarrassed and humiliated if I knew that anyone knew I was passing gas." She didn't buy my explanation that farting is healthy, that we all do it, and that her pain was being caused by holding it in. She told me she'd rather have the pain than have the "shame" of passing gas. (She couldn't even say the word *fart*.)

After recommending dietary changes to decrease her gas production, I referred Darlene to a psychologist, Dr. J. Kim Penberthy, who used behavioral techniques to get Darlene to face her problem head-on. As part of therapy, Darlene was presented with a challenging mental scenario: "If you passed gas right now, in the middle of this crowded hospital hallway full of people, what's the worst that could happen? Would people run away screaming and forbid you to come into this hospital again? Or would they smell something unpleasant and maybe move away from you a little?" Darlene acknowledged that the latter scenario was more likely.

After a few sessions of discussing her fears and why she had them, Darlene was ready for conditioning therapy. Dr. Penberthy took her to a bathroom in the hospital after lunch and had her pass gas in there. Darlene literally had to learn to do this in steps; she had to learn to relax her anal sphincter and let the gas out. She wasn't even aware that she was tightening her muscles and holding it in. Eventually Darlene learned not to suppress her bodily urges. She admitted that she still felt a little tremor of fear before she passed gas, but she was able to put this fear aside and take care of her body. "I'd rather deal with the few seconds of embarrassment than the hours of abdominal pain," she said.

Sometimes our fears about passing gas in public are too difficult to overcome. A patient named Claire was so embarrassed about her gas problems that she wouldn't even talk to my secretary about why she was calling to make an appointment. When I got on the phone, she whispered to me about her problems with gas. She used enemas regularly to ensure that she always had her bowel movements at home. Sometimes she even used laxatives. She told me she wanted to be "cleaned out" when she got to the office, so she didn't have to worry about passing gas or having a bowel movement in a public bathroom. She had been seeing a psychologist for over a year but had made little headway. She simply couldn't shake out of her head the notions that her mom taught her about what's "polite."

I've spent several appointments explaining to Claire the benefits of letting her bodily functions occur naturally, and I've warned her against tinkering with the timing of her bowel movements. "Chronic use of enemas and laxatives may have a detrimental effect on your GI tract and could cause you to become dependent on them to have a bowel movement," I told her.

Claire understands the logic of what I'm telling her, but she still needs to overcome her emotional reluctance.

SUPERSTRESSED BLOAT

You may have made the connection yourself: Being stressed can cause you to feel bloated. A household emergency, a fight with your spouse, or a harried day at work can cause you to do something that you're probably not even aware of doing: swallow air. Researchers at the University of Alabama at Birmingham found that thirty-eight healthy volunteers who had to do stressful tasks (listening to irritating noises and viewing unpleasant pictures) swallowed three times more frequently than those who engaged in relaxation exercises.

Whenever you swallow when you're not eating, extra air goes into your stomach and may eventually wind up in your intestines. If you do this excessively—when you're stressed—that extra air can cause your abdomen to expand. Stress can also make your intestines easily irritable so you feel more bloated even when normal amounts of gas are passing through your intestines.

In a follow-up study, the same researchers found that swallowing rates can be slowed through various relaxation techniques. When you're feeling stressed, take a ten-minute relaxation break by closing your eyes and breathing deeply, reading a few pages from a juicy novel, or gazing out the window. You can also try progressive muscle relaxation: Tense your feet and toes for five seconds, then relax them; next tense your ankles and shins for five seconds, then relax. Work your way up through all the muscles in your body. Finally, tense all your muscles at once and hold for five seconds, then relax.

Other ways to reduce air swallowing that's not caused by stress: Eliminate gum chewing, smoking, sucking on hard candies, drinking through straws or from bottles, and gulping large quantities of fluid.

LOVE HANDLES AND WEAK ABS

Having a combination of weak abdominal muscles and excess belly fat can lead to that bloated feeling. About 50 percent of newly gained fat appears on the belly, which leaves less room for the intestines to expand comfortably. Weak abdominal muscles add to the problem by not providing enough support. The result? Intestines full of food and digestive juices can sag and push forward, making you feel like your stomach is ballooning out. In a 1994 study researchers found that 40 percent of people who complained of bloating had gained ten or more pounds in the preceding year. Those who agreed to measure their waistlines daily had much larger fluctuations than a group of healthy volunteers. What's more, one-third of the bloating sufferers couldn't do a single sit-up.

Exercise can help you strengthen your abs and take off those excess pounds. You'll need to do a combination of steady exercise (walking, running, swimming, biking) and abdominal-strengthening exercises. Start slowly if you've been inactive, aiming for 15 to 20 minutes of exercise at a pace that makes you breathe hard but doesn't make you feel uncomfortable. To strengthen your abdominal muscles, improve your posture by standing up straight. That alone can help. You can also do modified sit-ups called crunches. Lie on your back with your hands behind your head or crossed in front of your chest; then raise your shoulders and head until your shoulders are four to six inches off the floor. (Pull your torso up with your ab muscles, not with your neck.) Lower and repeat five times. Work your way up to twenty-five repetitions, five or six times a week.

THE SPORTS TRAINING BLOAT

In my practice, I see a fair number of patients who are college athletes. These women exercise two or three or more hours a day, either running, biking, rowing, or swimming. Many complain of bloating and flatulence that occur either during exercise or, more commonly, between workouts. One study found that 71 percent of runners experience lower GI problems like flatulence, bloating, and diarrhea. Other studies have confirmed GI problems in endurance athletes.

Inappropriate training can contribute to gastrointestinal problems like gas and bloating. For instance, if you suddenly increase the intensity or duration of your workouts, you may develop GI symptoms as a result. To avoid this problem, increase gradually in small increments. If you're, say, a runner, you might want to increase your mileage by one or two miles a week, rather than eight or ten.

Eating a proper diet during training and competition is very important for maintaining good GI function. *Nancy Clark's Sports Nutrition Guidebook* by

THE PERCEPTION OF BLOAT

While I was writing this book, a twenty-five-year-old patient named Samantha, a medical technician, came to me complaining that she became extremely bloated every few months and that this bloating lasted for a few days to several weeks. When she first came to me, she grabbed her lower abdomen and said, "This is fat. I know that this bulge isn't bloat. But look at my upper stomach. This is bloated. Don't I look pregnant?" I had to admit that she did. She was standing and her stomach protruded outward, even though she wasn't overweight.

When Samantha lay down for an examination, however, I saw that her stomach was flat, and I didn't feel any distension or hear abnormal rumblings when I listened with my stethoscope. None of the tests that her previous gastroenterologist did (CT scan, ultrasound, MRI, colonoscopy) found any evidence of excess gas in her intestines. When Samantha came to me on a "nonbloat" day, she asked me if I noticed that her stomach was flatter. I told her I saw no difference from the last appointment, when she had felt very bloated. "Do you think I'm crazy?" she asked. I said, "Absolutely not. I believe that you have a real perception of gas in your intestines. For whatever reason, this perception is enhanced at certain times, which causes you to push out your stomach to ease the discomfort."

With gastrointestinal problems, I find that validation of symptoms is extremely important. I gave Samantha's symptoms real meaning, even if I couldn't necessarily make a firm diagnosis. I also helped her evaluate her diet and lifestyle to see if any bloating factors could be contributing to her problem. Samantha found that when she walked on the treadmill and worked out with light weights, she felt less bloated. So I encouraged her to do this, especially on her "bloated" days.

Nancy Clark, M.S., R.D. (Human Kinetics Publishers, 1990) is a great resource for nutritional guidance.

THE CRASH DIET BLOAT

I've told you already that I'm not a fan of crash dieting. Cutting your intake to less than 1,000 calories a day isn't a safe way to lose weight, and chances are you'll start gaining the weight back the minute you get off the diet. Here's one more reason why crash diets should be chucked onto the waste heap of failed weight-loss practices: They can lead to bloating. In a 1996 survey conducted by researchers at the University of North Dakota School of Medicine in Fargo, more than 45 percent of women who said they routinely went on strict diets and had irregular eating habits suffered from frequent bloating, compared to 20 percent of those who said they rarely or never dieted.

This phenomenon may relate to constipation. If you're constipated, you're likely to feel bloated. Skipping meals on a crash diet sets your body up for constipation since your digestive tract is a creature of habit, expecting food at certain times and in certain amounts. It can be thrown off kilter when it never knows when or how much food to expect. Also, many women who crash diet don't drink enough fluids, which aggravates constipation and bloating.

If you want to lose weight, I strongly urge you to lose the pounds gradually, cutting your daily intake by 250 to 500 calories. If you're determined to go on a more restrictive eating plan, make an all-out effort not to skip meals. Eat the same number of meals, but decrease the size of your portions. Have one bowl of bran cereal at breakfast instead of two. Your digestive tract can't work properly unless food comes through at least two to three times a day.

HIGH-ALTITUDE BLOAT

Feeling bloated after a long airplane flight is a common problem. At high altitudes the lower air pressure can cause intestinal gas to expand. Some people are more sensitive to this than others. Making bloating worse is the fact that you're probably stressed from traveling, and you've been stuck in one position for a long time, eating high-fat foods that you're not used to as well as carbonated beverages.

When you're on a plane, walk up and down the aisle a few times after you've finished eating. Walking will help move food and gas out of your digestive system. Also, make a conscious effort not to stray too far from your usual diet. You may even want to pack your own lunch or dinner. (This is practical nowadays, since many airlines have cut out meals as a cost-saving device.) Choose juice or water over soda, and avoid fatty foods, which slow digestion, leaving you feeling fuller longer.

Mountain climbers and those who visit high-altitude cities like Breckenridge, Colorado (which is above nine thousand feet), can also experience this problem, along with altitude sickness. If you experience bloating at high altitudes and other signs of altitude sickness, talk to your doctor about getting the prescription medication acetazolamide (Diamox), which makes it easier to tolerate thinner air. People usually take it one or two days before they reach a high altitude and continue it for the duration of their stay. You can also try an over-the-counter product containing simethicone (such as Gas-X, Extra-strength Phazyme-125, and others).

ARE YOU LACTOSE INTOLERANT?

Nearly 50 million American adults have lactose intolerance, a condition in which the body cannot digest significant amounts of a sugar, called lactose, found in milk and other dairy products. The condition occurs when the body is unable to manufacture adequate amounts of lactase, an enzyme needed to break down and digest lactose. If lactose gets through the stomach and small intestine without being digested, it makes its way to the colon, where colonic bacteria ferment it. This results in gas production and excess fluids, causing bloating and diarrhea. As many as 75 percent of all African Americans, Jews, Native Americans, and Mexican Americans develop this condition as adults, and nearly 90 percent of Asian Americans are also affected. (People of northern European descent are less likely to have lactose intolerance.)

The important thing to realize is that lactose intolerance usually develops in adulthood, so you may have

developed the condition without being aware of it—
even if you've always been able to tolerate dairy products. (As babies, we need our mother's milk to survive,
so our bodies must be able to digest lactose. As we get
older, we rely on milk less and less, so the amount of
lactase that our bodies produce declines.)

The symptoms can be mild or acute but usually
involve nausea, cramps, bloating, gas, and diarrhea,
which begin thirty minutes to two hours after eating
or drinking a food containing lactose, such as milk,
cheese, yogurt, ice cream, or sour cream. Your doctor
can diagnose lactose intolerance through a blood test
that measures your blood sugar levels after you ingest a
lactose liquid or through a hydrogen breath test.

This condition is easily managed: You can moderate
your intake of dairy products. How much dairy is it okay
to have? Only you can figure that one out. Basically, you
can have as much lactose as you can tolerate without experiencing uncomfortable gas symptoms. Most people
with lactose intolerance can tolerate two servings of
dairy products spread throughout the day (two cups of
milk or a few ounces of cheese and a cup of yogurt), according to a study conducted by Dr. Michael Levitt.
Avoiding lactose altogether is tough, given its presence
in many of the foods we eat (yogurt, pizza, cheese), and
many women rely on milk products to boost their calcium intake for osteoporosis prevention.

If you like eating dairy products but don't like the
effects of lactose intolerance, you can buy lactose-free
milk at the supermarket. You can also buy over-the-
counter drops, caplets, and chewable tablets containing

lactase (Lactaid, Dairy Ease, and others) to take with lactose-rich foods. When taken with a dairy meal, the lactase supplements will digest the milk sugar in the small intestine, allowing absorption and preventing it from traveling to the colon, where it can cause all the problems. Follow the instructions on the package to determine how much lactase to take. Dosage is determined by the amount of lactose in a particular food. For a guide to the amount of lactose in foods, log on to Lactaid's website at www.lactaid.com.

You can make your own lactose-free milk by adding a few drops of over-the-counter lactase to a quart of milk. After twenty-four hours in the refrigerator, lactose content is reduced by 70 percent. The process works faster if the milk is heated first, and adding a double amount of lactase liquid produces milk that is 90 percent lactose free.

MEDICATIONS THAT CAUSE BLOAT

If you're chronically bloated but aren't sure why, check the medications or supplements that you're taking. Common medications that might cause bloating include:

- fiber supplements, such as psyllium (Metamucil) and methylcellulose (Citrucel)
- calcium supplements (because they induce constipation), such as Tums, Rolaids, Caltrate, and Os-Cal
- iron supplements

- cough syrups and other liquid medications sweetened with sorbitol, mannitol, or fructose, such as Robitussin, liquid acetaminophen (Tylenol), and ibuprofen (Motrin)
- hormone replacement therapy (which slows motility)
- birth control pills (which slow motility)
- benzodiazepines like alprazolam (Xanax) and clonazepam (Klonopin)
- narcotics (which disrupt motility), such as acetaminophen plus codeine (Tylenol #3) or acetaminophen plus oxycodone (Percocet)
- tricyclic antidepressants such as amitriptyline (Elavil) and nortriptyline (Pamelor)
- calcium channel blockers such as verapamil (Calan) and nifedipine (Procardia)
- laxatives
- lactulose (used for treating constipation), such as Kristalose and Chronulac

AVOIDING FOOD CULPRITS

For many of us, gas and bloating are caused by some dietary offender. Often the solution lies in cutting back on a certain food or avoiding it altogether. When bacteria in your colon come into contact with undigested carbohydrates, gas is formed. Your digestive tract has a harder time breaking down certain forms of carbohydrates and these are the most likely to cause excess gas. You may want to consider avoiding, or at least moderating your intake of, the carbohydrate-rich foods discussed below.

DO YOU HAVE DIABETES?

Sometimes bloating can result from a slowdown in the movement of food through the intestinal tract. Gastroenterologists call this a motility disorder. The most frequent motility disorder I see is in patients with advanced diabetes. Uncontrolled blood sugar can damage the nerves that propel the GI tract. Usually the first sign of this occurs in the stomach, with delayed stomach emptying. Diabetics who have this motility disorder, called gastroparesis, may experience bloating, reflux, nausea, and vomiting. A complication of gastroparesis is the overgrowth of bacteria in the small intestine. In general, we shouldn't have any bacteria in the small intestine, although we do have bacteria in the colon to aid in digestion. With gastroparesis, food can ferment in the upper GI tract as a result of slow motility, which results in an abnormal bacterial colonization of the small intestine. This can cause problems with absorption of foods, resulting in excessive gas and bloating.

Sorbitol

Eating even small amounts of this sweetener, found in many "sugar-free" gums, candies, and cookies, can cause excessive amounts of gas. If you already have problems with gas and bloating, I recommend avoiding this substance. Check the labels of sugar-free products to see if they contain sorbitol. Cough syrups like Robitussin and other sweetened medications like liquid Maalox antacid often contain large amounts of sorbitol. (Check the label for inactive ingredients.) If you're sensitive to sorbitol, you should also avoid mannitol, another low-cal sweetener that is a source of gas.

Fructose

This fruit sugar—found in large quantities in soft drinks and other sweets made with "high fructose corn syrup," as well as figs, dates, prunes, grapes, and honey—may pass undigested through the small intestine and enter the colon. When bacteria in the colon break this sugar down, gas is released as a by-product. (Interestingly, research has shown that those who suffer from malabsorption of fructose or sorbitol are likely to suffer not only from bloating but also from depression. Those who cut their intake of these foods not only improve bloating but also improve their mood.) Some fruits, like apples, also contain high amounts of pectin, a fiber that produces gas.

A Sudden Switch to a High-Fiber Diet

If you suddenly increase your fiber intake from, say, 5 grams a day (the amount found in two pieces of fruit) to the recommended 25 grams a day (adding, say, a bowl of bran cereal and half-cup servings of broccoli, carrots, and lentils to your normal intake), you may experience a lot of gas until your body adjusts. The reason is that your colon may lack the good bacteria needed to digest the fiber. It may take a few weeks for these good bacteria to build up. In the meantime you can take a gas-relieving remedy or switch over slowly, adding just one fiber-rich serving a week to your diet.

Refined Flour

White bread, noodles, and other products made with refined flour are now known to increase the production of
gas and cause bloating by increasing water retention.
Many of my patients are shocked to learn that their
morning bagel may be causing gas. Only rice flour is not
associated with increased gas production. Whole oats
and whole-wheat flour may cause some gas, but they are
thought to cause significantly less gas than refined flour.

Beans and Legumes

Probably the most notorious gas producers, beans and
legumes contain difficult-to-digest starches and complex
sugars known as oligosaccharides. Use canned beans or
dried beans that are thoroughly cooked. Undercooked
beans have more oligosaccharides. Also, discard the cook-
ing water, since it contains some indigestible sugars. You
can also try Beano, an over-the-counter enzyme that digests oligosaccharides. It comes in drops or tablet form.
Take five drops per serving of beans or legumes, or three
tablets per meal.

Cruciferous Vegetables

Cabbage, brussels sprouts, broccoli, and cauliflower
contain similar starches, which also make them heavy
gas producers.

OVER-THE-COUNTER MEDICATIONS FOR REDUCING GAS AND BLOATING

Over-the-counter (OTC) remedies for gas and bloating fall into two general categories: those that improve upper GI gas (the kind that causes belching) and those that improve flatus (which occurs in the lower GI tract). Before using any OTC medication, read the instructions carefully for the proper dosage. Take them after meals when symptoms occur. Pregnant women shouldn't use any medication without the advice of a physician.

Gas pain without heartburn: Try a medication with simethicone, such as Gas-X, Extra-strength Gas-X, or Extra-strength Phazyme-125. Simethicone disrupts or breaks up the bubbles in the stomach or lower bowel, which helps the gas be more readily expelled by belching or passing flatus. It does not make intestinal gases dissolve or disappear.

Gas pain with heartburn: You need a product containing a combination of simethicone and antacid. Maalox Antacid/Antigas, Fast-Acting Mylanta, and others contain this combination.

Lower abdominal gas pain/flatulence: A number of remedies can help bring relief. Activated charcoal tablets such as Absorb Charcotabs and Charcocaps can help absorb excess gas in the intestinal tract. If you suffer gas from lactose intolerance, Lactaid in caplet or drop form can help reduce symptoms.

If you're looking for a natural approach, peppermint is a great soother of gas. You can buy peppermint tea in health food stores or make your own infusion: Mix 1 to 2 teaspoons of dried leaves into 8 ounces of hot water. If you have heartburn, you shouldn't drink peppermint tea since it produces a chemical in the stomach that can relax the esophageal sphincter. Take a peppermint tablet that's enteric coated, which means the tablet won't be broken down until it reaches the intestines. *Note: If you're pregnant, don't drink peppermint tea, since peppermint has been linked to miscarriage.*

WHEN TO SEE THE DOCTOR

Persistent bloating can sometimes be a sign of something more serious, such as an intestinal obstruction, an ulcer, inflammatory bowel disease, or in rare cases ovarian cancer. Consult your doctor if you have lengthy or frequent bouts of bloating (lasting longer than ten days or occurring several times a week) or bloating accompanied by any of the following:

- sharp stomach pains
- vomiting
- diarrhea or constipation
- fullness and pressure in the abdomen
- back pain
- unexplained weight loss

From time to time your digestive tract will react to different things in different ways. You may be able to

RED FLAG BLOATING FOODS

If you have a problem with gas and bloating, you may not be able to tolerate certain "gassy" foods. You may need to avoid these foods in your diet or moderate your intake to prevent the development of symptoms. The following list was developed by Steven Peikin, M.D., a gastroenterologist at Cooper Hospital in Camden, New Jersey, who served as the nutrition adviser for this book. It will help you know which foods to steer clear of and which foods to allow in your diet.

MAJOR RED FLAGS FOR INTESTINAL GAS

Fruits
apricots
grapes and raisins
prune juice

Legumes
beans
lentils
peas
soybeans

Vegetables
broccoli
brussels sprouts
cabbage
cauliflower
corn
turnips

Other
milk and milk products,
    except lactose-reduced or
    lactose free
nuts
red wine
sorbitol-containing foods
    (chewing gum, hard
    candy, soft drinks, etc.)
wheat germ

RED FLAG FOODS THAT CAUSE GAS
IN SOME PEOPLE

Vegetables
asparagus
avocado
carrots
celery
cucumbers
eggplants
green peppers
lettuce
onions
potatoes
radishes
sauerkraut
scallions
shallots
tomatoes
zucchini

Fruits
apples, applesauce, apple
 juice
bananas
berries
citrus fruits
dried fruits
melons
peaches
pears
prunes

Other
graham crackers
pastries
popcorn
potato and corn chips
soft drinks
wheat products

tolerate your favorite lentil dish one week but get gassy from it the next. The most important step you can take to reduce gas and bloating is to maintain a consistent diet day in and day out. Keep your fiber intake stable at around 20 to 25 grams a day, and make sure you drink adequate amounts of fluid. Opt for moderate activity on most days of the week rather than an intense bout of exercise over the weekend. Get enough sleep, and take some relaxation time for yourself. I've just written you a prescription for good gastrointestinal health—as well as overall health. You can apply this advice to any GI symptom you're having—like constipation, which I cover in the next chapter.

CHAPTER
....
6

CONSTIPATION—
THE DAILY STRAIN

Being a woman in today's world means being an efficient multitasker. We have to juggle so many things these days—a job, kids, aging parents, household responsibilities—sometimes all at the same time. It's no wonder many of us can't take the time to go to the bathroom. Far too many women have an added stress in their lives, the strain of having a bowel movement.

Constipation is one of the most common complaints I hear about from women in my practice. For many of us, it may be only an intermittent problem. But for numerous women, constipation is chronic. They experience abdominal bloating, fullness, and even low back pain from infrequent bowel movements. And they struggle with hard, rocklike stools while straining at the commode.

Constipation sufferers may learn to cope with the problem with self-help measures. My patients tell me how they eat five prunes a day or drink apple juice, or they increase their fiber intake with fruits and vegetables.

Life's Little Luxuries

"Being in the bathroom by myself is a luxury that I can indulge in only after my kids are asleep. I frequently find myself in the bathroom with one or more of my kids, and sometimes my one-year-old toddler climbs on my lap when I'm sitting on the toilet. I just try to get in and out of there as fast as I can. Sometimes I feel the urge to have a bowel movement, but I put it off because I'm too stressed."

—**Carey D.**, mother of three children under seven, who has occasional constipation

Many of them have tried over-the-counter laxatives and stool-softening suppositories, and some of my patients have resorted to enemas. I'm frequently asked which products are safe to use over the long term.

Several of my patients have discovered "tricks" that work for them. Some shift positions on the commode or insert their finger into their vagina and press backward toward the rectum. Others use their fingers to press up on the tissue between the vagina and the anus to enhance defecation. Some of my younger patients have tried herbal remedies or colonics.

Constipation has reached almost epidemic proportions in the United States, probably as a result of our lifestyle, our diet, and our hormones. The increase in our consumption of processed foods and the decrease in our activity levels probably play a role in the rise in constipation among American women. I'm basing my theories on the fact that constipation is much lower in developing countries where women are more physically active and eat a plant-based diet. What's more, more of us are overweight now than ever before, and being overweight doubles a woman's risk of constipation.

At least four or five million people in the United States suffer from chronic constipation, according to data from nationwide research surveys. In one study, researchers found that as many as 28 percent of our population suffer from occasional constipation (that's nearly 55 million people). Another study found that constipation afflicts 21 percent of women and 8 percent of men. Although I can't tell you which data are the most accurate, I can safely say that constipation afflicts women more often than men and that more of us are constipated today than we were in the past.

In the most basic sense, constipation simply means trouble having bowel movements. Your stools may be very hard, making them so difficult to pass that you have to strain. Or you may feel like you still need to have a bowel movement after you've already had one. Your mother may have told you that "normal" means having a bowel movement every day, but there's no golden rule about how often you should go. I've seen perfectly healthy women who have only one or two bowel movements a week. The general rule of thumb, though, is that anything between three bowel movements a day and three bowel movements a week falls within the "normal" range. And more important, I tell my patients that if their bowel habits aren't causing them any trouble, they're probably fine.

You, of course, should know what's "normal" for you. If you begin to have fewer bowel movements than previously, you may be getting constipated. Although you can live for years with constipation without suffering any major health effects, it's a drag on your quality of life to spend hours in the bathroom or feel cramped and bloated from not being able to empty your bowels. Constipation is usually a sign that you need to make a change, usually in your diet and in your activity level.

WHY WOMEN ARE PRONE TO CONSTIPATION

No one knows for certain why women tend to get constipated more often than men, but in many women there are several reasons involved. As we lead busier and busier lives, we take less time to walk to places and spend more time in our cars driving. Family meals around the table have faded into relics as more of us skip meals or eat on the run. Women also go on fad diets more often than men, which can leave us depleted of fiber or fluids. I myself am guilty of not drinking enough water. When I'm in the middle of a busy clinic or chauffeuring my kids to soccer or tae kwon do on the weekends, I often leave my water bottle at home. Sometimes it seems that taking time to drink water only means making time to find the bathroom.

We also don't make time to have bowel movements. Because we are more often on the run these days, it just isn't convenient to go when we have the urge. Women also take more vitamins and supplements like calcium and iron, which can be constipating. Another cause of constipation may be female hormones. Your hormonal fluctuations of estrogen and progesterone may make you constipated at certain times of the month, often during the latter half of your menstrual cycle, when these hormone levels are at their highest. Some birth control pills have also been associated with constipation.

Of course, pregnancy is notorious for bringing on constipation. As I discussed in Chapter 2, pregnancy causes your progesterone levels to soar, which in turn causes your digestive tract muscles to slow down. This causes food to move more slowly through your GI tract, triggering bloating and constipation. If you take a calcium or iron supplement or a prenatal vitamin that contains these minerals, you're even more prone to constipation.

Even after giving birth, your constipation troubles may not end. A day after delivering my son (who is now eleven), I remember lying in my hospital bed while the nurse told me that she wanted me to have a bowel movement before I went home. I had just pushed out a seven-pound baby and was swollen, torn, and stitched up "down there." I absolutely couldn't imagine pushing out stool! I cringed at the thought. My nurse offered me stool softeners to take home, which I happily accepted. I did manage to have a bowel movement in the hospital, but I can tell you that my bodily urges had to overcome my mind's reluctance.

Having an episiotomy or vaginal tear during childbirth can indeed cause painful bowel movements during the first few days when you're still very sore. Straining can put pressure on the suture line, and you may feel the urge to suppress your bathroom urges. Holding back for a day or two causes less fluid in the bowel, which causes harder movements that are more difficult to pass. This can set you up for constipation.

This experience can be even worse if you have a cesarean section (C-section). After any abdominal surgery, including a C-section, your bowel contractions slow down significantly for one or two days. You may feel bloated but unable to pass gas or have a bowel movement. These bowel contractions resume naturally on their own, but some women may find it takes a few days.

If you have one of these procedures during childbirth, don't shy away from stool softeners or laxatives that may be offered to you by your doctor or nurse midwife. These can be extremely helpful as you flinch and ease your way through that first bowel movement.

Constipation sometimes continues through your child's first few years. If you're nursing, you have to dramatically increase your fluid intake; if you don't drink enough, you could get constipation in addition to lowering your milk production.

What's more, in the midst of meeting the demands of a baby, many new moms find that they simply can't take the time to go to the bathroom. This can be a bad pattern to get yourself into. If you put off your urges when you have them, you may have to "retrain" yourself to respond to these natural stimuli. Keeping stool in your colon for longer periods of time allows more water to be absorbed from them, making them harder or more pelletlike and more often requiring more straining to pass.

Hormonal changes that occur during menopause can also result in the onset of constipation. When estrogen levels decline, vaginal tissues may become very dry. The colon too relies on mucus to lubricate the stool, which may decrease with menopause.

Pregnancy, not emptying your bladder enough, and gynecological disorders like uterine fibroids can also lead to constipation by increasing a woman's risk of developing pelvic floor dysfunction. This very general term describes a weakening in the pelvic floor muscles, which I discussed in Chapter 2. Some of my patients tell me that they feel like everything's just falling down "down there." Pelvic floor dysfunction may affect the normal angle of the rectum, the muscles that aid in defecation, or the relaxation of the anal sphincter.

The condition can also result in rectal prolapse (where rectal tissue protrudes out of the anus with straining) or a rectocele (a small pouch that protrudes from the rectum into the cavity of the vagina), both of which can definitely interfere with defecation. A rectocele can enlarge and trap stool within it, making it very difficult to pass. Rectoceles may require treatment with surgery, which can be successful at alleviating the constipation. I discuss this in more detail in Chapter 16.

Sometimes constipation can be caused by reluctance—subconscious or not—to pass stool. This condition—called rectosphincteric dyssynergia—occurs when a person has the urge to have a bowel movement but actually squeezes shut the anal sphincter instead of relaxing it to allow the fecal matter to pass. Stool flow becomes obstructed, which causes constipation. The problem can occur as a result of childbirth, surgery to the pelvis or perineum, painful hemorrhoids, or a psychological cause. I've seen patients who are constipated due to stress from sexual abuse. They don't even realize that they're tightening these muscles and are reacting subconsciously to their trauma.

MEDICAL CAUSES
OF CONSTIPATION

Although constipation is a symptom, not a condition, it can sometimes be caused by an underlying medical problem. I emphasize, though, that such cases are the exceptions, not the norm. The vast majority of the time constipation is brought on by deficiencies in diet and activity levels. Still, your doctor may want to rule out the possibility that your constipation is caused by one of the following conditions, especially if lifestyle changes aren't alleviating your symptoms.

Hypothyroidism

Low thyroid hormone levels caused by a low-functioning thyroid (hypothyroidism) can slow gut motility and affect stool liquidity, thus causing constipation. Since thyroid disorders are so common in women, we commonly check for hypothyroidism with a medical history, physical exam, and routine blood test whenever a woman comes to our clinic with constipation.

Irritable Bowel Syndrome (IBS)

Chronic constipation can be a part of IBS, a condition I discuss in Chapter 13.

Chronic Diseases

Certain chronic diseases like scleroderma, muscular dystrophy, or Parkinson's can cause constipation by slowing gut motility. Diseases that are associated with high calcium levels (for example, hyperparathyroidism, multiple myeloma, or sarcoidosis) can also worsen constipation. Severe diabetes can affect the nerves of the enteric nervous system and can result in constipation.

Genetic Predisposition

Severe constipation can be genetic and run in families. If your mom tended to be frequently constipated, you may have that same predisposition. Constipation beginning in early childhood might also suggest a congenital disorder such as Hirschsprung's, where an inborn genetic error causes a lack of nerve cells in a short segment of the lower colon. This condition results in an obstruction to normal bowel movements and often requires surgical correction.

Obstructions

True obstruction from tumors or even adhesions from prior surgeries can block the intestinal tract. Patients who have had portions of their colon removed during surgery for colon cancer or inflammatory bowel disease may develop constipation from scar tissue that narrows the width of the colon.

ARE YOU DEPRESSED?

This is one question I frequently ask patients who come to see me with constipation. I often get a surprised look in response. In fact, depression and constipation often go hand in hand. No one knows for sure why this is true, but twice as many women suffer from depression as men—and they're also more likely to suffer from constipation. One theory is that depression causes a big slowdown in the body. People tend to eat less because they lose their appetite. They move around less, especially if they're bedridden. Decreased movement and decreased food intake can lead to decreased peristaltic contractions, which sets you up for constipation.

Depressed people also tend to have lower levels of the feel-good neurotransmitter serotonin. Researchers believe this may be a major reason why depression occurs. What's fascinating, though, is that 95 percent of serotonin is located not in the brain but in the GI tract. Studies suggest that serotonin is released from the intestinal wall and triggers peristalsis, which moves food through the digestive system. So it could be that depressed people also have less serotonin in their digestive tract, which triggers constipation.

The American Psychiatric Association defines depression as the presence of five or more of the following symptoms within a two-week period (not accounted for by drug abuse or bereavement):

- depressed mood/loss of interest or pleasure
- significant weight gain or weight loss without dieting
- insomnia or hypersomnia (too much sleep)
- mental agitation, agitated mood

- fatigue or loss of energy
- feelings of worthlessness or excessive guilt
- diminished ability to concentrate
- recurrent thoughts of death
- suicidal thoughts

If you think you're experiencing depression, see your doctor for a referral to a mental health professional.

If you're concerned that your constipation may be caused by one of these medical conditions, be sure to mention it to your doctor during your appointment.

CONSTIPATION COMPLICATIONS

As I previously mentioned, constipation is usually just a nuisance with no real long-term complications. But it can lead to trouble if you don't manage it well. If constipation becomes very severe, a colon obstruction can occur from impacted stool and may eventually lead to fecal incontinence. Constipation is associated with a higher risk of urinary tract infections. Straining associated with hard bowel movements can also increase your risk of anal fissure and hemorrhoids (see Chapter 16).

Constipation can also increase your chance of developing diverticulosis, little pouches that form along the outer surface of the colon wall. Excess straining can cause weak spots in the colon to bulge out and become diverticula. About half of all Americans ages sixty to eighty have diverticulosis, and almost everyone over eighty has it. The leading theory is that a low-fiber diet is the main cause of diverticular disease, but this hasn't been proven. What we do know is that the rates of diverticulosis are highest in industrialized nations where people eat more processed foods like white bread, cookies, and pasta made from refined, low-fiber flour. The disorder is rare in certain African and Asian countries where people eat high-fiber vegetable diets.

Although most people with diverticulosis have no symptoms, some may have constipation, bloating, abdominal pain, or tenderness around the left side of their lower abdomen. Treating diverticulosis usually involves increasing the amount of fiber in the diet. Your doctor may also recommend that you take a fiber product such as Citrucel or Metamucil once a day. Until recently many doctors suggested avoiding foods with small seeds such as tomatoes or strawberries because they believed that the seeds could lodge in the diverticula and cause inflammation. But this recommendation is now considered to be controversial, and no evidence supports it.

On occasion, the diverticula may become infected and inflamed—a condition called diverticulitis—causing fever, nausea, vomiting, chills, or severe abdominal pain. Diverticulitis usually requires treatment with antibiotics and in severe cases may require hospitalization and possibly surgery.

WHAT YOU CAN DO
TO GET THINGS MOVING

As with other digestive symptoms, constipation has a lot to do with a person's diet and lifestyle habits. You can have a big impact in helping to alleviate your constipation by adding more fiber to your diet (in the form of fruits, vegetables, and whole grains), drinking more fluids, and increasing your activity level. You may also benefit from the occasional use of an over-the-counter remedy for constipation.

Start with Fiber

I can't emphasize enough how important fiber is to prevent constipation. Getting 20 to 25 grams of fiber each day can help form soft bulky stool. Dietary fiber may have other added health benefits like lowering cholesterol and helping prevent heart disease and diabetes and possibly certain types of cancer.

Fiber can be either soluble or insoluble, and most fiber-rich foods contain varying amounts of both. Soluble fiber dissolves in fluids found in the colon and forms a gel. It acts like a sponge, absorbing fluid as it moves through your lower GI tract, which results in softer, bigger stools—and often less straining at the toilet. Soluble fiber also sops up bile acid and cholesterol in the intestines, which helps lower cholesterol levels in the blood. Apples, pears, strawberries, beans, lentils, and oat bran are all high in soluble fiber. Insoluble fiber doesn't dissolve in intestinal fluids but soaks up water, adding bulk. This makes it easier for the intestines to move waste matter out of your system more quickly. Whole grains, wheat bran, carrots, spinach, and potatoes all are rich in insoluble fiber.

To reach your daily fiber goal, eat at least five servings of fruits and vegetables each day. Fruits and vegetables that are high in fiber include apples, broccoli, berries, brussels sprouts, beans, figs, carrots, oranges, cauliflower, pears, peas, and prunes. You should also replace white bread with whole-grain bread, and replace white rice with brown rice and beans. Look for whole-grain cereals that contain at least 3 grams of fiber per serving, which is listed on the food label. You can also try adding a quarter-cup of wheat bran to foods like cooked cereal, applesauce, or meatloaf. If food fiber doesn't work for you, it's fine to use a fiber or bulk supplement that contains a natural plant fiber such as psyllium seed husks (found in Metamucil).

If you're increasing your fiber, start slowly on the order of 4 or 5 grams per day. This will help prevent bloating, cramping, or gas that can occur if fiber is added to the diet too quickly. Your body will adjust to the extra fiber within a few days to a week. You can then continue to add fiber until you're up to a level that makes you more regular. *Note: It's important to drink more fluids when you increase the amount of fiber you eat to help move the fiber through your colon. When you increase your fiber intake, drink at least two more glasses of water a day.*

Increase Your Fluid Intake

You've probably heard that the golden rule of thumb is to drink eight 8-ounce glasses of water every day. I'm certainly not going to argue with that recommendation, but I will say that if you follow it, you'll probably spend a good part of your day running to the bathroom to urinate. If you're constipated, increasing the amount of fluid you get (in the form of water, juices,

A GUIDE TO FIBER-RICH FOODS

Fruits	Apple	1 medium	= 4 grams
	Peach	1 medium	= 2 grams
	Pear	1 medium	= 4 grams
	Tangerine	1 medium	= 2 grams
Vegetables	Acorn squash, fresh, cooked	3/4 cup	= 7 grams
	Asparagus, fresh, cooked	1/2 cup	= 1.5 grams
	Broccoli, fresh, cooked	1/2 cup	= 2 grams
	Brussels sprouts, fresh, cooked	1/2 cup	= 2 grams
	Cabbage, fresh, cooked	1/2 cup	= 2 grams
	Carrot, fresh, cooked	1	= 1.5 grams
	Cauliflower, fresh, cooked	1/2 cup	= 2 grams
	Romaine lettuce	1 cup	= 1 gram
	Spinach, fresh, cooked	1/2 cup	= 2 grams
	Tomato, raw	1	= 1 gram
	Zucchini, fresh, cooked	1 cup	= 2.5 grams
Starchy Vegetables	Black-eyed peas, fresh, cooked	1/2 cup	= 4 grams
	Lima beans, fresh, cooked	1/2 cup	= 4.5 grams
	Kidney beans, fresh, cooked	1/2 cup	= 6 grams
	Potato, fresh, cooked	1	= 3 grams
Grains	Bread, whole-wheat	1 slice	= 2 grams
	Brown rice, cooked	1 cup	= 3.5 grams
	Cereal, bran flake	3/4 cup	= 5 grams
	Oatmeal, plain, cooked	3/4 cup	= 3 grams
	White rice, cooked	1 cup	= 1 gram

Source: United States Department of Agriculture, USDA Nutrient Database for Standard Reference. Available at www.nal.usda.gov/fnic/cgi-bin/nut_search.pl.

and clear soups) may help. It's certainly necessary when you increase your fiber intake. Use your best judgment and make an effort to get adequate liquids at every meal and after exercising to prevent dehydration.

Get Active

Exercise is really a cure-all for most minor digestive problems. I've already recommended it for reflux and bloating, and now I'll extend the recommendation to constipation. Lack of exercise can lead to constipation, though experts aren't exactly sure why. What we do know is that getting active through walking, biking, or just taking the stairs more can help keep your digestive tract running smoothly.

Don't Ignore Your Natural Urges

Ignoring the urge to have a bowel movement may eventually cause you to stop feeling the urge, which can lead to constipation. You may postpone bowel movements because of emotional stress or because you're too busy with work or with your children. All I can say is that you need to listen to your body. When your body gives you the signal to go, head to the nearest bathroom. You shouldn't have to strain excessively.

Once you've had a bowel movement, get up and stop straining. This may sound obvious, but women who have hemorrhoid problems often tell me that they feel like they still have more to push out once they're finished. They strain sometimes for several minutes after they've made a bowel movement, which can aggravate their hemorrhoids. Hemorrhoids themselves can make you feel like you still have a little bit of something in the anal canal that needs to come out. It ends up as a vicious circle: You strain because you feel like something is still there, and you cause the hemorrhoids to get even bigger. More often than not, all of that effort results in only a pea-size piece of stool.

My advice? Don't waste your time and effort on that last little bit of stool. Once you're finished, you're finished. If you feel like you still have to go after you've already gone, you may be feeling a little bit of gas. Whatever stool that's left will come out next time and won't cause you to get constipated.

Eat Regular Meals—Especially Breakfast

Eating three meals a day can help you avoid constipation by keeping your gastrocolic reflex stimulated. This reflex causes your colon to contract, giving you the urge to move your bowels about thirty minutes after you finish eating. It works in your favor when you're trying to prevent constipation. (Some people who suffer from IBS have an exaggerated gastrocolic reflex that sends them heading to the bathroom as soon as they begin a meal.)

Your body doesn't give the signal to go very often, but when it does, it's usually after eating. It's especially important to eat something (even if it's just a cup of coffee or piece of fruit) at breakfast, when this reflex tends to be strongest. On the flip side, skipping meals or drastically cutting your calorie intake on a fad diet can wreak havoc on your digestive tract and lead to constipation. When you eat only once or twice a day, your digestive

DID YOU KNOW?

The use of laxatives increases with age. In U.S. population surveys, three percent of young adults reported using a laxative at least once a month compared to seven percent of people over 65 who said they used laxatives three to ten times a week. In a British survey, 23 percent of women age 60 to 69 reported using laxatives on an occasional basis; one-quarter of them said they used them more than once a week.

Why do elderly people use laxatives more often? Do they get more constipated? Actually, no, not in a technical sense. What's really happening is that they may have to strain more than they used to in order to pass a bowel movement. They associate this straining with constipation, even though they're able to have at least three bowel movements a week. The increase in straining among the elderly may be related to their decreased food intake (which produces smaller stools), reduced mobility, medication use, weak abdominal and pelvic muscles, or chronic illness.

I think that this population probably uses laxatives far too frequently. The problem lies in the misperception that straining equals constipation. This isn't always the case—especially if a soft bowel movement can be passed—and doctors need to make their elderly patients aware of this fact.

tract learns to expect less food, less frequently; as a result, your gastrocolic reflex may become weak or even disappear altogether. You may lose the urge to move your bowels and may develop constipation as a result. Constipation can linger even after you stop dieting. If the reflex doesn't return on its own, you need to go through bowel retraining, which I describe on page 208.

Try an Over-the-Counter Laxative

If fiber, fluids, and activity don't do the trick, it's okay to take an occasional laxative. When I go to my local grocery store, I'm always amazed at the huge number of GI products on the shelves. The laxative section is no exception. "Easy," "natural," "thorough," and "comfortable relief" are common terms in this section. Several different types of laxatives are available and are classified by their mode of action on your digestive tract.

Bulk fiber laxatives add volume and fluid to the stool. Some of these products, including Metamucil, Konsyl, Effer-Syllium, and Perdiem, contain natural plant fibers like psyllium seed husks. Others like Fiber-Con contain calcium polycarbophil. Citrucel contains the fiber methylcellulose. All of these forms of fiber have similar modes of action: They add nonirritating bulk to the stool and promote normal elimination.

Stool softeners like docusate sodium (Colace, Surfak, and others) contain moistening agents that help keep stools soft for easy, natural passage. They aren't technically laxatives.

Lubricants grease the stool, enabling it to move through the intestine more easily. Mineral oil and glycerin are the most common lubricants.

Saline laxatives work by increasing fluid in the GI tract. They include magnesium compounds like magnesium hydroxide (Milk of Magnesia, Haley's M-O) and magnesium oxide.

MY PERSONAL RX
FOR CONSTIPATION

Here's what I use when I get occasional constipation. I recommend this "prescription" to my patients as well. You can get both products over the counter in your local drugstore. Magnesium oxide is usually found in the vitamin section, and docusate sodium (Colace and others)—you can buy the generic—is found with other digestive health remedies.

- One or two 400-milligram tablets of magnesium oxide, twice a day
- One 100-milligram docusate sodium (such as Colace) capsule, twice a day

The magnesium oxide tablets serve as a laxative by increasing fluid in your stool. The docusate pill serves as a stool softener, which helps make stool easier to pass. Both are available in generic, over-the-counter form at your local pharmacy. You can substitute milk of magnesia (also a laxative) twice a day instead of the magnesium oxide tablets, but I find most of my patients prefer the tablets over the bitter-tasting liquid.

I actually learned about using magnesium oxide tablets as a substitute for milk of magnesia from a woman family practitioner during a round-table discussion of common GI problems that I was supposed to be leading! This combination treatment is relatively mild, with few or no side effects, and should help alleviate constipation within a day or two.

Stimulant laxatives act directly on the colon to make it contract. Some, like Ex-Lax, contain sennosides, active compounds from the herb senna. Others, like Correctol, Dulcolax, and Fleet Stimulant Laxative, contain the active ingredient bisacodyl.

One note of warning: Laxatives that contain phenolphthalein (which used to be in Ex-Lax) have recently been taken off the market because they may cause cancer. Avoid any laxative that you may have kept in your medicine cabinet that contains the chemical phenolphthalein.

If you're pregnant, check with your physician before taking any laxative. Bulk laxatives are generally considered to be safe during pregnancy. Lubricant, saline, and stimulant laxatives pose more risk to the pregnant mother or fetus.

In terms of how fast they work, stimulant laxatives produce the quickest results. One company used to advertise that you took a pill at night and had a bowel movement in the morning. Suppository stimulant laxatives can work even faster. Bulk and saline laxatives can take a few days to get things moving. In general, the stronger and harsher the laxative, the faster you get results.

There's been some debate as to whether the continuous use of laxatives can damage the bowel and ultimately make you more dependent on laxatives. I've heard arguments on both sides from gastroenterologists who specialize in this area of research. Some claim that laxatives cause no harm, while others say you should exercise caution and not use laxatives for more than two weeks at a time. I myself agree with the latter approach, especially when it comes to stimulant laxatives. I tell my patients to start with the gentlest laxatives first, like a bulk laxative and/or stool softener. They can graduate up to magnesium oxide tablets. If these don't work, I

COLONIC CLEANSING: DOES IT WORK?

Constipation and irregular bowel movements result in stool remaining in the colon for long periods of time. So wouldn't it make sense to have your colon cleansed on a regular basis if you suffer from constipation? Wouldn't a big clean-out help get things moving again? Like spring cleaning, isn't a regular cleansing good for you? Women in my clinic pose these questions to me from time to time and more often lately since colonics seem to be much more in fashion. The arguments may make sense in theory. But I can tell you that in practice colonics don't alleviate constipation. In fact, they can do more harm than good.

Colon cleansing with a high colonic treatment entails flushing the colon with 10 to 20 gallons of water under gentle pressure by way of a rectal applicator. The trouble is, your colon is a healthy organ filled with beneficial bacteria that aid in digestion and help your body process stool properly. Colonics clear out not only old stool and food remnants but also colonies of these beneficial bacteria. Alternative health practitioners will claim that colonics rid your body of toxins. In reality, they rid your colon of much-needed vitamins and electrolytes (salts such as potassium, sodium, and magnesium) as well as good bacteria.

Overall I am very wary of colonics. You have no quality assurance that the person performing the procedure is competent and that the equipment is clean and sterilized. Less-than-clean equipment can result in infectious diarrhea. What's more, inserting a substance such as coffee into your

colon may be downright dangerous. Certain chemicals found
in coffee and other colonic treatments can be irritating to the
colon lining and may cause colitis (inflammation of the
colon) in some people. Bottom line: I'm not a believer in
colonics, and I recommend avoiding them.

would then recommend trying a stimulant laxative, but
I emphasize that this type of laxative shouldn't be used
for more than two weeks continuously. Call your doctor
if your constipation continues unabated. I provide
more details on laxatives in Chapter 13.

Enemas, Anyone?

Most of us aren't eager to use enemas, but they're safe
and can be very effective in treating constipation. A
simple tap-water enema can distend the rectum, simulating the normal stimulus that triggers defecation. For
your convenience, a Fleet enema, available in your local
drugstore, can also be used.

Complementary and Alternative Therapies

Here are some home remedies that my patients have
found helpful. These are a mild way to get things moving if you don't want to use pharmaceutical laxatives
right away.

- Stewed or soaked prunes, one to three a day, have a
  slight laxative effect.
- Flax meal—1 heaping teaspoon in 8 ounces of

apple juice—provides fiber and soothes the digestive tract. You can add flax meal (ground flaxseed) to oatmeal, breads, and soups as well. Follow with an additional 8 ounces of water.
- Warm lemon water taken before meals stimulates digestion.

BOWEL RETRAINING OR BIOFEEDBACK

As I mentioned in Chapter 1, the anus has two valves or sphincters that prevent stool from leaking out involuntarily. You have control over the external sphincter. The act of pushing out stool opens this sphincter and enables you to control the timing of your bowel movements. Ignoring your body signals for too long can sometimes cause you to lose your ability to recognize when it's time to move your bowels. You may forget how to use your anal muscles to get the external sphincter to relax and open.

If you have this problem, try going to the bathroom at the same time every day when a bowel movement is most likely to occur, a method called *bowel retraining*. You may have the best results about thirty minutes after breakfast or after a cup of caffeinated coffee (caffeine stimulates the GI tract).

When you begin bowel retraining, take your time in the bathroom, but don't sit and strain. You may not feel the urge at first, but if you've just eaten, your bowels are primed to move into action. Any large meal can serve the purpose of bowel retraining if breakfast isn't a good time. Your gastrocolic reflex kicks in soon after you've eaten, and you'll have an easier time moving your bowels.

If bowel retraining on your own doesn't work, you might benefit from biofeedback therapy. I frequently refer constipation patients for biofeedback, which, under the guidance of a professional, can help them learn to relax their anal sphincter and move their bowels. Biofeedback for constipation often involves hooking a patient up to a monitor to measure muscle contractions along the external anal sphincter. The person is told to push down as if she were defecating, and the biofeedback machine measures the muscle tension. Often a woman pushes with her belly but tightens the sphincter muscle, which squeezes the sphincter shut and prevents the passage of stool. She may not be aware she is doing it. Biofeedback can help her find the correct muscles to push in order to enable her sphincter to relax and open.

In many hospitals, biofeedback is performed by a clinical psychologist and is usually part of a therapy program that includes other techniques, like behavioral therapy. Insurance frequently doesn't cover biofeedback alone, so many institutions (including the University of Virginia Hospital) fold biofeedback sessions into the overall therapy program, which is covered by insurance. For more information on biofeedback and for help finding a competent practitioner, you can contact the Association for Applied Psychophysiology and Biofeedback at (303) 422-8436 or www.aapb.org.

A WORD ON HERBS

Many of my patients tell me they take herbal laxatives for their constipation, in the mistaken belief that these "natural" products are safer and gentler on their system than Ex-Lax or a Fleet enema. The truth is, they usually aren't. Some herbal products can be harmful if you fail to use them properly. For instance, you may think you can drink limitless amounts of senna tea because, after all, it's a tea, not a medicine. But the herb senna actually contains powerful compounds, called sennosides, that act like stimulant laxatives. In fact, sennosides are the active ingredient in Ex-Lax and other OTC laxatives, which have controlled amounts because they're regulated as drugs. Herbal products, on the other hand, are considered to be food, so they aren't subject to the same stringent regulations.

I'm not going to tell you never to take a natural alternative remedy for constipation. Bulk fiber supplements are certainly safe. But if you're going to try an herbal stimulant laxative such as cascara, senna, or aloe vera, exercise caution. Follow the instructions on the package, and never take more than what's recommended. As with other stimulant laxatives, don't take herbal stimulant laxatives for more than two weeks at a time. *Don't take any of these herbs while you're pregnant or nursing unless you get your doctor's okay.*

WHEN TO SEE THE DOCTOR

Before coming to see me, most of my patients self-medicate for constipation by increasing their exercise and fiber intake and occasionally using a stool softener or laxative. If constipation has been a chronic problem for you and remains a problem a month after implementing self-help measures, you should probably make an appointment with your doctor. The American Gastroenterological Association has developed practice guidelines to help doctors distinguish between those patients who suffer from occasional constipation and those who probably need medical intervention. The guidelines define *chronic constipation* as fewer than three bowel movements per week and the presence of two or more of the following symptoms during the past year, lasting a total of three months or more, more than 25 percent of the time:

- straining when having a bowel movement
- lumpy or hard stools
- the sensation of incomplete evacuation
- a feeling that there's some obstruction or blockage
- a need for a manual maneuver to facilitate bowel movements, like inserting a finger into the rectum

Red Flag Warning Signs

You should see your doctor immediately if you have any of the following warning signs associated with constipation:

- blood in the stool
- excessive pain with defecation
- complete inability to pass stool
- nausea, vomiting, severe abdominal distension or bloating (which could indicate an obstruction)
- unexplained weight loss
- change in caliber of stool (if they become pencil thin)

DIAGNOSTIC TESTS
FOR CONSTIPATION

Most people don't need extensive diagnostic testing for constipation and can be treated with lifestyle and diet changes without a thorough evaluation. If you're young and have mild constipation, your doctor may need only to take a medical history and perform a physical exam. The tests your doctor performs depend on the duration and severity of your constipation, your age, and whether you have any of the red flag warning symptoms.

A physical exam may include a digital rectal exam with a gloved, lubricated finger to check for lesions in the anus or rectum, anal sphincter tone, or blood in the stool (see Chapter 8 for more details). If you have severe symptoms, your doctor may order the following tests:

Colonoscopy

A colonoscopy involves viewing the rectum, colon, and lower part of the small intestine to locate any problems. The night before the test you must drink a special liquid to clear out your colon. You may be lightly sedated during the exam, in which a flexible tube with a lighted camera on the end is inserted into the colon. This test allows your doctor to carefully examine the lining of your colon and rectum. Any abnormal areas can be biopsied during the procedure.

Colorectal Transit Study

The colorectal transit study, reserved for those with chronic constipation, shows how well stool moves through the colon. On specific days you swallow a capsule containing small plastic markers. The movement of these markers through the colon is monitored with an abdominal X-ray, taken several days after the capsule is swallowed. During the course of this test you'll be instructed to eat a regular diet and to avoid any laxatives.

Anorectal Function Tests

Anorectal function tests can diagnose constipation caused by abnormal functioning of the anus or rectum. One test, called *anorectal manometry,* evaluates anal sphincter muscle function by inserting a catheter or air-filled balloon into the anus. The catheter or balloon is then slowly pulled back through to measure muscle tone and contractions.

Defecography

Defecography is an X-ray of the anorectal area and lower segment of the colon that evaluates the completeness of stool elimination, identifies anorectal abnormalities, and evaluates rectal muscle contractions and relaxation. During the exam the radiologist fills the rectum with a soft barium paste that is the same consistency as stool. You then sit on a toilet seat positioned inside an X-ray machine and relax and squeeze out the solution. Afterward your doctor studies the X-rays for anorectal problems that occurred while you emptied the barium paste.

Barium Enema X-Ray

The barium enema X-ray is a study to look at the rectum, colon, and lower part of the small intestine. It may show intestinal obstruction and Hirschsprung's disease, a genetic disorder indicated by a lack of nerves within the colon. As with the colonoscopy, you have to clean out your colon the night before this exam. During the exam a chalky liquid enema is inserted into the colon and X-rays are taken; you may feel some abdominal cramping while the enema is in your colon.

MEDICAL TREATMENT
FOR CONSTIPATION

Your medical evaluation will determine the best treatment for you. If your constipation isn't being alleviated by over-the-counter remedies, you may need a prescription-strength treatment. Many "older" remedies—like fiber, glycerin suppositories, or sorbitol pills—still work well, and your doctor may prescribe one of those. But several new treatments for constipation have recently become available or will soon be available by prescription.

Lactulose (Kristalose, Chronulac Syrup, Duphalac)

Lactulose is a synthetic sugar that is poorly absorbed by the GI tract and as a result increases the water content of stool, helping to combat constipation. Most patients find that Kristalose is easier to swallow because it doesn't have the sickeningly sweet and thick consistency of Chronulac or Duphalac. These are osmotic laxatives, which means they increase the water content flowing into the colon, thereby softening stool. The one drawback is that they take 24 to 48 hours to produce the desired effect. Another drawback is that these synthetic sugars can be digested by colonic bacteria, resulting in gas and bloating.

MiraLax (Polyethylene Glycol, or PEG)

MiraLax is an osmotic laxative that is basically a smaller dose of the powder you mix with water for the traditional colon cleansing right before a colonoscopy. To take this preparation, mix one capful of powder into a cup of water once or twice daily.

Tegaserod (Zelnorm)

Tegaserod is a new medication that was recently approved by the FDA for women with IBS where constipation is the predominant symptom. It stimulates serotonin receptors in the GI tract, resulting in increased motility, increased intestinal secretion, and decreased gut sensitivity to pain. Women who take this medication report an increased number of bowel movements, stools that are softer and easier to pass, and less gas and bloating.

Now that you know how to deal with constipation, you'll see in the next chapter how to deal with the opposite problem: diarrhea. Unfortunately, to treat diarrhea, you *can't* just do the opposite of what you do for constipation, like eat less fiber and get less exercise. Diarrhea has a host of causes and can be fairly complicated to evaluate and treat. But it does have one thing in common with constipation: It usually means something isn't quite right in your diet or lifestyle. All of these gastrointestinal symptoms, from gas to constipation to diarrhea, indicate that you need to reevaluate your lifestyle. Chances are, you're not living as healthfully as you could be. That's why I'll keep saying this over and over again: Use your gut as your guide to good health.

DIARRHEA—DEALING
WITH THE RUNS WHEN
YOU'RE ON THE RUN

Aɴɴ, ᴀ ᴛʜɪʀᴛʏ-sɪx-ʏᴇᴀʀ-ᴏʟᴅ mother of two, knew the location of every bathroom in town. She needed to, because she had chronic diarrhea that sent her racing to the bathroom several times a day to avoid an accident. When she first came to see me at the clinic, she actually made light of her problem and asked me to quiz her on local public bathrooms. I said, "Route 29 North," and she said, "I usually stop at the Kroger grocery store. I pull into one of the parking spaces saved for 'new moms,' and the bathroom is right at the front of the store. I can pretty much make it in time if I'm less than three minutes away." I laughed at her joke, but we both realized that she had a very real problem that was severely interfering with her life. Ann told me that her diarrhea began after an episode of bronchitis three months earlier. Since then she'd had diarrhea every day, often first thing in the morning after her cup of coffee.

Each day after her initial run to the bathroom, Ann told me, she often had to go again in twenty minutes.

Sometimes she kept feeling the urge to go and didn't know when she could get out of the house. She'd canceled several outings with her friends at the last minute because she felt tied to the toilet. Dinner parties with her husband were the most stressful times. An hour before she left for a party, she took two Imodium and prayed that she could get through the evening without an accident.

When Ann came to see me, we discussed all the possible reasons for this unrelenting diarrhea. I told her she might have a chronic bacterial or parasitic infection that could still be lingering. Another possible culprit: the Advil that she had been taking on a regular basis for her headaches. She was also taking medication for an underactive thyroid, and I wanted to explore whether her Synthroid dose might be too high, since too much thyroid hormone speeds up the function of the GI tract. But first I needed to rule out more serious disorders like colitis.

After doing some blood tests and performing a colonoscopy, I learned that Ann's diarrhea was triggered by a form of colitis that was caused by the antibiotics she had taken to clear up her upper respiratory tract infection a few months earlier. The antibiotics that she was treated with had knocked out the bronchitis but had also killed off beneficial colon bacteria and allowed harmful bacteria, called *Clostridium difficile,* to colonize and damage the intestinal wall. As a result, Ann had developed a type of colitis that was causing her severe diarrhea.

Fortunately, her condition was treatable with another antibiotic called metronidazole. This knocked out the *C. difficile* and completely cleared up her diarrhea. On her follow-up visit, Ann happily reported to me that her bowel habits were back to normal, and she no longer frequents all the bathrooms in town.

DEFINING DIARRHEA

Diarrhea is a very loose (pardon the pun) term when used by patients who experience this symptom. One of my patients, Marsha, described her diarrhea as four to six bowel movements a day. Linda, another patient, told me she had diarrhea in the form of one stool a day that was always loose and often watery. Edna told me her diarrhea was so bad that she started having fecal incontinence at the age of fifty-four and now has to wear a pad every day.

Labor Pains

"The first time I was in labor I was surprised when I suddenly felt the intense urge to go to the bathroom in the middle of a painful contraction. I plodded over to the toilet and had a swoosh of diarrhea during my next contraction. I felt the most relief and control over my contractions just sitting on the toilet letting my bowels empty out. I did this until I felt the urge to push. My baby was born thirty minutes later—on the table, not in the toilet! I have now come to expect diarrhea during my labor. I consider it a sign that my body is working with me to get the baby out."

—**Debbie,** mother of three

DIARRHEA OR
SOMETHING DIFFERENT?

A condition called hyperdefecation can mimic the symptoms of diarrhea, causing cramping and loose stools, with frequent or watery bowel movements. But not enough stool is produced to cause the side effects that commonly occur with diarrhea, like dehydration or an electrolyte imbalance.

Kathy, one of my patients with irritable bowel syndrome (IBS), has "diarrhea" every time she eats spicy food or when she's really stressed out. She told me that on a bad day she'll have ten watery bowel movements. But when I really questioned her about her bowel habits, she told me she'll pass a few cups of watery stool first thing in the morning, but by the last few episodes in the late afternoon, she passes only a few tablespoons of stool and usually more gas. And she never has diarrhea that wakes her up in the middle of the night. Kathy, like most people with diarrhea-predominant IBS, complains of diarrhea symptoms but really has hyperdefecation. Changes in the consistency or frequency of her bowel movements can be due to an increased gut transit time or increased intestinal secretions. In developed countries like the United States, IBS remains the number-one cause of hyperdefecation in women.

Hyperdefecation can be triggered by stress—the kind that makes you rush to the bathroom right before a job interview. When you're stressed or anxious, you may experience an increase in colonic motility, which can cause loose stools or diarrhea. And this can happen to any of us, not only those with IBS.

Researchers don't know exactly how stress brings about these changes. Likely a combination of factors—both in the brain's central nervous system and in the gut's enteric nervous system—causes an increase in peristalsis and secretions from the lower GI tract. A specific factor that appears to be important in this pathway is corticotropin-releasing factor (CRF). CRF is released in the brain during episodes of stress and stimulates the release of adrenal corticotropic hormone (ACTH) from the pituitary gland and, ultimately, cortisol by the adrenal gland. Studies in humans have shown that giving intravenous CRF results in increased sigmoid colonic motility, similar to the effects of fear and stress. This is an area of active research, and several studies are currently under way to try to determine the factors involved in this reaction.

Female IBS sufferers who are sensitive to hormonal fluctuations during their menstrual cycle may develop diarrhea or hyperdefecation at certain times of the month. I find that I develop looser stools on the first day of my period, though I wouldn't classify this as diarrhea. I've seen many patients, especially IBS sufferers, who find themselves rushing off to the bathroom several times a day—during a particular phase of their menstrual cycle—with explosive bowel movements and cramping. As I detailed in Chapter 2, oral contraceptives that supply a steady dose of hormones throughout the month may alleviate this problem.

Although hyperdefecation doesn't measure up to the quantity of stools produced with diarrhea, I don't want to discount it as a real problem. It can destroy your quality of life if you're always afraid to be far from a bathroom. You can try some of the diarrhea remedies in this chapter or in Chapter 13 to manage your symptoms. If you don't get relief within two weeks, you should consider seeing your doctor. There are a number of new therapies in clinical trials that might benefit you.

Just what constitutes diarrhea? Even doctors have a tough time answering this question. If you go by the traditional medical definition, diarrhea is defined by the amount of stool passed in a day; more than 300 grams of stool. (That's almost a half pound, which is quite a bit.) The problem with a quantitative definition like this is that some people who eat a large amount of fiber might produce that amount of stool without having diarrhea. What's more, other people may have diarrhea in the form of loose watery stools and cramping, without producing 300 grams per day. So now the medical definition has expanded to include the frequency of bowel movements. In general, if you have more than three stools a day, you may have diarrhea.

Most of the time diarrhea occurs as an acute, self-limited bout and is caused by a specific offender. You may have eaten something that contained a harmful bacterial toxin, or you may have contracted an intestinal virus.

Normally, the colon secretes very little fluid. The colon, in fact, functions mainly to absorb water from our stools. But when an infection or toxin invades the gut, defensive mechanisms are set into action. Gut secretions and motility increase tremendously to try to expel the offenders, which results in diarrhea. In the majority of cases, you probably never pinpoint the exact cause because your diarrhea clears up within a day or two. The average adult suffers from a diarrhea bout four times a year. For most people, it's not serious and resolves on its own without treatment.

For others, though, diarrhea can be a long-term, chronic disorder (which means it lasts more than four weeks) and is caused by a specific gastrointestinal disease or other chronic condition. Patients with Crohn's disease may have intestinal inflammation that results in diarrhea. Severe long-term diabetes can change intestinal motility and bacterial flora, causing diarrhea. People with food intolerances that make them unable to digest food components like lactose (a milk sugar) or gluten (a protein in wheat and other grains) may suffer from chronic diarrhea. Surgery involving the gastrointestinal tract can also lead to diarrhea by changing how quickly food moves through the intestinal tract or by changing the release or absorption of certain digestive secretions such as bile.

THE THREE MAIN TYPES OF DIARRHEA

Diarrhea occurs due to a disturbance in your large intestine that is caused by one of the following three things.

Osmotic Diarrhea

A shift in the osmotic or fluid pressure in the membrane lining the intestine can cause fluid to rush into the intestine. This lining normally allows fluid and nutrients to pass in and out. Your body prefers balance and strives to create an equal fluid pressure on both sides, through a process called osmosis. Food particles that cannot be absorbed through the intestinal wall into the bloodstream (like lactose or gluten in those who have an intolerance to these nutrients) exert osmotic pressure and cause water from the bloodstream to cross the lining to try to balance the fluid concentration on both sides. This excess fluid produces diarrhea. Many laxatives (like milk of magnesia) work on this principle as well. They put additional osmotic particles into the gut, causing more water to be channeled into the intestines, which liquefies stools. The key to osmotic diarrhea is that it won't occur if you don't eat any food, drinks, or supplements that will bring it on. If you stop ingesting the culprit that causes this diarrhea, your symptoms should go away or at least improve dramatically.

Secretory Diarrhea

When food passes into your intestines, the cells lining them absorb fluid and nutrients and pass them into the bloodstream. With secretory diarrhea, these same cells secrete electrolytes like chloride or bicarbonate into the GI tract. Water follows these electrolytes into the GI tract and results in diarrhea. Infection is the most common cause of secretory diarrhea. Certain bacteria such as *Vibrio cholerae, Salmonella,* and *Escherichia coli* (a common cause of traveler's diarrhea) give off toxins that can stick to the intestinal lining, causing cells to secrete massive amounts of fluid into the intestine. This results in the voluminous watery diarrhea that's typical of food poisoning. Unlike osmotic diarrhea, secretory diarrhea isn't hindered by fasting. Another very rare cause of secretory diarrhea is a tumor that secretes substances that markedly increase intestinal secretions of fluid. Treating such a tumor may require surgery or medication to decrease intestinal secretions and motility.

COMMON CAUSES OF BACTERIAL FOOD POISONING

ORGANISM	COMMON FOOD OFFENDERS	AVERAGE TIME FOR SYMPTOMS TO OCCUR AFTER EATING	TYPICAL SYMPTOMS	TYPICAL DURATION OF ILLNESS
Bacillus cereus	fried rice, cream, pudding, meatballs, boiled beef, BBQ chicken, spaghetti sauce	2–9 hours	vomiting, crampy abdominal pain, diarrhea	half day to 1 day
Campylobacter jejuni	milk, chicken, beef	24–72 hours	fever, diarrhea (occasionally bloody), headache, muscle aches, vomiting	7 days
Clostridium perfringens	usually pre-cooked then reheated beef, turkey, chicken	8–14 hours	diarrhea, crampy abdominal pain	1 day
Escherichia coli	salads, undercooked beef	24–96 hours	nausea, crampy abdominal pain, diarrhea (occasionally bloody)	3 days
Listeria monocytogenes	milk, soft cheeses, raw vegetables, cole slaw, poultry, beef, pork, shrimp	Variable	fever, headache, abdominal pain, nausea, diarrhea—more severe in pregnant women	variable: can be short-lived or life-threatening
Salmonella	eggs, meat, poultry, dairy products	24 hours	nausea, fever, abdominal cramping, diarrhea (occasionally bloody)	3 days
Shigella	milk, salads (potato, tuna, turkey), ice cream, contaminated water	24 hours	crampy abdominal pain, fever, diarrhea (often bloody)	variable: antibiotics are indicated for most
Staphylococcus aureus	ham, canned beef, cream-filled pastry, custard	3 hours	nausea, vomiting, cramping, diarrhea	1 day
Vibrio parahemolyticus	raw/cooked fish or shellfish; rarely with salt water or salted vegetables	12 hours	explosive watery diarrhea, nausea, vomiting, headache, abdominal cramps	3 days
Yersinia enterocolitica	chocolate milk or raw milk, ice cream, pork	72 hours	fever, abdominal cramps, diarrhea	7 days

Many of these bacteria are also transmitted person to person by the fecal-oral route

Motility Disorders

The normal contractions or wavelike motions of the GI tract, called peristalsis, propel the intestinal contents from the mouth to the anus. Certain diseases, such as hyperthyroidism, can increase the motility or secretion of the gut, resulting in diarrhea. Intestinal motility is important for cleansing your intestines and preventing stagnation of fluid or overgrowth of bacteria. Certain diseases such as diabetes, Parkinson's, and scleroderma can affect the nerves and muscles of the intestine, slowing motility and giving bacteria the opportunity to multiply where they shouldn't be present—in the small intestine. Bacteria in the small bowel can set up an inflammatory reaction that damages the villi, hairlike structures lining the intestinal walls that are vital for nutrient absorption. This results in weight loss and diarrhea due to malabsorption.

INFECTIOUS DIARRHEA

Bacterial Infections

Along with viruses, bacteria are the most common cause of acute or temporary diarrhea. Several types of bacteria (*Vibrio cholerae, E. coli*) found in contaminated food or water produce a toxin that causes intestinal cells to release salt and water. The amount of fluid overwhelms the colon, making it impossible to reabsorb the fluid, causing secretory diarrhea. Other bacteria (*Shigella, Salmonella, Campylobacter*) can directly bind to the colonic mucosa, resulting in colitis and an inflammatory diarrhea that may be bloody. Bacteria are frequently transmitted in tainted foods: *Salmonella* and *Campylobacter* bacteria live on chicken and turkey, while *E. coli 0157:H7* is a deadly bacterium transmitted through cattle feces. Although most cases of bacterial infection are self-limited and one's own immune system can battle them, antibiotics may be needed in serious or prolonged cases. You should call your doctor immediately if you have bloody diarrhea, or diarrhea accompanied by severe abdominal or rectal pain, or a fever of 102 degrees Fahrenheit or higher. Any diarrhea that lasts more than three days may also require antibiotic treatment.

Viral Infections

Along with bacteria, viruses are the most common cause of diarrhea in both adults and children. They account for 30 to 40 percent of acute diarrhea cases in the United States. You might call viral diarrhea a case of the stomach flu, but actually this is a misnomer. Viral diarrhea is caused, not by a flu virus, but by any of various other culprits such as *rotavirus, Norwalk virus, enteric adenovirus, astrovirus,* and *torovirus.* Norwalk virus has caused epidemics of diarrhea in communities, camps, nursing homes, and hospitals; recently it was the culprit that caused the numerous outbreaks of diarrhea on cruise ships. It can contaminate drinking water supplies and shellfish (raw clams or oysters) and can be transmitted easily from person to person. Astrovirus has been associated with outbreaks of diarrhea in day-care centers. Rotavirus also causes a large number of cases of diarrhea in children. Adults usually acquire the disease from a sick child. Vomiting and diarrhea usually resolve after five to seven days, but some children can continue to shed virus in their stools for up to eight weeks after their illness has resolved.

Generally, viruses temporarily damage the lining of the small intestine, which interferes with fluid absorption and causes diarrhea. Like most bacterial diarrhea, viral diarrhea tends to be short-lived and controlled by our own immune systems. Antivirals generally aren't necessary to treat these infections, which usually clear up on their own within a few days.

Parasite Infections

Parasites can enter the body through contaminated food or water and make their home in your digestive tract, inflaming the intestines and interfering with the absorption of fluid and nutrients. Amebic dysentery, caused by the parasite *Entamoeba histolytica,* is a common culprit, causing colonic inflammation and diarrhea particularly in developing countries where water supplies are contaminated with the parasite. Another common water supply contaminant is *Giardia lamblia,* commonly found in mountain streams or untreated well water. *Giardia* infects the small intestine, resulting in an inflammatory process that hinders the normal absorption of nutrients and causes diarrhea, gas, loss of appetite, abdominal cramps, and bloating, which can last for a few days to a few weeks. If you're planning a wilderness camping trip, it may be a good idea to bring along a portable filter that can remove parasites from water (camping stores sell them), or boil water for at least one minute before you drink it.

Cryptosporidium has been found in contaminated water supplies in this country. Efforts are under way in many major cities to improve water-filtration techniques in public tap water supplies. Chlorine is added to kill off this parasite, but occasional outbreaks have occurred in recent years. Often parasite infections clear up on their own without any treatment. A drug called metronidazole (Flagyl) can be prescribed and is very effective against some parasites.

CONDITIONS THAT INCREASE DIARRHEA RISK

Immunosuppression can significantly increase a person's risk of developing infectious diarrhea from bacteria, viruses, or parasites. Patients with AIDS, those receiving chemotherapy for cancer, and those receiving immunosuppressive medications (organ transplant patients or those with lupus erythematosus, rheumatoid arthritis, or other chronic inflammatory disorders) have a higher incidence of developing complications from infectious diarrhea since their bodies are less capable of fighting off the invading organisms. In one recent case that made newspaper headlines, transplant patients who were visiting a well-known amusement park became violently ill with *Salmonella* food poisoning from eating tainted roma tomatoes.

Some GI conditions can increase your risk of developing diarrhea that's not associated with a bacterial or viral infection. Crohn's disease and ulcerative colitis produce bloody diarrhea associated with pus and abdominal pain. (Chapter 14 focuses in detail on these

MICROSCOPIC COLITIS

Janet R., a fifty-eight-year-old English professor, came to me several months ago complaining of chronic diarrhea. She travels abroad frequently with her husband and assumed she picked up a stomach bug in her recent trip to Africa. She was taking over-the-counter Imodium tablets but became constipated. The minute she stopped taking the Imodium, her diarrhea returned.

"I find that I can't go anywhere without first scouting out where the bathroom is," she complained. "A few times I didn't make it in time and had an accident. I was horrified and had to ask a friend to run to my house to get me a change of clothes." Janet found herself racing to the bathroom six to eight times a day and frequently woke up in the middle of the night having to make a bowel movement.

I decided to perform a colonoscopy to determine the cause of Janet's diarrhea. Although her colon looked normal during the endoscopic exam, I took a few biopsy samples because I suspected that she actually had a form of inflammatory colitis—not an African stomach bug. My suspicions were confirmed when the biopsy showed that Janet had collagenous colitis.

Collagenous colitis and lymphocytic colitis are two forms of inflammatory bowel disease with normal or near-normal endoscopic appearance of the colon. The diagnosis is made by looking at a biopsy specimen under the microscope; hence these two diseases fall under the category of microscopic colitis. This form of colitis often causes chronic diarrhea. It usually begins in middle age and strikes women more often than men. It is frequently associated with arthritis, celiac disease, and other autoimmune disorders. In fact, whenever I see a woman over forty with chronic diarrhea, I almost always take a colon biopsy to rule out microscopic colitis. Diarrhea usually occurs because of reduced absorption of fluid in the colon due to inflammation caused by this disease.

Once I diagnosed Janet, her treatment was fairly simple. I told her to halve her dose of Imodium, which she found resolved her diarrhea without giving her constipation. (Other patients with this condition may need a more complicated treatment regimen like anti-inflammatory drugs or corticosteroids to control their diarrhea.)

inflammatory conditions.) Bowel inflammation may also be associated with autoimmune diseases. Systemic lupus erythematosus, Behcet's disease, and other autoimmune disorders can cause colonic ulceration that results in inflammatory diarrhea.

YES, DIARRHEA CAN BE CONTAGIOUS

I want to make it clear that food poisoning (which can be caused by a virus, bacterium, parasite, or their toxins), as well as other acute bouts of diarrhea, can be extremely contagious. Most parents know this from experience, having come down with a bout of diarrhea when it was going around their child's preschool. If you have a "stomach bug," I strongly recommend that you avoid sharing utensils and cups with other family members, and avoid preparing meals for your family (especially young children). I encourage thorough hand-washing for all family members when someone in the household is sick with an infectious diarrhea. Scrub your hands briskly with antibacterial soap and water for five minutes, including under the nails. If this isn't a practical option, wear rubber gloves when handling food.

MEDICATIONS THAT
CAUSE DIARRHEA

Almost any prescription drug can cause diarrhea as a side effect. If you look in the *Physicians' Desk Reference*—the main resource that doctors use for information on prescription medications—it's nearly impossible to find a medication that doesn't list diarrhea somewhere in the "side effects" profile. Some over-the-counter products can also cause diarrhea. Several liquid medications contain sorbitol or fructose, which may induce an osmotic diarrhea. Antacids like Maalox and laxatives like milk of magnesia contain magnesium, which can trigger diarrhea because magnesium isn't easily absorbed by the digestive tract. Nonsteroidal anti-inflammatory pain relievers (e.g., aspirin, ibuprofen, naproxen sodium) may cause colonic ulcers that result in inflammatory diarrhea.

Medication-induced diarrhea usually sets in around twenty-four hours after you begin taking the drug. On occasion, the diarrhea may be short-lived and resolve after you take the medication for a few weeks. If you are taking a medication and have continued diarrhea, ask your doctor if the medication could be the cause.

The Antibiotic Risk

Whenever you take a course of antibiotics, you have a good chance of developing diarrhea. This may be a side effect of the antibiotic itself, as in the case of potent antibiotic therapy for the eradication of *H. pylori,* the bacterium that causes ulcers. For example, the antibiotic erythromycin mimics a natural substance, motilin, and causes diarrhea by increasing gut motility.

Another more important cause of antibiotic-associated diarrhea is a secondary superinfection of the colon. In these cases, diarrhea occurs because an antibiotic has wiped out all the normal flora that live in your intestines, including the good bacteria that prevent the overgrowth of yeast and harmful bacteria. When an antibiotic destroys your defenses, new, harmful bacteria can increase in number and colonize rapidly, causing diarrhea.

The culprit behind antibiotic-related diarrhea (as in Ann's case) and colitis is a nasty bacterium called *Clostridium difficile.* This bacterium is usually undetectable in the stool of healthy individuals, but when normal bacteria are suppressed by antibiotics, this one grows and multiplies and can quickly cause problems. It gives off a toxin that damages the lining of the colon (causing a form of colitis) and can cause fever, lower abdominal cramps, and diarrhea that can occasionally be bloody. If not treated, the colitis may progress, and the patient may, in rare cases, develop a bowel perforation that requires surgery to repair.

Mild diarrhea caused by antibiotics may be alleviated with over-the-counter probiotic tablets that contain live, beneficial bacteria that keep harmful bacteria in check (see page 249). Most diarrhea improves after you stop taking the antibiotic. If you develop fever or if your diarrhea persists after your antibiotic course is finished, your doctor may order a stool test to look for *Clostridium difficile* toxin. Test results may take several days, but if you're very ill, your doctor may start you on the metronidazole (or another antibiotic called vancomycin) regimen even before the results are available.

C. difficile diarrhea usually clears up within three to five days after beginning the antibiotics. Be aware, though, that up to 25 percent of people with *C. difficile* diarrhea experience a recurrence after going off metronidazole or vancomycin. They may require retreatment with the antibiotic that worked to clear up the diarrhea until the bacterial infection is completely resolved.

Weight-Loss Remedies

Certain kinds of over-the-counter diet pills contain stimulants that speed metabolism, which can lead to diarrhea by increasing colonic motility. Health food stores carry diet remedies that contain ma huang or ephedra, a stimulant that can cause diarrhea. Weight-loss teas containing senna or cascara (which are laxatives) can cause diarrhea if taken in large enough quantities. Even caffeine can be a cause of diarrhea when it's added in high amounts to weight-loss products. Some manufacturers even put thyroid hormone (often from horses) into their products, a powerful stimulant that can increase intestinal motility, causing diarrhea.

FOOD INTOLERANCES
AND MALABSORPTION

An inability to fully absorb or digest a particular food can be a major cause of diarrhea. Women with these food intolerances may develop a specific nutrient deficiency or significant weight loss. Not to be mistaken for a food allergy, a food intolerance means that a particular food causes you some sort of gastric distress. An allergy occurs when your body mounts an immune response to the food.

Our bodies require a number of enzymes, hormones, and bile (produced by the stomach, small intestine, pancreas, and liver) to assist in digestion of food; poor digestion can occur if one or more of these components is missing. For example, adults who develop diarrhea, cramps, and flatulence from drinking too much milk usually have an intolerance to milk—not an allergy. Their bodies lack an enzyme needed to digest the milk sugar lactose, so lactose goes undigested into the colon, where it gets fermented by bacteria. This reaction causes gas, bloating, and diarrhea. (On the other hand, babies who develop these symptoms in reaction to milk, especially if accompanied by a rash, may have a true allergy to milk proteins mediated by their immune system. All infants have enough lactase, the enzyme needed to break down milk sugar.)

Malabsorption generally implies a defect in the intestinal lining that won't allow the absorption of nutrients and water. Inflammatory diseases (celiac sprue and Crohn's disease) and certain infectious diseases (*Giardia* infection and small-bowel overgrowth) are all examples of disorders that can injure the small-intestinal lining and

MEDICATIONS ASSOCIATED WITH DIARRHEA

Here is a short list of common medications that can cause diarrhea. If you believe one of your medications is causing diarrhea, consult your doctor.

- most antibiotics
- nonsteroidal anti-inflammatory drugs, such as ibuprofen (Advil, Motrin, Nuprin) and naproxen sodium (Aleve, Naprosyn)
- other anti-inflammatory agents, such as gold salts (auranofin, brand name Ridaura) to treat rheumatoid arthritis, or 5-aminosalicylic acid (Asacol, Pentasa, Rowasa) to treat inflammatory bowel disease
- blood pressure medications, such as propranolol hydrochloride (Inderal)
- antacids (especially those containing magnesium), such as Maalox and Mylanta
- colchicine (used to treat gout)
- stomach acid reducers, especially H_2 receptor blockers such as cimetidine (Tagamet) and PPIs such as omeprazole (Prilosec), esomeprazole (Nexium), pantoprazole (Protonix), rabeprazole (Aciphex), and lansoprazole (Prevacid)
- theophylline (Theo-Dur), a medicine to treat asthma, chronic bronchitis, and emphysema
- vitamin and mineral supplements (especially those containing magnesium)
- herbal products containing senna, cascara, licorice root, buckthorn, dandelion root, yellowdock, or fennel seed, all of which act as laxatives
- misoprostol (Cytotec) (the "morning after" pill; also used to prevent ulcers in patients with gastric ulcers caused by nonsteroidal anti-inflammatory drugs who need to remain on these drugs)

ultimately hinder the absorption of food. Patients with pancreatic disease, like chronic pancreatitis, may also have maldigestion because they lack the pancreatic enzymes needed to break down fats and proteins into their smaller components for absorption, resulting in diarrhea.

Malabsorption isn't always caused by diseases. We can sometimes bring it on ourselves unintentionally, with the foods we eat. Some diet products—such as soft drinks, chewing gum, and candies—contain poorly absorbable sugars such as mannitol, sorbitol, and xylitol. Wow! potato chips contain olestra, a poorly absorbable fat. Although these products allow us to enjoy snack food without the consequences of increased blood sugar (sorbitol) or increased fat intake (olestra), they may carry a hefty price tag—in the form of diarrhea.

FOOD ALLERGIES

Gina came to my clinic last month complaining of diarrhea and abdominal cramping whenever she ate spaghetti or chili. She was convinced she had an allergy to tomatoes, garlic, or onions. Many of my patients genuinely believe that food allergies are the cause of their GI symptoms—when they usually have a food intolerance, as was the case with Gina. Truth is, food allergies are very rare in adults. Bona fide food allergies trigger an immune system reaction. Your immune system attacks the offending food by releasing histamine and other chemicals that increase inflammation. Allergic reactions can cause itching, hives, flushing, wheezing, and diarrhea. The reaction usually happens pretty rapidly after eating the food.

Food allergies are most likely to occur in babies. Up to eight percent of infants under the age of three are allergic to some food, usually milk. The allergy can manifest itself as diarrhea, vomiting, colic, blood in the stool, asthma, or an allergic dermatitis. Fortunately, most children "grow out of" their food allergies by age ten. Sensitivity to peanuts, nuts, and seafood, however, may remain into adulthood. Beware of medical quacks who say they can determine food allergies by examining a blood test or stool sample—they can't. You need to see an allergist with a medical degree, who will probably need to do a skin scratch test with several possible food allergens or a complex food elimination diet to find the culprit.

In adults, the most common food allergy disorders are celiac sprue (see the box on page 239) and oral allergy syndrome. Oral allergy syndrome causes a reaction at the site of contact, the same way poison ivy causes a local skin reaction. Whenever an offending food is eaten, an allergic reaction occurs rapidly in and around the mouth, with severe itching and swelling of the lips, tongue, palate, and throat. The reaction resolves fairly quickly. Oral allergy syndrome most commonly occurs after eating fresh fruits or vegetables (melons, bananas, potatoes, carrots, celery, apples, hazelnuts, mangoes, and kiwi). People who are allergic to ragweed or birch pollen are more likely to have this syndrome.

Certain chemicals in foods can cause reactions that mimic an allergic response. Fermented cheese, pork sausage, canned tuna, and sardines all contain histamine, a chemical released by the body in response to an allergic reaction. This chemical in foods can cause

CELIAC SPRUE: DO YOU HAVE IT?

Celiac disease is an inflammatory disorder of the small intestine that is triggered by exposure to gluten (wheat protein) in people who have a genetic predisposition to the disorder. The inflammatory condition causes a marked decrease in the absorptive surface area of the small intestine and results in a malabsorption of nutrients. Many patients with celiac sprue have minimal or no symptoms and often go undiagnosed.

The disease is most common in western Europe (occurring in one in a thousand people), particularly in those of Celtic heritage. It is also found in countries where Europeans have migrated, such as the United States and Australia, but the overall prevalence tends to be lower (one in three thousand in the United States). It rarely affects people of purely African or Asian descent.

Genetic factors play an important role in the risk for celiac disease. About 95 percent of patients with celiac disease have a specific inherited, immunologic marker, HLA DQ2 or HLA DQ8. Diagnosis generally involves the use of a blood test to look for antibodies against certain proteins. Endoscopy is often necessary as well, and a small-bowel biopsy can be obtained to confirm the diagnosis.

Celiac disease is associated with a number of other disorders, including a skin disorder called dermatitis herpetiformis, Type 2 (adult-onset) diabetes, thyroid disease, inflammatory bowel disease, and rheumatoid arthritis. It can also cause a host of GI symptoms, including diarrhea (due to malabsorption), flatulence, bloating, and weight loss. Celiac sufferers may develop anemia (due to a malabsorption of iron, folate, and/or vitamin B_{12}) and osteoporosis (due to a malabsorption of calcium and vitamin D).

Of particular concern to women, celiac disease can lead to fertility problems if left untreated. Lack of periods (amenorrhea) occurs in one-third of affected women of childbearing age—possibly due to weight loss caused by celiac sprue or possibly from other unknown causes. The disease can also lead to infertility, spontaneous and recurrent miscarriages, and a higher risk of having a low-birth-weight baby.

Treatment of celiac sprue requires following a gluten-free diet for life. This means avoiding all foods containing wheat, rye, and barley gluten. Patients can use only rice, corn, maize, buckwheat, potato, soybean, or tapioca for flours or starches. This dietary regimen can be extremely challenging. It means no bread, cake, pasta, pizza, cookies, or cereal. Wheat flour can be used as a filler in anything from gravy to medications. Celiac patients learn to become avid label readers.

I know this regimen can be difficult, but the payoff is big: Removing gluten from the diet usually leads to rapid healing of the intestinal lining. Symptoms disappear, and patients gain back their lost weight. UVA has a wonderful Celiac Sprue Support Group, which was started by our dietitian, Carol Parrish. Other important resources for patients include:

Celiac Sprue Association
P.O. Box 31700

Omaha, NE 68131-0700

tel. (402) 558-0600

fax (402) 558-1347

www.csaceliacs.org

National Digestive Diseases Information Clearinghouse

2 Information Way

Bethesda, MD 20892-3570

tel. (800) 891-5389

digestive.niddk.nih.gov/diseases/pubs/celiac/index.htm

Celiac Sprue Research Foundation

P.O. Box 61193

Palo Alto, CA 94306-1193

tel./fax (650) 251-9865

www.celiacsprue.org

Gluten Intolerance Group

15110 10th Avenue SW

Suite A

Seattle, WA 98166-1820

tel. (206) 246-6652

flushing, itching, and hives similar to an allergic reaction. Phenylethylamine, found in chocolate, aged cheese, and red wine, can cause migraines in susceptible people. Those who are sensitive to the food additive monosodium glutamate (MSG) can develop headaches, shortness of breath, or dizziness in response to eating a Chinese meal. Nitrates in smoked meat and cheese can cause GI upset, headache, and hives. All of these, though, are intolerances, not allergies.

SURGICAL TREATMENTS

Surgery involving the gastrointestinal tract can often lead to diarrhea. After bowel resection, food can move more quickly through the intestinal tract, and a loss in absorptive surface area can cause malabsorption. This is common after surgery to treat a stomach ulcer or inflammatory bowel disease. Diarrhea following gastric bypass surgery is also very common. As I explained in Chapter 3, gastric bypass speeds stomach emptying, so food isn't absorbed as well. Sugar and fats may pass undigested into the small intestine, where water and fluid are pumped in to regulate osmosis. This increase in fluid and motility causes diarrhea.

A patient named Sandy came to see me two months after gallbladder surgery for gallstones. After her gallbladder was removed, her abdominal pain symptoms subsided, but now she had developed diarrhea. When she came to the clinic, Sandy didn't even make the connection that her diarrhea might be related to her surgery.

She was surprised to learn that 20 percent of people develop diarrhea after they have their gallbladder removed. The gallbladder functions to store bile. Bile is produced by the liver and is an important substance in the absorption of fat. If the gallbladder is gone, between meals when there is no fat to bind to the bile, bile salts can reach the colon, where they trigger the release of fluid and increase motility, causing diarrhea. One particularly effective treatment for this kind of diarrhea is the prescription drug cholestyramine (Questran), which binds bile salts.

CLEARING UP THE PROBLEM

Try an OTC Remedy

Your first instinct when you have diarrhea is probably to reach for a package of over-the-counter antidiarrhea medication like loperamide (Imodium), attapulgite (Kaopectate), or bismuth subsalicylate (Pepto-Bismol). These products can indeed help ease symptoms (by decreasing stool frequency and liquidity and reducing cramps) in many people. But some physicians believe that antimotility agents like Imodium shouldn't be used for at least the first day or two of your symptoms if you're unsure about what is causing your diarrhea. For two common causes of diarrhea—bacterial and viral infections—loose, frequent stools are the body's way of flushing out the invading bug. Some experts believe the antimotility agents slow the process and can keep germs around, actually making the problem last longer. There is little scientific data to support this theory, however, so just be judicious with these agents when you have diarrhea. If you don't really need them, don't take them, but if you're suffering from your diarrhea, they may really help to make your symptoms better.

Replace Fluids and Electrolytes

One of the most important things you can do when experiencing diarrhea is to drink plenty of fluids. This

A DELICATE ISSUE

Like many women, Edna had seen commercials for Depends undergarments while watching her favorite soap operas. The fifty-eight-year-old mother had never dreamed, though, that she would one day need to wear them herself. "I thought I was done with diapers thirty years ago, when my two-year-old was potty-trained, and I certainly never thought I'd be wearing them again," she told me.

Edna's problem with "accidents" began about five years earlier. She was able to wear minipads and had occasional streaks of stool. Over time her symptoms worsened, and she had to wear Depends every day. "I can wear only baggy clothes because I don't want everyone to know I'm wearing diapers," she complained. She'd had several accidents and always had an extra set of clothes with her. Edna came to my clinic complaining of diarrhea. When I questioned her further, it was clear to me that her problem was less about diarrhea than an inability to control her bowel movements.

Many patients with fecal incontinence seek medical attention, believing that their problem is diarrhea. Their stools may be loose, but their problem is not about intestinal fluid or electrolyte absorption—it's more a mechanical issue due to some malfunction in the working of the anal sphincter. In my clinic, if a patient complains about diarrhea, I always ask about fecal incontinence. Understanding that Edna's problem was more about her anal sphincter allowed me to focus on specific diagnostic testing and treatment options. Edna's problems are now under control, and she no longer needs to wear an adult undergarment. For more information about fecal incontinence and possible therapies, see Chapter 16.

will help prevent dehydration, the excessive loss of fluid and electrolytes, such as potassium and magnesium, that commonly occurs with diarrhea. Your body needs these electrolytes to function properly. Absorption from the gut is significantly increased if the water is combined with salt and nutrients. Salty liquids that contain protein or sugars, such as chicken and beef broth, may be better choices.

When patients have diarrhea, I'm not a big fan of athletic replenishment drinks such as Gatorade. These drinks are made to replace minimal fluid losses that can occur with sweating, but they don't contain enough salt and potassium to replace the fluid losses that come with significant diarrhea. If sports drinks are the only thing you have close by, then you should supplement them with salty foods such as pretzels or crackers.

Oral rehydration therapies such as Pedialyte (Rehydralyte, Resol, Ricalyte), sold in local drugstores, are usually cheaper than sports drinks and are far more effective because they contain the proper amount of electrolytes and nutrients mixed into the fluid. If you have trouble keeping food down, sip the liquid slowly, in small amounts. How much you need to drink depends on how frequently you're having bowel movements, but a good rule of thumb is at least two cups of fluid each hour.

Go Easy on Food

Eat bland, nonfatty foods that are easily digested, like baked or boiled potatoes, plain pasta, cooked carrots, crackers, and baked chicken without the skin. Stay away from dairy products since diarrhea temporarily disrupts the body's ability to digest lactose. Avoid caffeine, which can stimulate gut motility, and red meat and spicy foods. You should also moderate your intake of

IS THERE BACTERIA IN YOUR SALSA?

Sometimes food poisoning can come from the most surprising of sources. A study in the June 2002 issue of the *Annals of Internal Medicine* looked at *E. coli* contamination in tabletop sauces from Mexican restaurants in Guadalajara, Mexico, and Houston, Texas. In the sauces (pico de gallo, guacamole, and salsa) these investigators found that 66 percent of the sauces from Guadalajara were contaminated versus 40 percent from Houston.

The bigger difference, however, was in the level of fecal contaminants: The Guadalajara sauces had levels more than a thousand times greater than the sauces from Houston. In Guadalajara all the sauces were sitting on tabletops at room temperature. In Houston all the sauces were brought to the tables and were cold to the touch. Temperature was thought to be one factor affecting the bacterial content of the sauces, but handling by multiple workers and reuse of the same sauce by multiple patrons probably contributed to the problem in Guadalajara. Guacamole was the most frequently contaminated sauce in both cities.

Most people believe that an acidic pH is protective against bacterial contamination, but this study refutes that notion. In Guadalajara restaurants the sauce containing the highest level of contamination with *E. coli* was the more acidic, tomato-based pico de gallo.

high-fiber foods, like fresh fruits and vegetables, which can be difficult for irritated intestines to absorb.

TRAVELER'S DIARRHEA

It can ruin any trip. If you travel to a third world country, you have about a fifty-fifty chance of developing diarrhea. Bacterial and viral agents are responsible for 50 to 75 percent of traveler's diarrhea that lasts less than two weeks. As the duration of diarrhea increases, the likelihood of a parasitic infection increases, although parasites are identified in only about a third of cases of chronic traveler's diarrhea. In some cases, no cause can be found. Diarrhea that begins more than a month after travel is likely not due to exposure during the trip.

The best way to avoid it? Stick to the saying "Boil it, peel it, cook it, or don't eat it," a rule that's advised by the Centers for Disease Control and Prevention. In more detail:

- Drink only bottled water (if you're the one who breaks the seal on it), carbonated soft drinks, and hot drinks like coffee or tea.
- Avoid raw or rare meat or fish.
- Don't drink tap water, including ice.
- Don't eat meat, chicken, or shellfish that isn't hot when it's served.
- Don't eat any raw fruits or vegetables unless they can be peeled or you peel them yourself.

Most episodes of traveler's diarrhea resolve during the trip or very soon after returning home. About five to ten percent of travelers have diarrhea that lasts over two weeks, and less than 3 percent have diarrhea lasting over four weeks. For episodes of nonbloody diarrhea, I recommend that if you know you're traveling abroad to a developing country, you bring small powdered packets of rehydration therapy. You can mix the powder into bottled water and use it to prevent dehydration if you develop diarrhea. You can find these powdered packets, called World Health Organization Oral Rehydration Solution, by contacting the manufacturer, Jianas Brothers, in Kansas City, Missouri, at (816) 421-2880. One note of caution: Bloody diarrhea with fever often signifies an invasive or inflammatory diarrhea that usually requires antibiotics. See a doctor immediately if you develop this symptom.

If you are considering traveling to an exotic locale, you can find specific recommendations for the country you're visiting posted on the Centers for Disease Control and Prevention website (www.cdc.gov/travel/food-drink-risks.htm). The site will tell you if you need certain vaccinations, which foods to avoid, and whether you should take along any medications as a precaution.

If you're fortunate to be near one, a travel clinic may also be useful. At UVA there is an excellent travel clinic run by a world-renowned infectious disease physician, Richard Guerrant. Many people who will be traveling to exotic countries come to this clinic beforehand to get all of the appropriate immunizations as well as tips for problems such as diarrhea. My husband, Tom, and I visited the clinic before traveling to Saudi Arabia, and Tom went there before going to India.

PROBIOTICS: AN ALTERNATIVE TREATMENT FOR DIARRHEA

Probiotics, a Latin term meaning "for life," are living bacteria that are formulated into a tablet or capsule as a dietary supplement or added to foods like yogurt. Some people swear by them as a side-effect-free way to prevent diarrhea, as well as a host of other GI problems, from IBS to inflammatory bowel disease. Extensive research is currently under way to try to prove these claims and to establish the types and amounts of bacteria that are beneficial for certain disorders.

Unlike bacteria that cause strep throat or gastroenteritis, probiotics are thought to benefit the body by taking up residence in the intestines and helping to maintain a healthy balance of bacteria. More than four hundred species of bacteria live in the digestive tract, and researchers believe that at least some of them thwart invading organisms by using resources that the bad bugs need or by producing chemicals that kill them.

Several studies have found a modest reduction in antibiotic-associated diarrhea in those who take a probiotic along with their antibiotic—reducing the risk, on average, by half, from 20 to about 10 percent. One study, using a probiotic containing the bacterium *Lactobacillus GG* in children who were taking antibiotics, found that those who took the probiotic had an 8 percent incidence of diarrhea compared to 26 percent in those who took a placebo.

Other studies have found that probiotics can help prevent traveler's diarrhea. A Danish study found that travelers to Egypt who took the probiotic VSL#3, a combination of *L. acidophilus, L. bulgarius,* bifidobacteria, and streptococci, reduced their risk of diarrhea from 71 to 43 percent.

PROBIOTICS: AN ALTERNATIVE TREATMENT FOR DIARRHEA (continued)

There's no shortage of probiotic products on the market. However, I can't tell you which are the most reliable because manufacturers of dietary supplements don't have to prove that their products actually contain what they've listed on the label. After analyzing fifty-five products labeled "probiotic," Belgian biologists recently found that only 13 percent contained all the bacteria types listed on the label. More than a third of the powdered products contained no living bacteria whatsoever. That's because bacteria have a short shelf life. They don't live forever in a tablet, and many capsules have to be refrigerated continuously to keep the bacteria alive.

The bottom line: It probably can't hurt to try a probiotic to prevent or alleviate diarrhea. Just realize that you may be wasting your money.

WHEN TO SEE THE DOCTOR

Diarrhea—even if it comes on suddenly—can sometimes be serious enough to warrant an immediate visit to the doctor or local emergency room. According to the National Institute of Diabetes and Digestive and Kidney Diseases, you should seek medical attention when you experience any of the following symptoms:

- blood, mucus, pus, or parasites in stools
- black-colored stools
- severe abdominal or rectal pain
- diarrhea that lasts for more than three days

- fever of 102 degrees Fahrenheit or higher
- signs of dehydration like vomiting, dizziness, or fainting

Black stools may be a sign of gastrointestinal bleeding, a serious condition that should be attended to promptly. But they can also be a harmless side effect of taking Pepto-Bismol. The bismuth in Pepto-Bismol can discolor the stool and make it turn black, and it can turn your tongue black as well. Bloody diarrhea has to be checked out by a doctor. It can be caused by anything from a relatively benign infectious diarrhea or a more serious bacterial infection, or it can be a sign of a bleeding ulcer or even colon cancer.

Use your best judgment. If you're doubled over in cramps and have wave upon wave of unremitting diarrhea, you may have a serious infection that requires immediate treatment.

Another consideration you should factor in is whether you've traveled abroad recently or have been camping. If you have done either, you may have contracted a bacterial, parasitic, or viral infection that needs prompt treatment. Likewise, if you've started a new medication, you should ask your doctor right away if that may be the cause of your diarrhea.

Even if you don't have severe symptoms, you probably don't want to neglect diarrhea symptoms that don't respond to home treatments within 24 to 48 hours. Diarrhea can cause severe dehydration if it continues unabated.

Part III

WHEN YOU
NEED A
DOCTOR'S HELP

PREPARING FOR YOUR
DOCTOR'S VISIT

So you think you need to see a doctor about your digestive problems. Now what? Well, you're going to have to take your symptoms—which you may have been dealing with in the privacy of your own home—public. You're going to have to talk about them with a medical professional.

I know that this may be hard to come to terms with. So many of my patients have talked to me about their symptoms in the barest of whispers because they're embarrassed to admit that they pass flatus or belch too much or spend hours straining to have a bowel movement. "I just haven't been able to talk to anyone about this" is a comment I hear again and again.

In order to get the help you need, though, you're going to have to talk about your symptoms. If you find a doctor who really listens to you and is sensitive to your needs, you'll have a much easier time opening up about your medical problems.

Not every woman with gastrointestinal problems needs to advance immediately to a gastroenterologist for treatment. Common GI problems like gastroesophageal reflux or irritable bowel syndrome are frequently handled by a visit to a primary care physician. If the problem doesn't go away or come under control under your practitioner's care, you may need to talk with your doctor about getting a referral to a specialist.

In most cases, the specialist to see for GI problems is a gastroenterologist. You may, though, benefit from an evaluation by a gynecologist if your GI symptoms are caused by pelvic floor dysfunction or endometriosis. If you have rectal prolapse or hemorrhoids, a colorectal surgeon may be the specialist to see. Your primary care physician, however, should discuss these options with you and help you determine which specialist to see for your particular problem.

FINDING A
WOMAN-FRIENDLY DOCTOR

I'm going to borrow a term that I've seen in women's magazines and say that you need a "woman-friendly doctor" when it comes to finding the right gastroenterologist. By "woman-friendly," I don't mean that you need to find a woman. Male gastroenterologists can be just as woman-friendly as female gastroenterologists. In fact, I can thank my mentor (and current vice president of the AGA), Dr. David Peura, for instilling woman-friendly values in me when I was a GI fellow training at the University of Virginia Hospital. He is a quintessential good physician. He is, of course, a first-rate diagnostician and practitioner, but beyond that he really listens to his patients. He shows them that he cares about them as individuals, validates their problems, and takes the time to explain things. I strive to be a good listener and a caring physician not because I was trained by a woman but because I was trained by a good clinician.

Of course, you can't exactly ask your prospective gastroenterologist if he or she is "woman-friendly." What you can do, though, is find out from your primary care physician if the gastroenterologist that you're being referred to has a practice with a large percentage of female patients. Those who treat mainly women are more likely to see the relation between GI problems and the menstrual cycle or pelvic floor dysfunction than those who treat mainly men.

Some GI doctors, like myself, are known to specialize in women's health. I want to emphasize, though, that you may need to find a GI doctor who has a particular subspecialty in your problem area. Patients who have advanced liver disease, for example, need to see a liver specialist or hepatologist. Other GI doctors specialize in perianal disease or inflammatory bowel disease. Your primary care physician should know if you need to see a general GI doctor or a subspecialist.

In this day and age of managed care, primary care physicians play a key role in making referrals to gastroenterologists. They should know something about the doctor to whom they're referring you. You can say to your doctor, "I'm interested in finding someone who is going to listen to me and who understands and knows what's important in women's issues." If you've developed GI problems since going through meno-pause, you may need to find a gastroenterologist who understands the connection between pelvic floor dys-function and bowel disorders. It's okay to ask your pri-mary care physician if you'll feel comfortable with this new doctor and if he or she is knowledgeable in the area in which you are having problems.

I also want to endorse the obvious: Seek out rec-ommendations from friends or family members. If your friend sailed smoothly through her colonoscopy, or your sister has a gastroenterologist who has helped her man-age her Crohn's disease, you may want to try the same person. Word of mouth is very powerful, and I can tell you that I get a lot of new patients through my old pa-tients' recommendations. If you know someone who is a nurse or physician, even better. He or she may have a connection or know someone who had a good experi-ence with a particular gastroenterologist. You can also call the gastroenterology department at a large hospital near you and ask them to make a referral.

Another excellent referral resource is the Amer-ican Gastroenterological Association. The AGA can provide you with the names of board-certified gastro-enterologists in your area. Check out their website at www.gastro.org.

Most important, trust your gut. On your first visit, you can get a general sense of how comfortable you are with this new physician. Your instincts are key in decid-ing if he or she is open to discussing your GI problems. And you can get a sense as to whether your doctor is up to date on women's GI health issues. Finally, and prob-ably most important, *communicate* with your physician.

This is a two-way street. I'm no mind reader. If I do something that's uncomfortable to you or if you are embarrassed to discuss something, *tell me*. It certainly isn't my intention to hurt you during an examination or to make you ill at ease.

PREPARING FOR YOUR FIRST VISIT

I recently saw a woman named Kerri for the first time. When I asked her to describe her abdominal pain, she gave me the vague response "It hurts like hell." She couldn't recall how often she had the pain or whether it was triggered by any particular foods. She told me she was on a pain medication for her arthritis, but she didn't remember the name. I had to tell Kerri that she was leaving me pretty much in the dark in terms of making a diagnosis.

Yes, your history is an incredibly important tool to help your doctor figure out what's wrong with you. As a doctor, I'm only as good as what you give me. I can't read your mind or plug myself into your GI tract to feel what you're feeling. You need to go to your doctor prepared to tell a story: the story of your gastrointestinal problems. If your symptoms began in your childhood, that's where your story should begin. If they began a month ago, begin there. Here's how to be an accurate storyteller:

- **Be as specific as possible when describing your symptoms.** Write down what it feels like when you're actually experiencing the symptoms. Use specific adjectives like burning, churning, aching, stabbing,

QUESTIONS TO ASK YOURSELF

1. What is the main problem taking me to the doctor? (Add any descriptors here that might be helpful.) _____

2. When and how often does this symptom bother me? _____

3. What brings it on (such as eating, fasting, positions, stress, bowel movements, etc.)? _____

4. What seems to make it worse? _____

5. What seems to make it better? _____

6. How long does it last? _____

7. What do I do to manage the problem? _____

8. Do I have any other symptoms (such as vomiting, abdominal pain, diarrhea, coughing, difficulty breathing, shortness of breath, or anything else)?

QUESTIONS YOU MAY WANT TO ASK THE DOCTOR

1. Can you tell me some of the possible diagnoses that may be causing my problem? _____

2. Do I need any medical tests to rule anything out or to pinpoint a diagnosis? _____

3. What should I do in the meantime to manage my symptoms while we're doing tests to determine a diagnosis? _____

4. If you're prescribing a medication, how does it work, and what if any are the side effects? _____

dull but always there. What makes the pain better? What makes it worse? Is it sharp? Is it dull? What side is it on? Be prepared to answer these questions.

- **Bring a list of questions that you want answered.** Think about what kinds of things you want to discuss with your doctor. Then write them down and bring the list to your appointment so you don't forget to ask them.

- **Bring a simple food and symptom diary.** I recommend that you keep track of your diet and symptoms on your calendar. For instance, if you had an attack of abdominal pain on a particular day, write down an adjective for what the pain felt like, how long it lasted, and when it happened. If you're constipated, make an *X* on your calendar. Doctors don't need paragraphs and paragraphs of information—just a sentence or two to describe how you were feeling that day. If you're computer savvy, keep the information in your Palm Pilot.

- **Bring along all the medications, herbal remedies, and vitamin/mineral supplements that you're currently taking.** Your doctor will want to see any prescription medications that you take, regardless of whether they're for your GI problems. I sometimes see patients who bring in a small tote bags filled with medications. Often they have some alleviation of their digestive disturbances once we whittle down the number of medications they use. Virtually all drugs can have digestive side effects, so my feeling is the fewer the better—unless you need a particular medication for a life-threatening condition like

If you suffer from abdominal pain, knowing where it occurs can help you pinpoint what may be causing the problem. This diagram can't replace a proper diagnosis from your doctor, but it can point to what chapter or chapters of this book you may want to read before your doctor's appointment. For instance, if you have right upper quadrant pain, you may want to read the chapters on gallbladder disease and reflux to familiarize yourself with these conditions. Your doctor will also want to know the location of your pain as precisely as possible.

If you have abdominal pain, providing a complete medical history to your doctor is the most important part of your evaluation. Your doctor will likely ask you about the following things:

- Character/intensity of the pain: You'll be asked to describe your pain (burning, gnawing, aching, tearing, crampy, boring, agonizing) and where it stands on a scale of 0 to 10, 0 being no pain and 10 the worst pain you've ever experienced.
- Location: Is it in a specific quadrant? Is it diffuse or localized? Does it radiate anywhere else, like to your back or flank?
- Chronology: How quickly does it come on? Has it progressed? Does it come and go, or is it constant? Has it been present for hours, days, weeks, months, or years?
- Aggravating and alleviating factors: What makes it better and worse—eating, bowel movements, position, stress, types of foods, medications, and so on?
- Associated symptoms: Is your pain associated with diarrhea, fever, vomiting, back pain, or some other symptom?
- Past medical history: Could your other medical problems shed some light on the cause of this problem?
- Family and social history: Does your family tree reveal any

clues as to your diagnosis? Are there any inherited diseases in your family? Do any of your family members have illnesses that put you at risk for certain disorders? Do your occupation, travel history, or social habits provide any clues?

Right Upper Quadrant: Pain in this area may indicate problems with the gallbladder, bile duct, or liver. Pain from gastritis (stomach inflammation), ulcers, reflux, or pancreatitis occurs just below the breastbone.

Right Lower Quadrant: The small bowel meets the large bowel in the lower right quadrant. Pain in this area may indicate appendicitis or Crohn's disease. Pain in either lower quadrant may be due to non-GI conditions like pelvic inflammatory disease, uterine fibroids, menstrual cramps, ovarian cysts or tumors, hernias, or ectopic pregnancy.

Left Upper Quadrant: Pain in this area can mean the involvement of the stomach, spleen, or colon. Constipation and/or irritable bowel syndrome can cause pain in this area. Pain around the navel can result from a partial obstruction in the small intestine from adhesions, pancreatitis, or gastroenteritis.

Left Lower Quadrant: Pain in this area usually involves the colon. Gas and constipation are common causes, followed by colitis or diverticulitis. Irritable bowel syndrome can cause pain in either lower quadrant but is more common on the left.

heart disease or diabetes. Your doctor will probably also ask you what form of birth control you're using and whether you take any nutritional supplements. I'm often shown one herbal product or another and asked whether it can cause any side effects. If I don't know, I'm honest with my patients. But I can usually find something about the product on the Internet.

- **Consider bringing a support person.** If you're particularly nervous about seeing a gastroenterologist or are embarrassed about telling your symptoms to a stranger, you may want to bring a loved one to your appointment. Your mom, sister, spouse, or daughter may be able to describe your symptoms more fully than you can if you're feeling uncomfortable. They can also take notes, so you can review what the doctor discussed with you after the conversation.

TRACKING YOUR GI PROBLEM

I often ask my patients to keep a symptom diary. As I've mentioned, such a diary provides valuable information to aid the doctor in diagnosing your problem. It also gives doctors an objective way to track how well various therapies are working. Tables are the easiest way to look at your problem over time. I prefer a table over a diary with page after page of information (which I'm not likely to read). The table on page 265 is only a sample. Once your physician has narrowed down the problem, he or she may have other data that he or she wants you to record.

THE GET-TO-KNOW-YOU CHAT

Now that you're prepared for your first appointment, here's what to expect on your first visit. This is, of course, based on how I conduct most of my first appointments. Gastroenterologists, like all doctors, vary in how they conduct an initial exam. Even in my clinic the level and intensity of questioning and physical examination varies based upon the severity or complexity of the patient's problem. For my patients I generally choose to do a full physical examination that includes an evaluation of all the major organ systems as well as the gastrointestinal system. Not all gastroenterologists do this, however, which doesn't mean they're giving subpar treatment. If you are concerned about a potential problem that your doctor may be missing, speak up

DATE AND TIME						
When did the pain start?						
Where is it located, and what does it feel like?						
What were you doing when it started?						
What did you eat in the 3 hours before?						
How did you manage the pain?						
Other?						

and ask if he or she is going to evaluate you for this problem.

If you are a patient coming to see me for the first time, you will first meet my nurse, Beth. She will escort you from the waiting area into a clinic room. There she will ask your height, then check your weight, blood pressure, pulse, and temperature. She will calculate your BMI. She will ask you about the main problem that brought you to the clinic today. She'll write down a list of your medications and ask about any medication allergies. She may ask you about your past medical history, occupation, habits, and family history. My secretary, Susan, will work very hard to get your medical records from your referring physician. I will look these over before meeting you and also review any lab or test results sent to me.

In the clinic room there is a desk with two chairs and an examining table. I generally like to meet my patients while they are fully dressed, and we sit at the desk to discuss their GI condition. I like to do this before you put on a gown because I feel we're on a more equal footing. After all, you're meeting me for the first time. I need to break the ice and develop a rapport with you before I can expect you to put your full trust in me. I may begin by asking you a few questions about what you do, how many kids you have, and whether you feel satisfied with the way your life is going (aside from your medical problems).

We'll spend the majority of the time focusing on the problem that brought you to the clinic. I usually launch into a detailed list of questions to get a complete medical history. What kinds of symptoms do you have? What makes them better? What makes them worse?

MEDICAL RECORDS, PLEASE

If you are being referred to a specialist, ask your primary care physician to fax over any pertinent test results or medical records. If you have old medical records from your childhood, for example, bring them along. If you have a family tree that details the people in your family and what diseases they've died from (like colon cancer), that's important. If you've had important X-rays and your doctor is getting a gastroenterologist's opinion about a mass in your pancreas or the stricture in your esophagus, try to bring the original X-rays with you. A picture is worth a thousand words and is much more valuable than a copy of the report.

Getting your X-rays really is an easy process. Most hospitals will allow you to check out your X-ray jacket or will give you copies of pertinent X-rays provided that you tell them who will be getting them. I generally give the X-rays back to my patients at the end of the clinic visit, but if I need to look at them with our radiologists, I'll keep them for a bit and send them back after I've finished with them.

If your primary care physician has been treating your GI problem up until now, you should get a copy of your chart so your gastroenterologist can see which medications have been prescribed and how well they worked for you. That way you won't have to start from scratch with a trial and error of different medications.

Did you have similar symptoms as a child? I'll want to know what your typical day is like: how many hours of sleep you get a night; whether you're stressed; and whether you eat three meals a day or just grab food on the run. I'll also want to know when your symptoms are more likely to occur, how long they last, and what, if anything, brings relief. If you have bowel problems, I'll ask you if you ever have a bowel movement in the middle of the night or whether you strain a lot when you have a bowel movement. I will generally review your past medical history and family history as well. We may discuss your medications or your habits or hobbies. I nearly always ask about diet and exercise. If you tell me you're watching your weight, I may ask if you've recently switched to fat-free or sugar-free snack foods. For instance, eating a lot of fat-free potato chips that contain olestra can lead to stool leakage and diarrhea. Sucking on sugar-free candies containing sorbitol can cause excess gas. These are just a few of the many questions that you'll be asked.

If you list a litany of symptoms that are troubling you, I may ask: If there is one thing you would like us to fix today, what would that be? This will help you focus on the primary problem. I also always ask: What are you afraid it is? I find that when I deal with my patients' fears head-on, I can alleviate a lot of anxiety. Cancer is usually the biggest fear, but often it is the least likely scenario. Finally, I will likely ask you about other symptoms you may be having, like fever, weight loss, chest pain, cough, urinary difficulties, and so on. In most cases, I will also ask about your gynecological history. How old were you when you started your periods? Do you have difficult periods? Are your periods regular? How were your pregnancies? Did you have vaginal deliveries or C-sections? Did you require an episiotomy or have a tear? Have you gone through menopause?

When? Did you have any associated symptoms like hot flashes, heat intolerance, or migraines?

THE PHYSICAL EXAM

After I have an adequate medical history, we'll move on to the physical exam. I'll ask you to change into a gown while I leave the room. With most new patients, I prefer to do a full physical exam. As it is important for me to understand your entire medical history, I feel it is equally important that I examine more than just your abdomen. I will look at your eyes and into your mouth. I will evaluate your teeth. I will likely palpate your thyroid and listen to your heart and lungs. I will examine your back and skin and check for swelling in your joints and ankles.

I will spend the majority of the examination evaluating your abdomen. I will start by looking for changes in the abdominal wall or scars from previous surgery. Next, I will listen to your abdomen with a stethoscope to evaluate your bowel sounds and to see if there are any extra sounds, like bruits—which sound like pulses of rushing water—that may signify narrowing of the arteries. I will then percuss your abdomen, literally tapping over different areas with my fingers. By so doing, I can get a sense of the size of your liver and spleen. In addition, I can tell if you have excess gas or fluid in your abdomen.

I'll then palpate your abdomen. If abdominal pain is one of your symptoms, I'll have you literally show me with your fingers how big the pain is and where it is located. I'll try to stay away from that area initially and

palpate other areas first. It's amazing what gastroenterologists can feel just by probing the abdomen. We
feel for masses or gas distension. We can feel hardened
stool, enlargement in different lobes of the liver, or even
an inflamed area of the intestine that could be indicative of Crohn's disease.

If your symptoms include rectal bleeding or significant constipation, I may do a thorough examination of
your perineum, the area around your labia and anus. I
will look for skin changes, inflammation, and evidence
of sexually transmitted disease like vaginal or anal
warts. I will specifically look at the perineal bar, the area
between the posterior part of the vagina and the ante-
rior part of the rectum. I'll look for evidence of bulging
that may indicate a rectocele (a small pouch that protrudes from the rectum into the cavity of the vagina) or
of significant pelvic floor dysfunction. I'll look for surgical scars from an episiotomy or evidence of tears
from a prior vaginal delivery.

At this point, I may also perform a rectal exam.
Here I will take a gloved, lubricated finger and insert it
into your rectum to evaluate for rectoceles, hemorrhoids, and anal fissures. With my finger in your rectum, I will ask you to squeeze, so I can check your anal
sphincter tone. I'll then ask you to bear down as if you
were having a bowel movement, so I can see if your
pelvic floor relaxes properly. I'll check for hidden blood
by doing a fecal occult blood test. Here I will take a
sample of stool and smear it onto a special card. We use
a chemical solution to "develop" the test, which tells us
if blood is present in the stool. I know that having a rectal exam may be the thing you most want to avoid dur-

ing a physical, so I try to get it over with quickly to keep embarrassment and discomfort to a minimum.

THE WRAP-UP

After the exam I'll leave the room again to let you get dressed and use the restroom if necessary. We'll then sit again at the desk to discuss my thoughts about your condition and our plan of action. I'll tell you about the treatment plan that I've outlined—if there is one—and what, if any, additional GI tests you need. I will try to write everything down so you will have a copy of the plan to take home with you.

My plan will be very specific. Besides detailing prescriptions for medications, it may outline an exercise regimen and make dietary recommendations. I might say, "Exercise (bike, walk, swim, do aerobics) for 20 to 30 minutes, 2 to 3 times a week."

I once heard former surgeon general David Satcher speak about his *Healthy People 2010* report. He said that physicians need to make diet and exercise as important to patients as medications. He suggested writing prescriptions for exercise, and I've taken that advice. I feel strongly that healthy living will lead to a healthier GI tract. I may write you a specific prescription to exercise, or I may even write you a referral for an exercise facility. I may write a referral for a nutrition counseling session with our staff nutritionist to map out your eating plan, because if you're out of shape, overweight, and living on junk food, I'm not going to be able to cure your GI problems no matter how many prescriptions I write.

My nurse, Beth, usually comes in for the wrap-up. After I've given you the overall picture of the plan, she furnishes you with the nitty-gritty. She will detail you on the blood work we might be checking. She'll tell you how to get to the lab. She'll tell you all about your endoscopy procedure if one is required: how to prepare for it, where to go to have it done, and when to expect the results. If we've come up with a diagnosis, she'll provide information in the form of pamphlets or available websites. If we plan to try a medication, she'll tell you about it and will give you drug information sheets about the benefits and possible side effects you might look for. She'll also tell you about how we'll follow up with you.

POSSIBLE BLOOD TESTS

We may take some blood to see if you have any underlying conditions that could be related to your GI symptoms. The results of these blood tests may take a few hours or a few weeks to come back. I may order a test to check your level of thyroid hormone, since an underactive thyroid can cause constipation, whereas an overactive thyroid can cause diarrhea. I may check your liver enzymes; this test can screen for a whole array of liver diseases, from hepatitis to fatty liver disease. If you're underweight or experiencing diarrhea, I may check for a nutritional deficiency like a low magnesium level or a vitamin D or B deficiency. I'll do a blood count, since an elevated white blood cell count may suggest an infection or inflammatory process; low levels of red blood cells tell me that you are anemic, which may indicate that you have an iron or other vitamin deficiency or bleeding in your GI tract.

Sometimes patients need to have an additional test like a colonoscopy, upper endoscopy, ultrasound, or barium X-ray to pinpoint the problem or at least rule out ulcer, colitis, or cancer. I want to emphasize that these tests aren't always necessary for making a diagnosis. I frequently can diagnose reflux, for instance, based on symptoms alone.

DIAGNOSIS OR NOT?

I wish I could tell you that after reviewing your medical history and conducting a thorough physical, your gastroenterologist will immediately be able to make a firm diagnosis. Unfortunately, that's not usually the case. If you're a reader of mystery novels, you know that a good detective puts together all the clues and tests a few theories before coming up with the solution. At the end of your first visit I will usually tell you what I suspect is going on, but until I have the results from the medical tests, I can't be 100 percent certain.

When it comes to treatment, solving your problem may take more than just a scribble on my prescription pad. As we'll discuss in the next chapters of the book, treatments for gastroesophageal reflux, irritable bowel syndrome, or inflammatory bowel disease—some of the most common conditions I see in my practice—often require a combination of medicine, lifestyle changes, and occasionally alternative therapy. I work together with my patients to find the best treatment plan to relieve their symptoms.

Your primary care physician and I will work together to improve your GI health. I can't emphasize enough how vital it is for you to have good communication with your doctor. If a particular medication isn't working to relieve your constipation, please tell me. We may consider an alternative treatment or a medication that works in a completely different way.

Establishing a strong, trusting relationship with your doctor is the key to getting the appropriate diagnosis. It will also help you navigate your way through the medical tests that you may need to pinpoint your diagnosis. In the chapters that follow, I will give details about the specific tests appropriate for each condition.

GERD—EFFECTIVE MANAGEMENT FOR A LIFELONG PROBLEM

IN PART II I TALKED ABOUT THE LINE that's drawn between a benign problem that causes you to have symptoms once in a while and a more serious medical condition that requires you to see a doctor for treatment. When it comes to heartburn, that line is a little fuzzy. For most Americans, heartburn is an occasional problem, a nuisance condition with no long-term consequences. But if you're prone to frequent or severe heartburn, you probably have a condition called gastroesophageal reflux disease (GERD). This just means that you get heartburn frequently enough for it to interfere with the quality of your life.

Truth is, gastroenterologists refer to all cases of reflux and heartburn as GERD, but for the purposes of this book, I will use the term GERD only when referring to a chronic problem that bothers you on a weekly or even daily basis. As I explained in Chapter 4, heartburn occurs due to a relaxed or weakened valve at the end of the esophagus, called the lower esophageal sphincter

(LES). An occasional bout of heartburn doesn't send most people running to the doctor. Heartburn that occurs after every meal, however, often does.

Nearly everyone experiences heartburn at some time or another. But more than 60 million American adults experience heartburn or GERD on a regular basis, at least once a month. About 25 million adults experience symptoms every day. In the United States, we spend billions of dollars a year on medications to manage heartburn associated with GERD. And GERD's impact isn't only on direct medical costs. The indirect costs associated with GERD include decreased quality of life, missed work days, and decreased productivity at work. If not managed properly, GERD can make you feel miserable, make it harder for you to function up to your full potential, and significantly decrease the quality of your life.

In most cases, I can assure my patients that their GERD has no long-term damaging health effects. But in some people GERD has more significant ramifications, like damage to the esophagus. Exposing sensitive tissue in the esophagus to stomach acid and pepsin can lead to esophagitis (inflammation), ulcers (erosions), and scarring (a stricture). People with severe GERD may have trouble swallowing (especially solid foods) and may even have food get stuck in the esophagus or be forced to regurgitate the food. They may also have bleeding from the inflammation and ulcers.

For unknown reasons, GERD is on the rise in women. In the 1970s male GERD sufferers outnumbered females by three to one. Now the number of female and male GERD sufferers is about equal. (Men, though, are two to three times more likely to have esophageal damage associated with their GERD and are ten times more likely to have a condition called Barrett's esophagus, which increases the risk of esophageal cancer.) This recent rise in GERD in women may be the result of a corresponding rise in obesity. Or it may be due to our fast-food lifestyles or to the fact that, juggling career and families, we have less time than ever before to take care of ourselves.

If you've been suffering from chronic heartburn for several months, your doctor will probably want to rule out certain gastrointestinal conditions. GERD is the most likely culprit, but you may have an ulcer or nonulcer dyspepsia, both of which I'll discuss in the next chapter. Your doctor may want to perform certain tests to help pinpoint your diagnosis or to look for any damage caused by reflux.

I should warn you, though, that finding an exact diagnosis for an upper GI problem can be tricky. With all the current TV commercials for acid-blockers, you might think that all heartburn woes are due to reflux. Chrissy, a patient of mine, assumed that a benign case of heartburn was the cause of her feeling nauseated after every meal. She tried all kinds of antacids and over-the-counter acid-blockers and reduced her intake of fatty foods and alcohol, but she got no relief. When I first saw her, she was convinced she had acid reflux. I did an upper endoscopy, which came back normal, so I assumed Chrissy probably did have reflux, since her only symptom was nausea. I prescribed a stronger acid-blocker, hoping that would do the trick. A few weeks later Chrissy came back to my clinic complaining that her symptoms were much stronger than before. When I examined her, I realized at once that she had more than nausea. She had a lot of abdominal discomfort on her right side. I immediately suspected gallbladder disease, and an ultrasound did indeed reveal gallstones. Chrissy had her gallbladder removed through surgery, and her symptoms cleared up immediately afterward.

I'm not saying that your heartburn symptoms aren't caused by GERD, but I don't want you to do any self-diagnosing. If you have a chronic problem with heartburn and other reflux symptoms, I urge you to get evaluated by your doctor.

WHAT IS GERD, AND WHY DO I HAVE IT?

GERD is a malfunction that occurs in a valve that separates your esophagus from your stomach. When you eat, food travels from your mouth down the esophagus to your stomach. At the end of the esophagus, it passes through a one-way valve called the lower esophageal sphincter (LES), the opening to your stomach. Normally, the LES opens just a few seconds after you swallow. It allows food to enter the stomach then shuts quickly. But sometimes it becomes so weakened that it stays open all the time, which causes severe GERD. Most of the time, though, the LES just opens too frequently (even in the absence of swallowing), causing acid and stomach contents to backwash, irritating the esophagus.

No one knows what causes the LES to malfunction; it could be aging or genetics. Some researchers have shown that reflux runs in families. Lifestyle also plays a big role: eating too much food or certain kinds of foods, being overweight, smoking, wearing tight-fitting clothes, taking certain medications, and so on. The severity of your heartburn depends on the amount of food you backwash and how much acid is mixed in, which varies from person to person. Some people have a problem of delayed stomach emptying, which causes more food to backwash since it stays in the stomach longer. Others may produce too much pepsin (a stomach enzyme) or too much stomach acid, both of which can backwash and irritate the lower esophagus.

Research has shown that GERD often goes hand in hand with *hiatal hernia*. A hiatal hernia occurs when the upper part of the stomach moves from its normal place in the abdominal cavity up into the chest through a widened opening in the diaphragm. The diaphragm, the muscle separating the abdominal organs from the chest, normally has an opening just wide enough for the esophagus to pass through. Without the support of the diaphragm, the LES is more likely to relax and cause heartburn symptoms. Many GERD sufferers have a hiatal hernia, and its size directly corresponds to the severity of symptoms. Studies show that a hiatal hernia functions like a pocket or a little reservoir that can collect acidic gastric juice. These contents can more easily backwash into the esophagus, causing reflux. Hiatal hernias can occur from the increased pressure caused by severe coughing, vomiting, straining to defecate, or sudden physical exertion. You're more likely to develop the condition if you're pregnant or overweight. It can also occur simply from aging. Many otherwise healthy

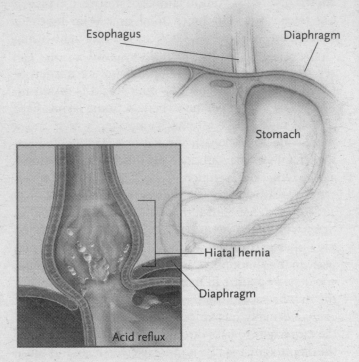

The stomach normally rests below the diaphragm. If it protrudes above the diaphragm, in what is known as a hiatal hernia, the LES is more likely to relax, resulting in acid reflux.

women over age fifty develop hiatal hernias. And guess what? As you age, your risk of developing GERD also increases.

Midlife spread may be partly to blame—in fact, I think it plays a major role. Consider this: The average woman gains about a pound a year from age twenty-five onward. This means by your mid-forties, you could be sporting twenty extra pounds. What's more, as you get older, your body fat tends to shift from your hips and thighs to your belly. Excess belly fat may increase pressure on your LES, increasing reflux episodes and putting you at greater risk of developing a hiatal hernia. (The rise in obesity may also be responsible for the increase in GERD in children. Childhood obesity in the United States has reached epidemic proportions, and today gastroenterologists prescribe more reflux medications for childhood GERD than ever before.)

Beyond treating GERD symptoms, most hiatal hernias don't require treatment. On rare occasions, your doctor may suggest surgical repair of a complicated hiatal hernia if you're experiencing vomiting or weight loss or if you have a hernia so large that food doesn't digest well but sits for long periods of time, causing ulceration and/or bleeding.

GERD AND PREGNANCY

Pregnancy is the number-one reason women develop GERD. Up to 80 percent of pregnant women experience heartburn at one time or another. Some, though, develop full-blown GERD, suffering from heartburn and reflux on a daily basis. Increased levels of progesterone and/or estrogen can cause a relaxation of the LES, causing it to open more frequently. Progesterone can cause delayed stomach emptying, which keeps food in your stomach longer, increasing the odds of reflux. What's more, the growing uterus and baby push all of your abdominal organs upward, making it easier for stomach contents to backwash. All of these things set the stage for chronic heartburn that can begin in your first trimester and last throughout your pregnancy. The good news is that 98 percent of pregnant women who have GERD report that their symptoms resolve immediately after delivery, according to research published in the *American Journal of Gastroenterology.*

Occasionally pregnant women are referred to me by their obstetricians. One woman, Michelle, came to our clinic almost weekly during the last two trimesters of her pregnancy because she had such severe reflux. Once she delivered her baby, she suddenly had no more heartburn, and the only time we saw her again was when she stopped by to introduce us to the fruit of her labor!

Since GERD during pregnancy is usually temporary, most pregnant women and their health care providers take a conservative approach to the management of symptoms. In general, diagnostic tests aren't necessary unless you have complications of reflux, like difficulty swallowing or bleeding. Treatment is conservative as well. Surgery is pretty much out of the question. Lying on your left side and raising the head of your bed can help you avoid nighttime heartburn. You can also try eating smaller, more frequent meals and avoiding certain heartburn foods. (See my heartburn prevention tips for pregnancy in Chapter 2.) You should also discuss with your health care provider which medications you can safely take during pregnancy. My colleague Kathie Hullfish, M.D., an obstetrician-gynecologist at the University of Virginia Hospital, says pregnant women can safely take an over-the-counter antacid like Tums or Maalox to relieve heartburn. An acid-blocker, like Tagamet-HB, Zantac-75, Pepcid AC, or Axid, can be used as a second line of therapy if the antacid isn't working, but check with your doctor before taking an over-the-counter formulation. If you're still having severe GERD symptoms, your physician may give you a prescription-strength acid-blocker that is safe to take during pregnancy.

GERD AND OTHER DISEASES

Sometimes GERD is associated with other health conditions. Women who suffer from the eating disorder *bulimia nervosa* often experience reflux symptoms from recurrent self-induced vomiting. About one-third of women who engage in this behavior have severe GERD that causes esophageal inflammation and erosions. On more than one occasion I've uncovered hidden bulimia in young women who come to me for GERD symptoms. Because these young women were of normal weight, no one suspected that they had an eating disorder. Bulimia victims often aren't underweight since they tend to binge on thousands of calories and then induce vomiting afterward.

GERD can also be associated with diabetes. Advanced diabetes can cause damage to the nerves of the intestinal tract, which results in the slowing of food moving out of the stomach. This delayed stomach emptying, known as *gastroparesis,* can result in reflux. Controlling blood sugar and treatment with prokinetic medications that increase stomach motility can help improve gastroparesis.

A whopping 70 to 90 percent of women who are afflicted with the nervous system disorder *scleroderma* develop GERD as a result of having the disease. This disorder, which causes a hardening and thickening of the skin, most commonly strikes Caucasian women ages forty to fifty. With advanced scleroderma the smooth muscle (which controls the coordinated peristalsis of the esophagus) and the LES are damaged. With an inability to clear food from the esophagus and a malfunction of the LES, esophageal reflux occurs unabated and often causes complications such as stricture formation or Barrett's esophagus.

Several years ago a patient named Jean was referred to me for help with her reflux symptoms. Jean had been diagnosed with scleroderma and for several years had been bothered by thick, taut skin over her fingers and face; dry eyes and mouth; and significant cold intolerance at her fingertips. Six months before she came to me she developed worsening heartburn and was treated with the acid-blocker Zantac. Jean tried altering her diet and raising the head of her bed, which helped her somewhat. Still, every time she drank a glass of water or juice and bent over to tie her shoe or to do some gardening, she would regurgitate a mouthful of hot liquid.

I decided to perform an endoscopy and found that Jean had a completely lax LES, with severe esophageal ulcers from continued reflux. I started her on a prescription-strength ulcer medication, which brought her the relief she sought and enabled her esophagus to heal. More recently Jean's esophageal motility and reflux have worsened, and she has had frequent episodes of aspiration pneumonia combined with chronic hoarseness and cough. I treated Jean with prokinetic agents to help her motility and with higher doses of acid-suppressing medications, with good results.

SYMPTOMS OF GERD:
THE NORMAL AND THE UNUSUAL

The hallmark symptoms of GERD are heartburn and regurgitation. *Heartburn* is that burning feeling that generally starts in the middle to upper abdomen—sometimes referred to as the *solar plexus*—and moves up into the chest behind the *sternum* (breastbone). Heartburn is most likely to occur after meals, when stomach acid levels rise. *Regurgitation* is the spontaneous return of gastric contents into the esophagus or above. Some people describe an acid or vomit taste in the back of their mouth, while others describe it as just "hot liquid" in their throat. You could also have reflux even if you don't have these classic symptoms. Other symptoms of reflux include:

- hoarseness
- chronic cough (Reflux can irritate the upper respiratory tract and trigger the cough reflex.)
- constantly clearing the voice
- bad breath
- thinning front teeth (Acid can strip away dental enamel in back of front teeth.)
- feeling that something is caught in the back of the throat (Generally, people point to the sternal notch, just at the base of the neck.)
- repeated bouts of pneumonia
- asthma (GERD strikes up to 80 percent of asthma patients, often triggering wheezing instead of heartburn as acid in the lower esophagus results in constriction of the bronchial passages in the lungs.)

- repeated bouts of bronchitis
- atypical chest pain (where heart disease has been ruled out)

Note: Hoarseness, throat clearing, and bad breath can be caused by the direct irritation of the throat by acid

IS YOUR SEX LIFE SUFFERING?

Severe heartburn symptoms can spring up at the most inconvenient times—like right in the middle of sexual intercourse. In a provocative study conducted by Scottish researchers, 77 out of 100 women with GERD reported that they experienced heartburn during intercourse. This study suggests that the problem is quite common. So if you suffer from heartburn during sex, don't be afraid to discuss it with your doctor.

No one really knows why sex brings on heartburn. One theory is that a hormonal release during orgasm causes a weakening of the LES. Other experts think the problem could be due to abdominal pressure that results from quick movements when you're lying prone. It could also be a simple problem of positioning. Lying flat on your back with your hips tilted upward could result in a gravitational flow of acid back up your esophagus. In fact, that was the theory that the Scottish researchers held. They recommended switching from a missionary position (with the woman on the bottom) to a female-superior position (with the woman on top). This switch alleviated reflux in 61 of the 77 women in their study who previously experienced symptoms during sex. Another option is to take an over-the-counter acid-blocker an hour or two before sex.

or pepsin in the backwash. Bronchitis or pneumonia can be caused when backwashed contents head back downward into the windpipe, instead of into the esophagus. Asthma and chronic cough can occur when a nerve reflex caused by the backwashing of food triggers a spasm in the windpipe or airway.

WARNING SYMPTOMS OF GERD

When heartburn is accompanied by one or more of the following symptoms, it may indicate a more severe case of GERD or a complication such as a stricture or esophageal cancer. They require a visit to your doctor for further evaluation—usually via an endoscopy to see if there's damage to the esophagus.

- difficulty swallowing
- food getting "stuck" in your esophagus that takes a long time to travel downward or must be regurgitated back up
- blood in your stool
- vomiting blood
- unexplained weight loss

GETTING DIAGNOSED

Unlike other GI diseases, no single test can give a definite diagnosis of GERD in most patients. In many cases GERD can be diagnosed by a careful medical history alone, where the patient recounts a history of heartburn and regurgitation. Some physicians argue that the symptom pattern for GERD is the most specific of any

GI disorder. In many instances I believe that diagnostic testing is not necessary. If your symptoms are classic and if you respond to reflux medications, you probably don't need to have a "test" to make the diagnosis. However, I do want to stress that if you have daily heartburn requiring continuous medication, or if you have warning symptoms of GERD, you probably need a diagnostic workup that includes one or more medical tests. If your diagnosis is in question, your doctor will probably suggest medical testing.

Of course, your first line of action will be a medical exam in which you describe your symptoms to your doctor. The more specific you can be about your symptoms, the better. In Chapter 8, I recommended keeping a symptom journal for a week before your doctor visit. Bring this journal with you to your appointment. Your doctor will ask you about your lifestyle habits (eating, drinking, smoking, and so on) and will perform a physical exam. Based on your medical history and the results of your physical exam, your doctor will be able to make a diagnosis. Medical tests can help confirm the diagnosis, determine the severity of your GERD, and detect the presence of any damage caused by the condition.

Several diagnostic tests can be used to evaluate GERD. You should know that there is no one gold standard test to diagnose GERD. All of these tests have their benefits and drawbacks.

Esophageal Endoscopy

This test involves inserting a small lighted tube into your upper GI tract. This flexible camera explores the lining of your mouth down into your esophagus, stomach, and the first part of your small intestine. The probe sends video images to a monitor, which allows your doctor to see problems as it passes through. These images will reveal specific details of your upper GI anatomy (such as the presence of a hiatal hernia) and will show irritated areas, ulcers, or inflammatory changes in your esophagus caused by the reflux. If needed, your doctor may snip off a tiny sample of tissue during the endoscopy to do a biopsy. This can be sent to a pathology department to be more closely analyzed under a microscope.

Your doctor may recommend endoscopy if you have a long history of symptoms, haven't received relief from standard medical treatment for GERD, or have atypical symptoms or warning symptoms. If you're over fifty, you may also be told you need an endoscopy since the risk of Barrett's esophagus (see page 293) is higher in people over fifty. Most gastroenterologists, myself included, believe that if a diagnostic test is warranted for GERD, the first step should be endoscopy. Endoscopy yields the most information and can help determine the severity of the disease, which can make a big difference in the long-term management of GERD.

Before your test, you may be given a sedative and your throat may be sprayed with an anesthetic, making it easier to swallow the probe. You shouldn't eat or drink anything for six to eight hours before the test. The day after the test, you may have a slight sore throat.

Limitations: Probably the biggest drawback of endoscopy is that it is invasive. In my experience, however, it causes no pain in the majority of patients. On average, it takes 10 to 15 minutes to perform. Endoscopy can't be counted on to "diagnose" GERD since 30 to 70 percent of GERD sufferers have a normal endoscopy. These patients have *nonerosive GERD*, meaning that the acid reflux causes symptoms but no noticeable damage to the esophageal lining. In addition, while endoscopy primarily shows anatomic abnormalities, it does not actually show the function of the LES.

pH Monitoring Test

Your doctor may want to specifically measure the number of times per day that you experience acid reflux by testing the pH or acid level of your esophagus. This is done by placing an extremely thin acid-measuring probe through your nasal passage into your esophagus for up to twenty-four hours. Since the probe is so thin, most patients feel little discomfort when the probe is in place. A liquid anesthetic is used to numb your nasal passages, so you feel no pain during the placement of the probe.

You keep the probe in place for a day while you follow your normal dietary and lifestyle routines. Every time you feel heartburn, indigestion, or an atypical symptom such as wheezing, cough, or chest pain, you click a button and record your symptoms in a diary. The test will tell you whether your symptoms correlate with increased acid backwash. For the duration of this test, you need to avoid acid-inhibiting medications, like acid-blockers and antacids, since they can affect the accuracy of the test. This test works best to correlate symptoms with acid reflux events and can be extremely useful if you have atypical reflux symptoms. The monitoring test can also be helpful in determining whether a medical treatment is working to prevent acid backwash. (If it is, your doctor may ask you to have the test while taking your acid-blocking medications.)

Ambulatory pH monitoring is the closest thing we have to a gold standard test to diagnose GERD. Your doctor may recommend having this test before you have surgery for your reflux to confirm that your symptoms really are caused by reflux and that surgery will help. In a new advance, a small pH monitoring sensor is placed on the inside lining of the patient's esophagus at the time of endoscopy, instead of the probe hanging out of their nose (an embarrassing thing to have showing for a day). If you need this monitoring test, ask your doctor about this new technique.

Limitations: The endoscopy is invasive, and the nose-monitoring probe can be uncomfortable and inconvenient for people to wear. Patients must be cooperative and capable of clicking a button at the onset of symptoms and completing the symptom diary. For the most part, this is not a first-line test—physicians generally recommend its use to confirm a more difficult diagnosis and specifically to correlate atypical symptoms to reflux events.

Upper GI Series

This test is a series of X-ray films to study the esophagus, stomach, and small intestine. As you swallow a barium milk shake, X-rays monitor the barium dye while it travels to your stomach, capturing any reflux action on film. The X-rays may also show whether you have a hiatal hernia. You should not eat or drink anything for six to eight hours before having this brief, painless test.

Limitations: Although this test is the simplest and least invasive, it is also the least reliable in terms of diagnosing reflux or its complications. Reflux events during this test don't necessarily indicate GERD. Also, because the barium only coats the lining of the GI tract, subtle findings (like Barrett's esophagus) may be missed. This test also does not allow physicians to biopsy the abnormal area, which they can do during endoscopy.

Esophageal Manometry

If your doctor suspects you may be a candidate for antireflux surgery, you may be given a more sophisticated test to measure the motility of your esophagus and the muscle tone of your LES. Esophageal manometry involves numbing your nose and throat with an anesthetic in order to pass a thin, lubricated tube down into your stomach. The tube device makes pressure measurements in the esophagus and stomach during and after wet and dry swallows. You're not allowed to eat or drink anything for 8 to 12 hours before the test, which takes about thirty minutes. You may have a slightly sore throat after the test.

Limitations: Esophageal manometry is seldom used as a first-line test for GERD sufferers because it is invasive. It may be important to surgeons prior to antireflux surgery, to ensure that esophageal motility is normal before the construction of a new LES (which is called a wrap). Additionally, this test may be useful for a small number of patients whose reflux is caused by a completely relaxed, permanently open LES.

FEAR OF GERD

When it comes to GERD, my patients' biggest fear is: Will it shorten my life span or cause long-term health effects? Many are also concerned about the cancer risk because of recent media reports of an increased risk of esophageal cancer in patients with GERD.

As I've discussed, in most cases GERD has no long-term damaging health effects. In very rare cases, however, esophageal damage can lead to a condition called *Barrett's esophagus,* which causes cellular changes in the lining of the esophagus. If the condition continues unchecked, it may, on rare occasions, lead to a type of esophageal cancer called *adenocarcinoma*. People who have Barrett's esophagus need to have a follow-up endoscopy to monitor for these cell changes. The good news is that Barrett's esophagus is rare, and it is even rarer in women than in men. Men with GERD, for some reason, are twice as likely to develop these cell changes and are more likely to suffer esophageal cancer in general than women. They're also more likely to have esophageal damage associated with GERD. One theory is that men naturally produce more stomach acid than women and may have higher amounts of acid in their backwash than women. This could be due to genetics, or possibly female hormones may provide some protective benefit.

I do see Barrett's esophagus on occasion in my female reflux patients. One such case is Maggie, a fifty-four-year-old insurance agent. Before she came to see me, Maggie had suffered from reflux symptoms for decades. She had tried several prescription medications and had cut out chocolate, caffeine, and alcohol but still couldn't find relief from her symptoms. Her family doctor sent her to me for an endoscopy to see if she had any esophageal damage associated with her reflux. On her first endoscopy I found that Maggie had Barrett's esophagus and several small ulcers in her esophagus.

When I reviewed the findings with her, Maggie was extremely afraid of her risk of esophageal cancer. I told her that our first priority was to aggressively treat her esophagitis and to monitor her esophagus for changes leading to cancer. Just like cervical cancer, esophageal cancer generally does not occur suddenly, I explained, but generally progresses through stages of mild, moderate, and then severe dysplasia (cell abnormalities) before turning to cancer. I told Maggie that she needed periodic endoscopies to check for dysplasia, just like she needed periodic Pap smears to check for cervical cancer. I also prescribed medications (discussed on pages 302–303), which helped alleviate Maggie's symptoms and esophageal damage. She has had periodic endoscopy for several years now and fortunately has had no evidence of dysplasia.

So let's say your doctor says you have GERD but your endoscopy is normal. There are no ulcers or erosions, and no Barrett's esophagus. You still have acid reflux, but your esophagus is impervious to the onslaught of acid backwash. If I were your doctor, I'd tell you to relax. You have an extremely low risk of esophageal cancer or long-term damage to your esophagus. You probably don't even need to come back for a repeat endoscopy—unless your symptoms change dramatically. A long-term study of several hundred patients with GERD studied for over twenty-five years suggests that the majority of people do not progress beyond the stage of their initial diagnosis. The only time you need to worry is if your symptoms change or if you develop some of the warning symptoms that I described earlier. In this case, you need to have further medical testing, like a repeat endoscopy, to determine if your GERD has progressed.

TV commercials for GERD medications would make you think that everyone with GERD symptoms has damage to their esophagus. *This is simply not true.* Many—perhaps even most—GERD sufferers have symptoms that aren't life-threatening, even if they are a nuisance.

If you have no damage to your esophagus, you'll still have to deal with symptoms that are keeping you up at night, ruining your nights out on the town, or throwing a wrench in your sex life. If you fall in this category, I'm going to push you to make lifestyle modifications, because they can make a difference and even decrease your need for medication over time.

STEP 1: LEAD A GERD-HEALTHY LIFESTYLE

For most patients, GERD is a chronic disorder. It's something they manage, not cure. Like heart disease or diabetes, you *can* get GERD under control and keep your symptoms at bay if you follow the proper lifestyle measures. In Chapter 4, I provided a list of ways to prevent indigestion. All of these suggestions also help prevent GERD. I can't emphasize enough how important it is for you to change your lifestyle. To get GERD under control, you must lose weight if you're obese, and you must change your eating habits if you're overindulging in high-fat, high-calorie meals. Management may also include taking a prescription medication or combination of medications.

Many of the lifestyle changes that I'm asking you to make for GERD are the very same changes that promote healthy living in general. Are you thinking about losing weight or joining a gym? Great! Weight loss and exercise both can help alleviate GERD symptoms. I say this over and over again to women I treat for GERD: "A healthy body will lead to a healthy GI tract."

First, review the eight-point list of suggestions for preventing indigestion that begins on page 139. I realize that it's hard to do *everything* on this list. The good news is that you probably won't have to. Different people have different reflux triggers—see what works for you. Avoiding caffeine may make no difference, but reducing spicy foods may do the trick—or vice versa. You'll also need to keep in mind that improvement probably won't happen from making one change. Just avoiding chocolate, for instance, isn't likely to cure all your reflux woes. (Sorry, it's not that easy!) Most of my patients tell me that their biggest challenge was finding the right combination of lifestyle changes that made their GERD symptoms tolerable. Once they had their own ticket to relief, the rest was smooth sailing. You can also try the following GERD-specific strategies.

Embark on a Healthy Weight-Loss Plan

If you're overweight, you know you have to get to a healthy weight. Maybe your cholesterol or blood pressure levels are high. Or maybe you have diabetes or a family history of heart disease. You may have already heard a long lecture from your doctor on the virtues of keeping your weight down. If you have GERD, I can say almost without a doubt that your symptoms will improve dramatically if you lose excess pounds. So now you know. The question is, how can you lose weight and keep the pounds off permanently? Going on a crash diet isn't the answer. In fact, crash diets can make some of your digestive symptoms worse.

As I emphasized in Chapter 3, the key to healthy weight loss is a balance of diet and exercise. If you've had difficulty making changes on your own, ask your doctor to refer you to a nutritionist to help you devise an eating plan with the appropriate amount of calories and nutrients for healthy weight loss. And make a commitment to exercise. Most of us do better having an exercise buddy. Convince a friend or loved one to work out with you. In general, a healthy diet and exercise will take off pounds over the course of months rather than days. Set realistic goals. Initially, aim for reasonable weight loss—only five to ten percent of your current body weight—to ensure that you'll keep the weight off for good. Yes, you can improve your symptoms by losing just 10 to 15 pounds. If you've reached this goal, pat yourself on the back and keep going. Continuing with a regular exercise program is the best way to maintain your new healthier weight.

Go to Sleep on an Empty Stomach

A recent survey conducted by the American Gastroenterological Association found that three-quarters of GERD sufferers experience heartburn symptoms at night that prevent them from falling asleep or wake them up in the middle of the night. Avoid eating two to three hours before bedtime. Remember that it may take several hours for a normal stomach to empty. Lying down with a full stomach only tempts gravity to allow food contents to slide upward.

Consider Elevating the Head of Your Bed

Your doctor may also suggest that you elevate the head of your bed to avoid nighttime heartburn. This helps some of my patients. Others, however, find it uncomfortable and difficult to sleep with their head and chest raised. If you decide to try it, elevate your bed by raising the head four to six inches off the floor. (Stacking pillows won't help because you'll only be raising your head. You need to raise both your head and chest by raising the mattress.)

STEP 2: TRY AN OVER-THE-COUNTER HEARTBURN REMEDY

When I walk through the medicine section of my local grocery store, I'm amazed at the huge number of over-

HOW TO SHED POUNDS WITHOUT GOING ON A DIET

These recommendations are based on a series of syndicated articles written by Sally Squires, a reporter for the *Washington Post*, called "The Lean Plate Club."

- Eat at least five servings a day of fruits and vegetables.
- Drink five to eight cups of water a day.
- Write down every morsel of food that you put in your mouth. This proven technique works consistently for those who successfully lose weight and keep it off.
- Eat three servings a day of whole grains.
- Eat two servings a day of foods rich in healthy fats (such as olive oil, nuts, avocado, fatty fish such as salmon, tuna, and mackerel).
- Eat one low-fat vegetarian meal a day.
- Take a multivitamin.
- Exercise for at least twenty minutes a day.

the-counter heartburn remedies that are available. Americans spend $2 billion annually on them. Antacids are still the most popular; they immediately neutralize acid in the esophagus, and you experience relief within seconds of swallowing the antacid. The problem with antacids is that the heartburn relief they provide is short-lived, usually lasting only several minutes, so repeat doses may be necessary. Certain antacids also contain ingredients that can be problematic: Those that contain calcium may cause constipation, and those that contain magnesium can cause loose stools or diarrhea.

A new antacid chewing gum, marketed by Wrigley, by the name of Surpass, is now available over the counter in 600- and 900-milligram strengths. One recent study found that the antacid gum was more effective at reducing heartburn symptoms and providing sustained relief from symptoms than two antacid tablets of the same strength. The theory behind the gum is that it applies antacid to the esophagus continually over a period of time, unlike a tablet, which is chewed, swallowed, and gone.

Acid-blockers work by decreasing acid secretion from the stomach. Three H_2 blocker medications— cimetidine (Tagamet), ranitidine (Zantac), and nizatidine (Axid)—are available over the counter at half prescription strength. Famotidine (Pepcid) is now available in full prescription strength. A new over-the-counter product is omeprazole (Prilosec)—previously available only by prescription—which may provide better and longer symptom relief than other acid-blockers because it is a proton pump inhibitor (PPI) with a different mode of action than H_2 blockers (which I explain on page 302). Realize that all acid-blockers must be absorbed into the bloodstream to have their effect. They may take a little longer to work, but their ability to decrease acid secretion generally provides more complete and longer-lasting relief of heartburn and acid indigestion. These medicines are generally safe and are well tolerated; they have few, if any, side effects.

Bottom line: If you want fast relief, an antacid is the ticket. If you want longer-lasting relief, or if you want to prevent reflux from occurring before you go out for tacos and a margarita, an acid-blocker is your best bet.

Take it at least an hour before your big meal to prevent
the postmeal acid indigestion. You can also take a combination product (Pepcid Complete) that contains
both an antacid and an acid-blocker. In general, I recommend following the label and not using these products continuously for more than two weeks. If your
symptoms persist beyond that point, you should see
your doctor for a prescription medication.

STEP 3: USE A PRESCRIPTION DRUG IF NECESSARY

Several prescription medications are used to treat GERD.

INFORMATION ON GERD? DON'T COUNT ON TV

If you're like most people, you may have been introduced to
the term GERD from a TV commercial. In a recent survey, 53
percent of people said they learned about GERD from a TV
commercial, and 41 percent from a magazine or newspaper
ad. The worst part is that people aren't getting the correct information. When polled, fewer than 25 percent of people knew
that lifestyle modifications could lessen the symptoms and
were unaware of specific things they could do, like wearing
looser clothing or remaining upright after eating. The bottom
line is that you need to be wary of those glossy advertisements
for products promising to cure GERD. Be a savvy consumer,
and ask your doctor or pharmacist to explain what these medications really can (and can't) do and about any possible side
effects.

Reducing Stomach Acid

Blocking acid is a critical component in the management of GERD because it is acid that can do damage to the esophageal lining. H_2 acid blockers are available in prescription as well as over-the-counter strength. They work by blocking the histamine-2 receptor on the stomach parietal cell, the cell that makes gastric acid. In general, acid-blockers are useful for patients with mild to moderate reflux; they can reduce symptoms and heal inflammation in the esophagus. The medications work less well in those with more severe GERD.

Proton pump inhibitors (PPIs), which came on the market in the late 1980s, seem to work better in helping to manage severe reflux. These medications work by blocking the final step in stomach acid secretion, in which a pump within the parietal cell brings in potassium and pumps out hydrogen ions (acid) into the stomach. PPIs are extremely potent and result in a more prolonged suppression of gastric acid than H_2 blockers. In my experience, PPIs are the most effective medical therapy to control GERD symptoms and heal esophagitis. Several different PPIs are available—lansoprazole (Prevacid), pantoprazole (Protonix), rabeprazole (Aciphex), and esomeprazole (Nexium)—and all are very well tolerated with very few side effects. As I mentioned, omeprazole (Prilosec) is now available over the counter. The most common side effects reported are headache, dizziness, fatigue, diarrhea, constipation, and abdominal pain. These medications can also be safely used for long-term treatment of GERD if your doctor feels that maintenance therapy is necessary.

Increasing Motility

Because the cause of GERD is related to defects in the ability of the esophagus and stomach to move food through, medications that speed this movement, or motility, can be useful, although they have no effect on the secretion of stomach acid. One of these medications, metoclopramide (Reglan), can improve stomach emptying and esophageal clearance and increase LES pressure. Another, bethanechol (Urecholine) can increase LES pressure and stimulate esophageal clearance. In general, these medications are disappointing when used alone but may be helpful in augmenting GERD treatment with PPIs or H$_2$ blockers. The biggest downside to these medications is their side effects. Metoclopramide can cause tremor, agitation, and (rarely) more severe neurological side effects. Bethanechol causes dry eyes, dry mouth, and (rarely) urinary retention. A new medication being studied in clinical research trials for GERD is tegaserod (Zelnorm), which is currently FDA-approved for constipation-predominant irritable bowel syndrome. It appears to improve GI motility with fewer side effects than the other medications.

STEP 4: DISCUSS THE OPTION OF SURGERY

Surgery is certainly not the first treatment of choice for GERD, but it offers the best chance of a permanent cure for those who don't want to take medications chronically. I and most of my colleagues believe that surgery isn't necessary for the vast majority of reflux sufferers. Nevertheless, surgical therapy for GERD has seen a recent boom because of a new technique that allows the procedure to be done using a laparoscope. A surgeon can avoid making large incisions in the chest and abdomen by using a video camera attached to surgical equipment. A patient winds up with a tiny scar, stays in the hospital for a shorter time, and recovers in days instead of weeks.

In this procedure, called *laparoscopic fundoplication*, the surgeon creates a new LES by wrapping the top of the stomach (fundus) around the lower portion of the esophagus. This "wrap" strengthens the LES and makes it less likely for stomach contents to reflux back into the esophagus. If you have a hiatal hernia, this can be repaired at the same time. The surgery, which usually lasts two to four hours, is performed through several small incisions through which a laparoscope is inserted.

The downside to surgical therapy is that patients may experience trouble belching with their new LES, which can cause a buildup of excess gas that can cause bloating symptoms. (Surgery has improved in the last few years, and many surgeons are doing "partial" or "loose" wraps to avoid this complication.) Surgery also won't reverse Barrett's esophagus, which will still have to be monitored with periodic endoscopies. Also, the effects may not last forever. Reflux can recur five to ten years after surgery, requiring repeat surgery and/or medication. Before you consider this surgical procedure as your golden ticket to a life without reflux, talk to your primary care doctor, your gastroenterologist, and your surgeon to be sure this treatment is right for you. If you do opt for surgery, ask your gastroenterologist to refer you to a competent surgeon who has substantial experience with this particular procedure.

PROMISING NEW TREATMENTS
FOR GERD

In the next few years we'll see a number of exciting treatments for GERD emerge. At recent medical conferences I've heard about several that sound like they could transform GERD management—if they work. In one procedure a miniature suturing or stapling device is attached to an endoscope and used to tighten the LES. This serves to strengthen the valve and prevent reflux. Another up-and-coming therapy is the Stretta procedure. In this outpatient procedure a flexible catheter is inserted into the esophagus down to the level of the LES. Temperature-controlled radiofrequency energy is delivered to the LES, just below the surface lining, to create thermal lesions. As these lesions heal, the barrier function of the LES is improved, basically "toughening" the LES area so that it's less likely to relax, thereby reducing the frequency of reflux events. A third procedure employs Enteryx, a rubbery substance that is injected deep into the layers of the LES to create a mechanical barrier. Because these treatments are very new, only a limited number of doctors across the nation have received the specialized training necessary to perform them correctly. In addition, several clinical research trials are currently under way to

establish their long-term usefulness in the management of GERD.

GERD RESOURCES

**NATIONAL DIGESTIVE DISEASES INFORMATION
CLEARINGHOUSE**
2 Information Way
Bethesda, MD 20892-3570
tel. (800) 891-5389 or (301) 654-3810
digestive.niddk.nih.gov
This clearinghouse offers pamphlets and brochures about
GERD and the latest treatments.

AMERICAN GASTROENTEROLOGICAL ASSOCIATION
www.aga.org
Information about GERD and other digestive diseases for
patients and the general public.

GERD INFORMATION RESOURCE CENTER
www.gerd.com
This site, sponsored by AstraZeneca Pharmaceuticals
(which makes GERD medications), provides information
and graphic pictures on reflux, diagnostic tests, and
treatment procedures. It also contains a list of articles
on GERD and the latest research on managing it.

ULCERS—A CURE IS NOW POSSIBLE

FIFTY YEARS AGO ULCERS WERE blamed for the majority of stomach problems. People assumed they were caused by stress or spicy foods. Any burning or churning in the gut was blamed on an ulcer. Since doctors had no way of peering into the stomach or duodenum (the upper portion of the small intestine) without performing exploratory surgery, they just diagnosed an ulcer based on the symptoms.

They also didn't really know how to cure ulcers. My father-in law was told to drink a lot of cream when his ulcer was diagnosed in the 1960s. Others were told to avoid garlic and chili peppers. Some doctors even recommended making a career switch to a less stressful job.

Now we know these "cures" were all myths. Let me say this in black and white: Stress doesn't cause ulcers. Spicy foods don't cause ulcers. Milk doesn't heal ulcers.

Now that doctors have more high-tech diagnostic tools, like endoscopes, that can peer into the stomach and duodenum, we can definitively diagnose ulcers. We have determined what causes them and how to cure them. What we've learned is actually quite fascinating. First of all, ulcers are not as common as we once thought; endoscopy has shown that many people who have ulcer symptoms actually have nonulcer dyspepsia (see page 321) or GERD (see Chapter 9). Whenever I see an ulcer during an endoscopy, I call over my GI fellows to show them what it looks like. They may not see that many ulcers during their training, so I point them out when I find them.

An ulcer is an irritation or sore in the lining of the stomach or the duodenum that can cause abdominal pain. Like an untreated open wound, an ulcer that isn't treated can grow larger and deeper, causing problems like severe bleeding, a perforation (hole) in the stomach or duodenal wall, or an obstruction (blockage) that prevents the stomach from emptying.

So what is the proper treatment? Actually, we learned about fifteen years ago that the best way to cure an ulcer is with a strong acid-blocker and a course of antibiotics to kill the bacteria that cause ulcers. That's because about 50 to 75 percent of the stomach and duodenal ulcers that occur in Americans are caused by a stomach infection by the bacterium *Helicobacter pylori*. These nasty bacteria set the stage for an ulcer by causing trouble in numerous ways: They increase the amount of acid produced by the stomach; they weaken the barrier that protects the lining of the duodenum and stomach from acid; and they trigger the influx of inflammatory cells (to fight the bacterial infection), which can damage the mucus lining. Fortunately, *H. pylori* infection can be eradicated with a course of potent antibiotics, which can cure ulcers for good.

These bacteria have been on the decline in recent years. Older people are far more likely to carry them than children and young adults; about half of people over sixty are infected with *H. pylori* compared to 20 percent of people under forty. (Just a small percentage of those infected with the bacteria actually develop ulcers.) Older people probably were infected in early childhood from their food or water supply, or by person-to-person spread in families. In recent decades improved sanitation, less crowded living conditions, and more widespread use of antibiotics have all contributed to a lower rate of *H. pylori* infections in this country.

The vast majority of ulcers not linked to *H. pylori* are caused by chronic use of aspirin (any products with salicylic acid or salicylates such as Bayer, Excedrin, Bufferin, and others) or other nonsteroidal anti-inflammatory drugs such as ibuprofen (Advil, Motrin, Nuprin), naproxen sodium (Aleve), and ketoprofen (Orudis), which can be purchased over the counter or are available by prescription. These medications decrease the production of prostaglandins, chemicals that cause inflammation and trigger pain in arthritis and other conditions. Certain prostaglandins, however, protect the lining of the stomach and duodenum against injury from acid and pepsin. Aspirin and NSAIDs indiscriminately knock out the protective prostaglandins, leaving the stomach and duodenum vulnerable. This lack of protection can lead to an erosion of the stomach lining or to a deeper injury, an ulcer.

Even taking one baby aspirin a day (just an 81-milligram dose) to prevent heart disease can lead to an ulcer—especially if you're combining it with another NSAID for arthritis or back pain. Combining aspirin with another anti-inflammatory pain reliever can be particularly damaging to the lining of the stomach and duodenum. And you may be taking a pain reliever without even knowing it. Some over-the-counter products, like Alka-Seltzer and certain cold remedies, contain a pain reliever like aspirin along with other active ingredients. For this reason, I urge you to carefully read medication labels, and be careful not to combine aspirin with a second NSAID.

A very small percentage of ulcers are caused by medical conditions, including rare pancreatic tumors, Crohn's disease, chemotherapy drugs, or lymphoma. And in some cases, we don't know the cause of the ulcer.

Since we now know more about the specific causes of ulcers and how to treat them, we may expect ulcers to become even more infrequent over the next few decades.

SYMPTOMS OF AN ULCER

Pain is the most common symptom of an ulcer. It usually:

- is a dull, gnawing ache in the midabdomen, the epigastric area (just at the solar plexus)
- comes and goes for several days or weeks
- occurs two to three hours after a meal

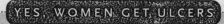

Women get ulcers about as frequently as men, but there are some interesting differences between the two genders. Men are more likely to develop duodenal ulcers, while women are more likely to develop gastric (stomach) ulcers, according to a 1998 study in the journal *Gut*. This gender difference, the researchers theorize, may be due to the fact that men naturally secrete more stomach acid and may be more likely to harbor *H. pylori*, both of which factors are more likely to cause duodenal ulcers. Women, on the other hand, are more likely to use NSAIDs on a regular basis to relieve arthritis, migraines, and menstrual cramps.

- occurs in the middle of the night (when the stomach is empty)
- is relieved by food

Other symptoms can include:

- weight loss
- poor appetite
- bloating
- burping
- nausea
- vomiting

Warning Symptoms

If you have any of these symptoms along with other ulcer symptoms, call your doctor right away.

- sharp, severe, persistent stomach pain
- bloody or black stools
- persistent vomiting
- bloody vomit or vomit that looks like coffee grounds

These emergency symptoms could be signs of a serious problem such as a perforation (a hole in the stomach or duodenal wall), bleeding (when the acid or ulcer erodes into a blood vessel), or obstruction (when the swelling from the ulcer blocks the path of food trying to leave the stomach).

MAKING THE DIAGNOSIS

If you have symptoms of an ulcer, there are a number of tests your doctor can perform to make the proper diagnosis.

Endoscopy

Doctors can detect not only an ulcer but also the presence of *H. pylori* by performing this test. You'll be put under mild sedation, and a thin, lighted tube with a camera on one end will be eased through your mouth and down your throat, so that your doctor can see the stomach and duodenum. Your doctor can then take photos of the ulcer or remove a tiny piece of tissue to view under the microscope.

The tissue sample can also be used to check for the presence of *H. pylori*. Your doctor may decide to do a rapid urease test to detect the presence of the enzyme urease, which is produced by the bacteria. Alternatively, the tissue sample may be examined under a microscope to look for the actual bacteria. A third option is a culture test, allowing *H. pylori* to grow in the tissue sample.

Endoscopy is the gold standard for diagnosing ulcers, but it's also more invasive and expensive (though it's usually covered by insurance) than other techniques.

Upper GI Series

This test is an X-ray of the esophagus, stomach, and duodenum. It can detect an ulcer but not as reliably as endoscopy. And unlike endoscopy, it doesn't yield a tissue sample to test for *H. pylori*, so you'll have to have a separate test to detect these bacteria.

Tests to Diagnose *H. pylori*

1. Breath Test This is the simplest and least invasive way to test for *H. pylori*. You swallow a capsule that contains a small amount of radioactive urea. (The amount of radiation is extremely small.) Ten minutes later you exhale into a balloon that contains a detector for radioactive carbon dioxide. If you are infected with *H. pylori*, the urease produced by these bacteria will break down the ingested radioactive urea into water plus radiolabeled carbon dioxide. This radiolabeled carbon dioxide is present in your exhaled breath specimen. If no bacteria are present, the urea isn't broken down but is expelled in the urine.

2. Blood Test   This test checks for antibodies to *H. pylori* and can tell you if you are or have ever been infected with the bacteria. This test is less expensive than the breath test but is also less reliable. That's because the test detects antibodies for *H. pylori* rather than the bacteria themselves. These antibodies can remain in your blood for years even after you've been treated for the bacteria. This means the test can't be used as a follow-up test to see if treatment worked to eradicate the bacteria. (You'll need to have a breath test for that.) Still, the blood test has a pretty good detection rate, and many of my colleagues use it.

TREATMENT OPTIONS

Treatment for an ulcer depends on its cause. If you have an ulcer and test positive for *H. pylori*, you'll need a combination of antibiotics and acid-blockers to get rid of the bacteria and treat the ulcer. If your doctor determines that your ulcer is caused by NSAIDs, you'll probably be given an acid-blocker to heal your ulcer and may need to switch to a different medication for pain relief. I've divided this section into two parts depending on the cause of your ulcer.

If You Have an Ulcer Caused by *H. pylori*

Curing *H. pylori* infection isn't an easy task. The bacteria are fairly resistant and require a combination of powerful antibiotics for about two weeks. The usual antibiotics prescribed are combinations containing clarithromycin (Biaxin), amoxicillin (Amoxil), metronidazole (Flagyl), or tetracycline (Achromycin, Sumycin). Your doctor may also advise you to take bismuth subsalicylate (Pepto-Bismol) or prescription ranitidine bismuth citrate (Tritec), which works in conjunction with the antibiotics to kill the bacteria.

Since antibiotics frequently have unpleasant side effects, you may experience any or all of the following while you're taking the drugs: nausea, vomiting, diarrhea, dizziness, headache, or yeast infection. Even if you're feeling lousy, though, it's very important for you to finish the treatment regimen. Noncompliance or incomplete therapy increases your chance of developing resistant strains of *H. pylori* that may be infinitely harder to eradicate. The good news is, once you've gotten rid of *H. pylori,* your risk of devloping future ulcers will be greatly diminished.

Along with antibiotics, you'll also need to take an acid-blocker to heal the ulcer. Acid-blockers include H_2 blockers such as cimetidine (Tagamet), nizatidine (Axid), famotidine (Pepcid), and ranitidine (Zantac). They also include the more potent proton pump inhibitors (PPIs) such as omeprazole (Prilosec), esomeprazole (Nexium), lansoprazole (Prevacid), rabeprazole (Aciphex), and pantoprazole (Protonix). Any of these medications can be added to the antibiotic regimen, and you can discuss with your doctor which is best for you. Realize, though, that during the two-week regimen to cure the ulcer you may need to take as many as twenty pills a day.

If the digestive side effects caused by the antibiotics linger after the therapy is complete, you may consider trying a probiotic. Probiotics are dietary supplements sold in health food stores that contain active bacteria that colonize the gut and keep bad bacteria in check. Antibiotics often kill off good bacteria, allowing bad bacteria or yeast to multiply and causing symptoms like diarrhea, vomiting, or yeast infection. I tell my patients to take a brand that contains upward of 100 million lactobacillus colonies per dose.

If You Have an Ulcer Caused by NSAIDs

If your doctor determines that NSAIDs are to blame for your ulcer, you'll be given an acid-blocker to heal the ulcer. Your doctor may discuss switching to an alternative pain medication that doesn't cause ulcers, or may choose to keep you on the acid-blocker indefinitely along with the NSAID to prevent ulcers from recurring in the future.

Healing the ulcer is pretty straightforward. It usually involves taking an acid-blocker (either an H_2 blocker or a PPI) for 6 to 12 weeks, depending on the choice of acid-blocker and whether the ulcer is in your duodenum or your stomach. If it is in your stomach, your doctor may also recommend a repeat endoscopy after you've completed treatment to be sure the ulcer has healed. If it hasn't healed, you may need to remain on acid-blocking medications for a few more weeks.

Switching to a different pain medication can be a little trickier. If your doctor determines that you need to remain on the NSAID that you were originally taking, you may be told to stay on an acid-blocker medication indefinitely to prevent another ulcer from occurring. Your doctor may also prescribe misoprostol (Cytotec), a "good" prostaglandin that helps to increase the protective factors in the lining of your stomach. *(Note: Misoprostol cannot be used in pregnant women or women who have a chance of getting pregnant, as it will increase the chance of abortion. In fact, it is now prescribed by some gynecologists to terminate first-trimester unwanted pregnancies.)*

Fortunately, other options for pain relief are now available, in the form of a new class of NSAIDs that appear much less likely to cause ulcers. These medications, called COX-2 inhibitors, target only those prostaglandins that are associated with inflammation and pain and not those that protect the lining of the stomach and duodenum. The COX-2 inhibitors currently on the market include rofecoxib (Vioxx), celecoxib (Celebrex), and valdecoxib (Bextra), among others. Researchers are currently testing other COX-2 inhibitors as well as other innovative products, like a new kind of aspirin that provides all the heart benefits and pain relief of aspirin without the gastrointestinal side effects. The medication was created by taking a regular aspirin and binding it to nitric oxide, which has protective effects on the lining of the digestive tract. These new medications may become available within the next year or two if studies validate their safety and effectiveness.

OTHER FACTORS INVOLVED IN ULCERS —AND THOSE THAT AREN'T

As we've seen, *H. pylori* infection and the use of NSAIDs are by far the biggest risk factors involved in ulcers. But, other factors can also come into play, setting the stage for an ulcer or preventing an existing ulcer from healing properly. Some factors, contrary to popular belief, play no role in ulcer formation, and I would like to dispel the lingering myths about them.

Factors That Are Involved in Ulcers

Medications: In addition to NSAIDs, other medications can increase your risk of developing ulcers: potassium chloride pills, bisphosphonates such as alendronate (Fosamax), and some cancer chemotherapy agents. Steroids, like prednisone, can increase your risk of ulcer complications such as bleeding and perforation.

Smoking: Beyond its other ills, this dangerous habit increases the production of acid in the stomach and decreases the secretion of acid-neutralizing bicarbonate from the duodenum. Smoking can also delay the healing of ulcers. Studies show that cigarette smokers have decreased prostaglandin concentrations in the stomach and duodenum—a necessary chemical for protecting the stomach lining from the damaging effects of acid.

Medical Conditions: A number of chronic illnesses have been associated with ulcers. About 30 percent of people with emphysema have ulcers, perhaps due to their smoking habit. Those who have Crohn's disease, hypercalcemia (high calcium levels), lymphoma (cancer of the lymph nodes), herpes simplex infection, cirrhosis of the liver, or chronic kidney failure are also at increased risk for ulcers.

H. PYLORI'S LINK TO STOMACH CANCER

What do you do if your doctor tells you that you have *H. pylori* but no signs of an ulcer? The answer is not so simple. The bacteria may have been detected by a blood test or during an endoscopy exam to evaluate heartburn or other upper GI symptoms. If no ulcer is found, a dilemma often arises about whether to treat the bacteria. Some doctors insist on treating the bacteria in any patient who is infected. But the combination antibiotic therapy can have uncomfortable side effects, like diarrhea and yeast infection. Additionally, specific strains of *H. pylori* may be more virulent than others and increase your odds of getting an ulcer. Thus, if you don't have an ulcer now and have never had one, your doctor may decide not to treat your case of *H. pylori* because it may never cause you any problems.

The debate over whether to treat is being fueled by new research findings linking certain strains of *H. pylori* to stomach cancer. In industrialized countries the incidence of stomach cancer has dropped along with a decline in *H. pylori* infections; in developing countries where *H. pylori* infections remain high, stomach cancer rates have also remained high, even as life expectancy rates have increased. Some experts contend that those who have nonulcer dyspepsia (ulcer symptoms without the ulcer) and have *H. pylori* can be cured of their symptoms if the bacteria are eradicated. This theory, though, remains unproven, and studies have had conflicting results.

Many of my patients with *H. pylori* are concerned that their infection will lead to stomach cancer. I assure these patients

H. PYLORI'S LINK TO
STOMACH CANCER (continued)

that this risk remains very low, but I also look at other factors to see if they're at higher-than-average risk. I take into account their family history (any close relatives with stomach cancer), whether they smoke cigarettes, and whether they eat a high-salt diet—all of which are risk factors for stomach cancer. I spend a lot of time weighing the pros and cons with my patients and tell them that the jury is still out over whether asymptomatic patients have to be treated. When it comes down to making the decision, I take an individualized approach that weighs the patient's own preference with her individual risk factor for stomach cancer.

Severe Medical Trauma: Being hospitalized with a serious trauma—such as extensive burns, major surgery, head trauma, or a major medical illness that leaves you in the intensive care unit—can cause a stress-related stomach ulcer by weakening the defenses of your stomach mucus lining.

Factors That Aren't Involved in the Formation of Ulcers

Alcohol: Although ulcers are more common in patients with alcohol-induced cirrhosis of the liver, alcohol has never been proven to cause ulcers. Wine and beer do cause an increase in stomach acid secretion, but this hasn't been shown to cause an ulcer. Imbibing, however, can make ulcers worse.

Diet: No study has convincingly linked diet and ulcers. The evidence that acidic or spicy foods cause ulcers is virtually nonexistent—though they can cause heartburn and indigestion. Doctors used to prescribe a bland diet or milk products for ulcers, but such diets have not been shown to have any benefit in preventing or treating them.

Emotional Stress: We've all heard that emotional stress causes ulcers, but this connection hasn't been proven in any studies. Emotional stress can increase stomach acid production, but that alone does not appear to be sufficient to cause ulcers. It may, however, contribute to ulcers in those who are already susceptible because of *H. pylori* infection or NSAID use. For instance, researchers found an increase in bleeding stomach ulcers among the population after a devastating earthquake occurred in Japan, killing thousands. They speculated that the emotional trauma may have increased the severity of ulcers in those who already had them.

WHAT IF YOU DON'T HAVE AN ULCER BUT HAVE ALL THE SYMPTOMS?

There's a diagnosis for this condition, and it's called *nonulcer dyspepsia*. Nonulcer dyspepsia—also known simply as dyspepsia—accounts for up to 60 percent of chronic indigestion symptoms like upper abdominal pain, heartburn, belching, bloating, nausea, or vomiting. In fact, dyspepsia afflicts about 25 percent of the

U.S. population at some point during their lives. Many women never seek medical attention for their symptoms.

Most chronic sufferers are diagnosed when they have upper GI symptoms for more than three months and have no chemical or anatomical abnormality. Basically, however, doctors diagnose this condition by ruling everything else out.

When a woman comes to see me complaining of persistent indigestion—with no clear-cut diagnosis—I usually order an ultrasound to rule out gallbladder disease and an endoscopy to rule out ulcer disease, GERD, or some other abnormality of the lining of the upper GI tract. I may also do a gastric emptying study to look for slow stomach emptying. Unfortunately, I can't come to the conclusion that a woman has dyspepsia until I'm certain that she doesn't have something else. Sometimes dyspepsia can be combined with another problem, like irritable bowel syndrome.

One note of caution: You can't diagnose yourself with nonulcer dyspepsia. Only your physician can do that, after ruling out other causes like ulcer, gallbladder disease, inflammation of the pancreas, and in very rare cases stomach cancer.

Dyspepsia can be a frustrating condition because you have all the symptoms of an ulcer but no ulcer. None of your tests show a specific diagnostic finding, which is both good news and bad news. The good news is that your symptoms probably won't cause damage to your digestive tract. The bad news is that your doctor can't treat and eradicate your condition in the way that ulcers are treated and eradicated. However, working with your doctor, your symptoms can be managed and perhaps even alleviated permanently.

I can comfort you by telling you that your symptoms are not in your head. Dyspepsia is a real condition, even though gastroenterologists can't see it with an endoscope. I can't tell you why you have the condition or why you're experiencing debilitating symptoms. But I can reassure you that your symptoms aren't life threatening.

The best treatment is self-help measures, like the ones I outlined in Chapter 4. For instance, you should avoid spicy and acidic foods as well as alcoholic beverages, all of which can irritate the stomach. You need to stop smoking and avoid NSAIDs. Take acetaminophen (Tylenol) instead, or ask your doctor if you can try an alternative pain reliever such as a COX-2 inhibitor, which may not cause as much stomach upset. You may also find relief from a prescription-strength acid-blocker medication.

Your doctor should also discuss your emotional well-being with you. Studies have shown that those who suffer from dyspepsia have higher rates of anxiety, depression, chronic tension, hostility, and a more pessimistic outlook on life. Researchers have found that psychological treatments like psychotherapy, behavioral therapy, relaxation therapy, and hypnosis can help improve dyspepsia symptoms in many sufferers.

I firmly believe that there's a strong connection between gastrointestinal health and mental health. In fact, the Women's GI Clinic works closely with a psychologist to counsel patients on their emotional well-being. Reducing stress, managing anger, and leading a happier life overall may be the key to overcoming digestive health problems that have no well-defined pathology. This doesn't mean that your dyspepsia is "all in your head." But in combination with other lifestyle measures, evaluating what is in your head may help you overcome your symptoms.

GALLSTONES—TO TREAT
OR NOT TO TREAT?

·

W HILE I WAS WRITING THIS CHAPTER, I entered an online women's health chat room to see what women were saying about their gallstone problems. A total of 377 women posted messages about their gallstone attacks. Here's what four of them had to say:

> It felt like I was being stabbed in the gut repeatedly—horrible pain, slightly easing, then horrible again. I had two gallstone attacks—both occurred after eating a rich meal—before I decided to have my gallbladder removed.—Analisa

> I had a terrible attack on a Monday morning at 2 A.M. The emergency room where I went didn't even *consider* that it might be gallbladder. They just gave me some sedatives and sent me home saying I had the flu and should check with my doctor. I went to my doctor's office the next day, and he sent me for an ultrasound, even though my attack had subsided. During the ultrasound,

the technician ran to get the doctor. Needless to say, I was on the operating table a few hours later having my gallbladder ripped out. My doctor told me I had stones blocking a duct that caused my gallbladder to become severely infected.—Jenny

I had one major gallbladder attack before I had my gallbladder removed. It sent me to the emergency room, and I told the doctor and nurses that I thought I was having a gallbladder attack since I have a strong family history of stones. But they treated me first as if I was having a heart attack since the symptoms are sometimes similar. I had pain in my chest, pain in the middle of my back, and shortness of breath. Finally, I was diagnosed by ultrasound and the real problem—a huge gallstone—was discovered.—Lauren

I'm only 17 and about 5 months ago I got a horrible stomachache, and it felt like my stomach was on fire. Then it felt like I had sore muscles on the inside and after about 15 minutes it went away. A month later, the same thing happened but it woke me at 2 A.M. and kept me up until 6 A.M. I was pale, feverish, and felt like I was going to be sick to my stomach. Finally I went to the doctor, and he did an ultrasound and found gallstones. The week before my surgery, I had a severe attack and threw up everything I ate, except crackers. I lost 8 pounds that week. Oh, and after the surgery, my doctor handed me my gallstones in a bag. I had 20. Now I don't have any attacks and

I'm able to hang out with my friends again.—
Tabatha

These women's tales about their gallbladder disease
are all harrowing. Their symptoms are well known to
twenty million Americans who have gallstones. Many
opt not to live with the pain. Every year more than half
a million Americans have surgery to fix the problem.
Gallstones—chunks of crystallized bile found in the
gallbladder—are far more prevalent in women than in
men. Nearly 25 percent of women in the United States
develop gallstones by age sixty, and up to 50 percent of
women have them by age seventy-five. (Most of these
cases, however, cause no symptoms and don't need to
be treated.) Gallstones can pose particular problems
during pregnancy and are more likely to cause symptoms than stones in nonpregnant women.

Why are gallstones more prevalent in women? I
and my colleagues believe that women are particularly
susceptible to gallstones due to the female hormones,
estrogen and progesterone. Research suggests that estrogen promotes the formation of gallstones by stimulat-
ing the liver to remove more cholesterol from the blood
to divert it into the bile. Progesterone decreases the
emptying of the gallbladder. These two factors make
conditions right for the formation of gallstones, which
are hardened chunks of calcium- and cholesterol-
enriched bile.

Another reason for the higher prevalence may be
weight fluctuations, which are more common in
women due to multiple pregnancies, obesity, and rapid
weight loss. In fact, it's pretty much a given that if you

lose more than 20 percent of your body weight in a rapid fashion (more than two pounds a week), you're going to get gallstones. Certain factors play a role in increasing your risk of gallstones. The typical person who gets gallstones is a woman who is over forty and overweight. You'll see how all these factors contribute to gallstone risk.

YOUR GALLBLADDER: HOW IT WORKS, WHAT IT DOES

Your gallbladder is a holding tank for bile, a fluid produced by your liver to aid in the digestion of fats. Bile flows from the liver into the gallbladder through the cystic duct and is composed mainly of water, bile acids, lecithin (an emulsifier), and cholesterol. The four-inch muscular-walled sac that is your gallbladder stores bile and makes it more concentrated, removing two to five cups of fluid a day until a few tablespoons of concentrated bile are left to be released during digestion.

As food enters your small intestine, a hormone called cholecystokinin is released, which signals the gallbladder to contract and deliver bile into the intestine. The force of the contraction propels the bile down into the common bile duct and then into the small intestine, where it emulsifies (mixes and breaks down) fats. This process allows fat molecules as well as fat-absorbable nutrients, including vitamins A, D, E, and K, to enter the bloodstream through the intestinal lining.

Most gallstones are formed because of an imbalance of cholesterol and bile in the gallbladder. Cholesterol actually makes up only five percent of bile, but in order for it to remain dissolved, it must be properly balanced with bile acids. If the balance tips toward more cholesterol and less bile acid, the fluid turns into a thick sludge. If the cholesterol becomes supersaturated in the sludge, crystals form gradually—sometimes over several years—and become stones that range in size from smaller than a grain of sand to larger than a golf ball.

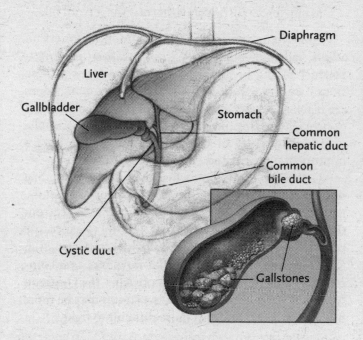

Your gallbladder stores bile and releases it into the intestine to aid in the digestive process. When stones develop in the gallbladder they can block the bile duct and cause painful distension, resulting in inflammation and/or infection.

You can develop excess cholesterol in your bile for one of the following reasons:

- Your liver secretes too much cholesterol into the bile.
- Your gallbladder's emptying mechanisms are defective so that the bile becomes stagnant and sludge forms, eventually forming stones.
- The cells lining your gallbladder lose their capacity to efficiently absorb cholesterol and fat from bile.

Sometimes, though far less common in American adults, gallstones are formed from calcified bilirubin, a product of the breakdown of red blood cells. These stones are known as pigment stones. Pigment stones are black or brown and often form in the gallbladders of people with chronic hemolytic anemia (for example, sickle cell disease) or cirrhosis. Some people have a mixture of pigment and cholesterol gallstones.

Gallstones cause pain when they obstruct the bile ducts, resulting in distension and spasm. A gallstone that obstructs the cystic duct (the duct that leads from the gallbladder to the common bile duct) can cause pain (called biliary colic), gallbladder inflammation (cholecystitis), and/or gallbladder infection. Less commonly, gallstones pass into and obstruct the common bile duct. These common bile duct stones may be more difficult to detect and also more difficult to treat.

ARE YOU AT INCREASED RISK?

If you maintain a healthful lifestyle that includes following a moderately low-fat, well-balanced diet, engaging in regular exercise, and keeping your weight steady, then you probably have nothing to worry about. If you're overweight or a yo-yo dieter, you're at increased risk, especially if gallbladder disease runs in your family. Here are some major risk factors:

Obesity

Research suggests that women who are morbidly obese have seven times the risk of developing gallstones compared to normal-weight women. A large clinical trial found that being even moderately overweight increases your risk for gallstones. The most likely reason is that obesity causes an increased secretion of cholesterol into the bile. It also decreases gallbladder emptying.

Pregnancy

Gallstones occur in up to 12 percent of pregnant women, but they seldom cause trouble. (Nearly 70 percent of those with gallstones during pregnancy have no symptoms.) Gallstones are more likely to occur in the second and third trimesters of pregnancy due to increasing levels of estrogen and progesterone and are usually diagnosed during a routine prenatal ultrasound. They occur more commonly in younger pregnant women and in those who have had more than two prior pregnancies.

Most of the time gallstones can be managed during pregnancy with increased fluid intake and pain medications. In most women the sludge clears up after pregnancy. Subsequent pregnancies, though, can increase the likelihood of permanent gallstones. If surgical removal of the gallbladder is required for severe symptoms, laparoscopic cholecystectomy is usually preferable during the first or second trimester to minimize the risk of premature labor.

Estrogen

Excess estrogen from oral contraceptives (especially those that contain high doses of estrogen) and hormone replacement therapy (see box) also increase a woman's risk for gallstones. *Note:* Low-dose oral contraceptives (the "mini-pill"), which are used in perimenopausal women who are still ovulating occasionally but don't

DOES HORMONE REPLACEMENT THERAPY CAUSE GALLSTONES?

As if it hasn't fallen far enough out of favor, hormone replacement therapy now has another risk associated with its use: gallstones. Women who take HRT are three times more likely to develop gallstones than women who do not, according to a 2002 study conducted by British researchers. The study, which followed more than 13,000 women for three years, accounted for other risk factors such as alcohol use, previous pregnancies, and being overweight. Researchers also drew a correlation between risk of gallstones and the length of time a woman took HRT: Women who took HRT for less than three years were 2.5 times more likely to develop gallstones, and those who took it for more than three years were four times more likely.

need full-strength birth control, are not associated with an increased risk of gallstone formation.

Rapid Weight Loss and Weight Cycling

Losing more than a pound or two a week causes the liver to secrete extra cholesterol into the bile. Ditto for fasting diets. Fasting decreases gallbladder emptying, causing bile to become more concentrated with cholesterol. As I said in Chapter 3 and emphasize to my patients: Losing weight on fad diets is detrimental to your GI health. Your body goes into a type of shock mode when you suddenly deprive it of calories and vital nutrients. A recent medical study showed that 28 percent of obese people who ate ultra-low-calorie liquid diets developed gallstones. Weight cycling, or yo-yo dieting, is also a risk factor. Case in point: Researchers who followed women for sixteen years found that those who lost and regained more than twenty pounds at least once had a 68 percent higher risk of gallstone surgery than women who lost the weight and kept it off or women who never lost the weight in the first place.

If you're overweight and want to reduce your health risks, by all means go ahead and begin a weight-loss program. But do it sensibly. You should be on a plan that contains at least 1,200 to 1,500 calories per day, which will take weight off gradually, about a pound a week. If you are morbidly obese and need to lose weight quickly, ask your doctor about a prescription medication called ursodeoxycholic acid or ursodiol (Actigall). This medication can be used to dissolve existing cholesterol gallstones and may help prevent gallstone formation in those who need to undergo rapid weight loss. (See "Nonsurgical Options" on page 351.)

Age

People over sixty are more likely to develop gallstones than younger people. By age seventy-five at least 35 percent of women and 20 percent of men have developed gallstones.

Ethnicity

Native Americans have a genetic predisposition to secrete high levels of cholesterol in bile and have the highest rates of gallstones in the United States. Among the Pima Indians in Arizona, 70 percent of women have gallstones by age thirty. Hispanics and northern Europeans have a higher risk for gallstones than Asians and African Americans.

Diabetes and Heart Disease

High total cholesterol levels alone do not increase one's risk for gallstones, but people with low HDL cholesterol (the so-called good cholesterol) or high triglyceride levels are at increased risk. Diabetes has not been clearly identified as an independent risk factor for the development of gallstones, but diabetics may be more susceptible to complications from gallbladder disease such as infections or perforation. Still, the medical consensus is not to recommend surgery in diabetics who have asymptomatic gallstones. Physicians generally take a wait-and-see approach and do careful monitoring, recommending laparoscopic cholecystectomy only when symptoms develop.

Cholesterol-lowering drugs like gemfibrozil (Lopid) and clofibrate (Atromid-S) also increase risk of gallstones because these medications actually increase the amount of cholesterol secreted in bile. Thiazide diuretics, which are used for high blood pressure, can also slightly increase the risk of gallstones.

CAN YOU PREVENT GALLSTONES?

Actually, you can. You may also be able to prevent small gallstones from getting larger and shrink the ones that you already have.

Lose Weight Slowly

Losing weight is the number-one thing you can do to reduce your risk of gallstones—provided you lose it slowly, no more than a pound or two per week. In fact, research shows that by losing weight you can actually shrink gallstones by lowering the amount of cholesterol in your bile. I provide guidance on getting to a healthy weight in Chapter 3.

Reduce Your Intake of Saturated Fats

Avoiding saturated fats (found in whole-milk dairy products, red meat, and butter) can certainly lower your risk of gallstones by lowering your cholesterol levels. Some studies have also found that even if you eat the same amount of fat, making a switch from saturated fats to monounsaturated fats (found in avocados, nuts, and olive and canola oils) can lower your risk of gallstones.

Increase Your Intake of Fiber

Soluble fiber acts like a sponge to sop up excess cholesterol in the intestines. All fiber-rich foods have a combination of soluble and insoluble fiber, but some have more soluble fiber than others. Apples, pears, strawberries, beans, lentils, and oat bran are all high in soluble fiber. For a more detailed list, see page 199.

Cut Back on Sugar and Other Refined Carbohydrates

Eating sweets and starches in excess amounts can cause a rise in your triglyceride levels. So can being overweight. Switching from refined carbohydrates (crackers, cookies, chips, brownies) to fruits, vegetables, nuts, and low-fat protein sources (fish, skinless chicken, lean cuts of beef) can help improve these levels.

Eat Vitamin C—rich Foods and Consider a Vitamin C Supplement

Vitamin C (ascorbic acid) breaks down cholesterol in the bile, and vitamin C deficiencies have been associated with a higher risk for gallstones. A 2000 study, which confirmed prior studies, also found that women who took vitamin C supplements had a reduced risk of gallbladder disease.

Drink Alcohol and Coffee in Moderation

Alcohol appears to have a protective effect against gall-stones. Women who drink moderate amounts of alcohol (one ounce per day, which is equivalent to two glasses of wine) reduce their risk of gallstones by 20 percent, according to one study.

Coffee also appears to have a protective effect. In a 2002 study, women who drank two to three cups of regular coffee daily (instant, filtered, espresso) had a 22 percent lower risk of developing the disease over twenty years than did women who were not coffee drinkers. Those who drank more than four cups a day had a 28 percent lower risk. I don't recommend going on a coffee binge, however. The benefits and risks of alcohol and caffeine consumption vary depending on an individual's health, so I wouldn't recommend either of them as a preventive measure.

Exercise

Along with its other benefits, regular vigorous exercise may reduce the risk of gallstones and gallbladder disease, even in people who are overweight. One study indicated that men who performed endurance-type exercise (such as jogging and running, racquet sports, and brisk walking) for thirty minutes, five times per week, reduced their risk for gallbladder disease by up to 34 percent. The benefit depended more on the intensity of activity than the type of exercise. Some researchers theorize that in addition to controlling weight, exercise helps normalize blood sugar and insulin levels.

Consider Nonsteroidal Anti-Inflammatory Drugs

Some data indicate that taking an NSAID, such as aspirin or ibuprofen, protects against the development of gallstones. Taking these drugs regularly, however, can lead to other gastrointestinal ills, like ulcers or dyspepsia. What's more, a recent study of more than four hundred chronic arthritis sufferers who took NSAIDs regularly reported no significant protection against gallstones. I have mixed feelings about NSAIDs. I think you need to discuss your own health profile with your doctor to determine if taking them is right for you.

INNOCENT OR UGLY?

Most of the time gallstones are found during tests for other problems. You may be walking around with gallstones and not even know it until poof! one appears on an ultrasound that you're getting for some other reason. For instance, a pregnant woman may have gallstones diagnosed when she has a routine ultrasound to assess the fetus.

Recently a forty-year-old patient, Tina, was having vague pain in her upper abdomen. Her doctor had referred her for an ultrasound, and the test showed that she had two gallstones. She came to me to discuss her situation because she didn't know whether she needed to have her gallbladder removed. After taking Tina's medical history, I really felt that her pain was classic for reflux. We treated her heartburn symptoms, and her pain resolved. On her next visit she said, "So now what should I do about those gallstones?" I told her that asymptomatic gallstones rarely cause problems, and—to Tina's relief—I didn't recommend surgery at this point.

Since Tina was obese, I counseled her on weight-loss measures and told her she would minimize her risk of gallstone attack if she modified her fat intake. I also listed the specific symptoms she should be aware of in case the gallstones ever gave her trouble.

More than 80 percent of people with asymptomatic gallstones wind up never having any problems. Determining whether to treat trouble-free gallstones can be a complicated matter that you need to discuss with your doctor. The American College of Physicians states that when a person has no symptoms, the risks of both surgical and nonsurgical treatment for gallstones outweigh the benefits. I generally take a wait-and-see approach except in very specific cases. If you fall into one of the following categories, your gallstones need to be treated even if they're asymptomatic:

- You're at risk for gallbladder cancer (for example, you have a calcified gallbladder).
- You're a Pima Native American.
- You have a gallstone larger than three centimeters (measured via ultrasound).
- You have large polyps on your gallbladder.

Note: One study reported that very *small* gallstones increase the risk for acute pancreatitis, a serious condition. Some experts therefore believe that gallstones smaller than five millimeters warrant immediate surgery.

The wait-and-see approach does involve certain

minor risks. Gallstones almost never disappear sponta-neously, except sometimes when they are formed under special circumstances, such as during pregnancy or fol-lowing sudden weight loss. At some point, then, asymp-tomatic stones may cause pain, complications, or both and require treatment. Some studies suggest that your age at diagnosis may be a factor in whether your gall-stones will eventually warrant future surgery. The prob-abilities are as follows:

- A 30 percent risk of future surgery for people diag-nosed with gallstones at thirty years old. (Younger people also have a somewhat higher risk of gall-bladder cancer.)
- A 20 percent risk of future surgery for people diag-nosed at fifty years old.
- A 15 percent risk of future surgery for people diag-nosed at seventy years old.

SIGNS OF A GALLBLADDER ATTACK

Classic gallbladder attacks are often triggered by meals. These are typical symptoms:

- You feel steady, severe pain in the mid- or right up-per abdomen (under the rib cage).
- You feel pain in the back, between the shoulder blades, or in the right shoulder.
- This pain occurs several hours after eating and wakes you up during the night.
- The intensity of the pain increases rapidly but dis-appears after one to five hours.

- Changes in position, over-the-counter pain relievers, and passage of gas do not relieve the pain.
- You experience nausea or vomiting.

Gallbladder attacks, known as *biliary colic* in medical lingo, most commonly occur when a gallstone lodges into the cystic duct. The pain resolves when the gallstone dislodges from the cystic duct and falls back into the gallbladder. The whole scenario can happen again if that stone or another one lodges into the cystic duct. Once you have one gallbladder attack, chances are good that you'll have another. Sometimes attacks occur years apart or only once, but this is less common than recurrent attacks spaced months or weeks apart. When a gallstone remains lodged in the cystic or common bile duct, inflammation and infection of the gallbladder (acute cholecystitis) develops. Acute cholecystitis can progress to gangrene or perforation of the gallbladder if left untreated. (Diabetics are at particular risk for this complication.) Urgent medical care, including the use of antibiotics, is necessary to treat infectious gallbladder complications. These complications can be avoided by seeing a doctor as soon as gallbladder symptoms occur.

RED FLAG WARNING SIGNS

You should see a doctor right away if you have any of the following symptoms during a gallbladder attack, since they may indicate an emergency situation:

- prolonged, severe pain and tenderness in the right upper abdomen

- fever and chills
- sweating
- yellowish color of the skin or whites of the eyes
- clay-colored stools

WHEN PROBLEMS HIT
YOUR PANCREAS

Another major complication of gallstones occurs when a stone blocks the small muscular opening, or sphincter, at the end of the common bile duct, called the *papilla of Vater*. At the papilla the bile duct and pancreatic duct join together to empty their contents into the small intestine (duodenum). If a stone lodges at the papilla, it can cause a backup not only of bile but also of pancreatic enzymes. This can irritate the pancreas, a digestive organ that makes and stores digestive enzymes and insulin.

If this happens, the pancreas can become inflamed, causing acute pancreatitis. (Gallstones and excessive alcohol intake account for 85 percent of patients who develop this condition.) Pancreatitis is signaled by severe pain in the upper abdomen that sometimes spreads to the back, lasting hours or even days. Other symptoms include a swollen, tender abdomen, vomiting, fever, and a rapid pulse. Eating even small amounts of food makes the symptoms worse. In severe cases, the pancreas can bleed during an attack, causing tissue damage and infection and releasing enzymes and toxins into the bloodstream, which may damage other organs, including the heart, lungs, and kidneys. This can make the disease life threatening.

If your doctor suspects you have acute pancreatitis,

you'll probably have a blood workup that checks your levels of pancreatic enzymes, calcium, sugar, and lipids. You may also have an abdominal CT scan or possibly an ultrasound to differentiate acute pancreatitis from other potential diagnoses.

GETTING DIAGNOSED

If you have a gallbladder attack, your doctor will probably want to order some blood tests to check the status of your gallbladder. Liver enzymes may be elevated with a bout of acute cholecystitis. A high white blood cell count may also indicate acute inflammation or infection.

In order to get a firm diagnosis of gallstones, your doctor will probably refer you for one of the following tests:

Ultrasound

Many gallstones can be seen with this simple, noninvasive procedure—it's the most commonly performed test to diagnose gallstones. Before the test you must not eat or drink for six or more hours. The test itself generally takes about fifteen minutes. You lie on a table, and a technician rubs some gel on your abdomen and runs a wandlike instrument over your upper abdomen. The sound waves emitted from the wand pass into your abdomen, bounce off your gallbladder, and get translated into an image that appears on a monitor. The stones appear on a screen as solid round objects.

Ultrasound can detect gallstones as small as two millimeters in diameter with an extremely high rate of accuracy. During the same procedure the radiologist can check your liver, bile ducts, and pancreas and quickly scan the gallbladder wall for thickening (characteristic of cholecystitis). Air in the gallbladder wall may indicate gangrene.

Cholescintigraphy

This noninvasive test may be useful if ultrasound does not reveal cholecystitis but the condition is still suspected because of your symptoms. Cholescintigraphy can take one to two hours or more and involves injecting a tiny amount of a radioactive tracer into your bloodstream. This material is taken up by the liver and excreted into bile. A special camera watches the tracer as it passes from the liver into the gallbladder. If the dye fills the common bile duct but does not enter the gallbladder, a gallstone may be blocking the cystic duct.

Oral Cholecystography

This is another noninvasive X-ray procedure that is useful for determining the structural and functional status of the gallbladder. It's usually done to give the surgeon more information before gallbladder surgery. The day before the test you will need to eat a fat-free meal and not eat or drink anything after dinner. Three hours after dinner you will swallow several contrast tablets at five-minute intervals. The contrast dye is absorbed by the intestine, excreted by the liver, and concentrated in the gallbladder.

During the procedure a technician will take X-rays of your gallbladder and liver. The contrast agent will highlight the stones. If a stone is lodged in the cystic duct, the gallbladder will not be seen, as the contrast will bypass it.

Endoscopic Retrograde Cholangiopancreatography (ERCP)

This invasive test involves passing an endoscope (a flexible scope containing a miniature camera and other instruments) through the mouth, past the stomach, and into the duodenum to the papilla of Vater. A catheter can then be passed through the papilla into the common bile duct, allowing X-ray pictures with an injection dye or therapeutic manipulations. ERCP provides an accurate diagnosis of common bile duct stones, but because it is an invasive procedure, it has more risks of complications than other tests and requires considerable skill. ERCP allows your doctor to see the bile duct and to remove small gallstones. This may require making a small incision at the papilla of Vater to widen its opening to allow the gallstones to pass. This is a complicated procedure to perform. If you need to have it, I recommend using a doctor with substantial expertise in this procedure.

Percutaneous Transhepatic Cholangiography

In this test a long, thin needle is inserted through the skin and into the liver to inject a contrast dye into the bile duct. The bile duct is then X-rayed. If necessary, a drainage tube can be left in place to drain bile into a bag outside the skin. This is generally a temporary option. If surgery is not an option, the hole from the skin can be enlarged over several weeks and stones can be removed this way. Obviously this is not a common way of removing stones, but it may be the choice in a patient who is too sick to undergo surgery or ERCP.

Three High-Tech Tests on the Horizon

Endoscopic Ultrasound (EUS), which I've begun performing fairly routinely, involves the insertion of an endoscope with an ultrasound wand attached on one end. EUS is being used more and more and may eventually serve as an alternative to ERCP. It's better than transabdominal ultrasound for looking at the pancreas and bile ducts because the ultrasound wand actually gets closer to these organs than ultrasound that scans through the tissue/fat/skin of the abdominal wall. The scope is designed to allow the passage of instruments that can actually perform the same functions as ERCP, such as the removal of bile duct stones.

Magnetic Resonance Cholangiopancreatography uses magnetic resonance imaging (MRI) and is proving to be very acurate in identifying abnormalities in the pancreas, gallbladder, bile duct, and pancreatic ducts. Like other MRI procedures, this test is expensive and cannot be performed in patients with pacemakers. It is also more difficult for patients who are claustrophobic.

Helical Computed Tomography uses computed tomography (CT) scanning to obtain images of the liver, pancreas, bile duct, and pancreatic duct. It takes less time than a standard CT scan and obtains clearer images.

GETTING TREATED

The type of treatment you receive and the timing of that treatment depend completely on your particular condition. If you are admitted to the hospital with acute cholecystitis, you will likely be treated with intravenous fluids and painkillers initially. If you show signs of a gallbladder infection, such as fever or a high white blood cell count, you will probably be put on antibiotics for 12 to 24 hours. Surgery to remove the gallbladder (cholecystectomy) is usually the next step, but your surgeon may wait one or two days to perform the procedure to allow any inflammation to improve or infection to resolve. If gallstones are found to be blocking

GALLBLADDER CANCER AND PORCELAIN GALLBLADDER

Gallstones are present in about 80 percent of people with gallbladder cancer. This cancer is very rare, however, even among people with gallstones. The exception is in people with so-called porcelain gallbladder. In this condition, the gallbladder wall becomes calcified and looks like porcelain on an X-ray. Prophylactic cholecystectomy is indicated to prevent the subsequent development of cancer, which may occur in up to 20 percent of cases. Whether gallstones themselves cause the cancer or whether some factor in bile is responsible for both conditions is unknown.

your common bile duct, you may require endoscopic retrograde cholangiopancreatography (ERCP) for diagnosis and treatment.

These, though, are the worst-case scenarios. The vast majority of people with gallstones don't have any symptoms. If symptoms do develop, most people have a mild attack that sends them to their doctor's office rather than the emergency room. If you're in this category, your doctor will probably refer you for an ultrasound to make a diagnosis of gallstones. Your doctor will then talk with you about several options for your care: monitoring without medical treatment, nonsurgical removal of the gallstones through medications, or surgical removal of your gallbladder.

SURGERY AND RECOVERY

If you and your doctor decide that your gallstones warrant the removal of your gallbladder, you'll probably have a procedure called a laparoscopic cholecystectomy. This type of "belly button" surgery is performed on hundreds of thousands of patients each year. Laparoscopic cholecystectomy requires general anesthesia, but most procedures are done as outpatient surgery.

The surgeon first creates space in your abdominal cavity by filling it with carbon dioxide, which flows out of a needle inserted through the navel. The surgeon will then make three or four small incisions in the abdomen to insert instruments and a laparoscope, a thin camera that displays the image of the surgery on a video monitor. This type of surgery is a little like a video game.

The surgeon manipulates instruments while watching through the laparoscopic camera. The surgeon's hands are never actually in your abdominal cavity—instead, they guide the instruments to do the cutting and the sewing.

The gallbladder is severed from the cystic duct and blood vessels and is then pulled through one of the incisions in the abdominal wall. The ducts and vessels are stitched closed, and the patient's wounds from the external incisions are usually sealed with strong surgical tape that eventually falls off in a few days.

Let me emphasize that laparoscopy has revolutionized gallbladder removal. First performed in 1987, it is now performed in nearly 75 percent of all cholecystectomies in the United States. Before that, open cholecystectomy (the removal of the gallbladder through an abdominal incision) was the standard treatment.

Laparoscopy has important advantages over open cholecystectomy: There is a short or no hospital stay; the incisions are small, and there is less postoperative pain; and it has fewer complications. This has become one of the most common surgical procedures performed on women. It can even be performed on pregnant women with low risk to the baby and mother.

Five to ten percent of the time a patient undergoing laparoscopy must be switched to an open cholecystectomy procedure. This could occur because the internal structures are not clearly visible (often because of scar tissue from prior surgery), or because unexpected problems crop up, such as bleeding that cannot be stanched. Surgeons sometimes find common bile duct stones, which may not be easily removed by laparoscopy. I want to emphasize that laparoscopy isn't as easy to perform as it sounds. You need a qualified surgeon who is competent in this technique. You should not be shy about inquiring into the number of laparoscopies the surgeon has performed. (It should be thirty or more.)

As with any surgery, you will need some time to recover from a laparoscopic cholecystectomy. For the most part, people experience mild to moderate pain for a few days and return to their full activities within a week. Some patients do experience a short adjustment period during which they have diarrhea. One of my patients recently told me that after the surgery she would be eating and then feel like she had to go to the bathroom right away. This diarrhea lasted three weeks. If your diarrhea lasts for more than a week or two, you should discuss it with your doctor.

Other than that, most women don't need to make any particular modifications to their diet or lifestyle following the surgery. When your gallbladder is removed, you lose the storage capacity for bile, but the bile will simply flow directly from the liver into the small intestine. What's interesting is that we haven't found any evidence that the total amount of bile produced by your body increases to compensate for this alteration. It's a baffling but lucky phenomenon: Patients with no gallbladders have gastrointestinal tracts that function completely normally (unless, of course, they happen to have some other GI problem). So you don't need to worry that you'll be threatening your digestive health if you opt to have the surgery.

NONSURGICAL OPTIONS

If you're reluctant to have surgery or if you have a serious medical problem that increases your risk from surgery, there are several nonsurgical treatments for gallstones. You should be aware, though, that recurrence of gallstones is very likely with these treatments.

Oral dissolution therapy is the most common nonsurgical option. Bile acids in pill form are used to melt gallstones. Ursodiol (Actigall) and chenodiol (Chenix) are both available by prescription and can help get rid of smaller cholesterol gallstones. Only about 30 percent of patients are candidates for oral dissolution therapy. The treatment can take up to two years to dissolve gallstones and can cost thousands of dollars per year. Generally stones will recur when the medication is stopped.

Contact dissolution therapy requires the injection of an organic solvent, methyl tert-butyl ether (MTBE), into the gallbladder to dissolve the gallstones. This procedure is technically difficult and is generally only performed at research hospitals.

Extracorporeal shock wave lithotripsy uses high-energy ultrasound shock waves through the abdominal wall to break up the stones. This therapy works best on small, solitary gallstones.

A small risk of gallbladder cancer is associated with gallstones. According to the National Cancer Institute, fewer than one percent of people with gallstones will develop gallbladder cancer, but in those who are diagnosed with gallbladder cancer, up to 80 percent have gallstones.

GALLBLADDER RESOURCES

AMERICAN GASTROENTEROLOGICAL ASSOCIATION
4930 Del Ray Avenue
Bethesda, MD 20814
tel. (301) 654-2055
www.gastro.org
At www.gastro.org/clinicalRes/brochures/gallstones.html
the AGA provides a brochure on gallstones with
information for both physicians and the public about
symptoms, treatments, research initiatives, continuing
medical education, practice management, medical
position statements, and public policy.

**NATIONAL DIGESTIVE DISEASES INFORMATION
CLEARINGHOUSE**
2 Information Way
Bethesda, MD 20892-3570
tel. (800) 891-5389 or (301) 654-3810
digestive.niddk.nih.gov
At www.niddk.nih.gov/health/nutrit/pubs/dietgall.htm
the clearinghouse provides information on dieting and
gallstones, including weight-loss programs that
minimize your risk of developing gallstones.

MEDLINE PLUS
www.nlm.nih.gov/medlineplus/ency/article/001138.htm
This site run by the National Library of Medicine
contains all you need to know about gallstones from
symptoms to causes and complications. It contains
illustrations and advice on when to call your doctor.

LIVER DISEASE—COULD YOU HAVE IT WITHOUT EVEN KNOWING IT?

WHAT'S A CHAPTER ON LIVER DISEASE doing in a book about digestive health problems? The liver isn't usually the culprit behind gas, constipation, or diarrhea. In fact, liver problems are often silent, causing few symptoms. Still, your liver is vital to good digestive health. It prevents toxins from entering your bloodstream; it stores sugar and other nutrients; and it helps manufacture bile for digestion—to name just a few things that your liver does.

Since the liver (as well as the gallbladder) is connected to the GI tract, gastroenterologists are trained to diagnose and manage liver disease. Unfortunately, far too few women with liver disease are being treated. Many go for years without being properly diagnosed because they aren't aware that they're at risk for having liver problems.

A patient named Anna recently came to my clinic because of unexplained fatigue. Anna, forty-two, is a nurse, so she is familiar with hepatitis and thought that her tiredness and loss of appetite might be attributed to liver problems. I took a blood test, and sure enough, Anna had hepatitis C. "Where could I have gotten it from?" she asked me. "I don't do drugs, and my husband and I are faithful to each other." She also told me she was never accidentally stuck with a needle and followed hospital safety guidelines very carefully. I asked Anna if she had *ever* done drugs at any point in her life. "Well, there was this one time about two decades ago when my husband and I went to a party and tried some sort of amphetamine. But that was the one and only time that I've ever injected any drugs, and I only shared with my husband." I told her that that one time was all she needed. It turned out her husband tested positive for hepatitis C as well. Both were treated with the drugs pegylated interferon (Pegasys, Peg-Intron) and ribavirin (Rebetol, Copegus). Anna cleared her infection with treatment. Unfortunately, her husband did not respond to the treatment, and we are now taking a wait-and-see approach to see if his liver damage progresses.

Hepatitis simply means inflammation of the liver. I want to dispel the myth that it's caused only by infections—it's not. It can result from many causes, including medications, excessive use of alcohol or illegal drugs, autoimmune diseases, fatty infiltration of the liver due to obesity, and genetic diseases—as well as from food-borne viruses and sexually transmitted infections. Cirrhosis—the end result of long-term inflammation from hepatitis—means the liver is scarred. This scar tissue can disrupt liver function and eventually cause liver failure.

Hepatitis makes the news when a celebrity is diagnosed with a form of the virus or has liver problems due to alcoholism. Several years ago actor Larry Hagman's bout with hepatitis due to his excessive use of alcohol made headlines. As I was writing this chapter, TV talk show host Larry King interviewed Pamela Anderson about her recent diagnosis of hepatitis C. She told him about the shock of learning that she had contracted her disease from her ex-husband, who hadn't told her he had it. Country singer Naomi Judd recently announced that she had been cured of hepatitis C after her second round of interferon therapy. These celebrities are helping to increase awareness of hepatitis, and hopefully more women are having themselves tested for this common liver disease.

I can't tell you how many times I've diagnosed liver disease in women who tell me, "I can't have a problem with my liver, I'm feeling fine." Like high blood pressure, you can have the condition and not know it until specific tests are done. If left undiagnosed, liver disease can cause severe problems and can even be life threatening. Some people go on to develop liver failure or liver cancer from liver disease that advances unchecked.

The good news is that most liver diseases are treatable if you are diagnosed before extensive and permanent damage occurs. First, you need to know if you're at risk.

RISK FACTORS

You're at risk for liver disease if you fall into any of the following categories:

- You have a family history of liver disease.
- You drink more than two alcoholic beverages a day on a regular basis.
- You had a blood transfusion before 1992.
- You engaged in intravenous drug use or inhaled an illegal drug, even once.
- You are overweight or you have high lipid levels or diabetes mellitus.
- You engage in high-risk sexual behavior: unprotected sex with multiple partners or with those who have sexually transmitted diseases.
- You're a health care worker, and you are exposed to blood products or suffered a needle-stick accident.
- You have tattoos or body piercing.

HOW YOUR LIVER WORKS

Weighing in at close to three pounds, your liver is your body's largest internal organ, lying underneath your rib cage. Its size underscores its importance.

I like to think of the liver as the "brain" of the digestive tract. All of the nutrients and everything else you ingest (drugs, preservatives, bacteria, etc.) are absorbed from the small intestine and are sent, via the portal vein, to your liver. Liver cells (known as *hepatocytes*) are among the most specialized cells in the body.

Your liver is a master synthesizer, taking simple substances and combining them into larger units. Hepatocytes make the vast majority of proteins circulating in your bloodstream from amino acids, the building blocks of protein. Some of the proteins your liver produces are called binding proteins; they bind to vitamins, hormones, and drugs and transport them throughout the body. One protein, called vitamin D–binding protein, transports, as you probably guessed, vitamin D. Thyroid-binding globulin binds specifically to thyroid hormones. Another protein, called albumin, binds and transports many different substances. Proteins needed to prevent bleeding are made in your liver. Liver cells make bile (which helps to digest fats) and play a major role in the breakdown and synthesis of cholesterol.

As if all this weren't enough, your liver also serves as a large storage tank. Hepatocytes coordinate messages from throughout your body to determine which nutrients your brain and muscles need immediately and which should be stored. Using signals from hormones and nerves, liver cells can change blood sugar (glucose) into a storage form (glycogen). When your body needs energy, the liver converts glycogen back into glucose. The liver also stores vitamins (such as vitamin A, folate, and B_{12}) and minerals (such as iron and copper) until they're needed in other areas of the body. And it regulates hormone levels such as insulin and estrogen in the blood.

Your liver works as a powerful purifier, transforming harmful chemicals into harmless substances. Toxic substances such as drugs and alcohol are inactivated by the liver. What's more, some drugs may be activated (rather than inactivated) by the liver before they can begin working.

While the liver helps your body by detoxifying foreign substances like ethanol (in alcoholic beverages) and nicotine (in cigarettes), it may damage itself in the process. Detoxification of ethanol, for example, can lead to liver injury and ultimately to cirrhosis or scarring. Your liver also breaks down toxins produced by the body itself, like ammonia, which is manufactured in the intestines when food is digested.

SYMPTOMS OF LIVER DISEASE

Jaundice

The most obvious sign of liver disease is jaundice. This condition occurs when the liver isn't functioning properly and fails in its handling of bilirubin, a waste product made from the breakdown of old red blood cells. Normally bilirubin is carried to the liver, where it undergoes chemical changes before it is transferred to the bile and eventually excreted from the body. Having excess bilirubin in the blood can be a sign that your liver isn't functioning properly or can indicate a benign disorder called Gilbert's syndrome (see box on page 362). Elevated bilirubin levels, which can be measured on a routine blood test, often cause signs of jaundice. These are:

- yellowing of the skin and whites of the eyes
- dark urine
- clay-colored stools (sometimes)
- abdominal pain (sometimes)

The Subtle Signs

Jaundice is the most obvious sign of liver disease, but it doesn't always occur. Unlike diseases in other organs, liver disease may cause only subtle, nonspecific signs.

You may have one or two of these symptoms from time to time that have no relation to liver disease. Moreover, liver disease can also be silent and produce none of these symptoms.

- unexplained fatigue
- mild abdominal pain in the right upper quadrant
- menstrual irregularities (cessation of periods, less frequent periods, pain with periods, or irregular bleeding)
- reduction in appetite
- fuzzy thinking (being in a mental fog)
- itchiness of the skin
- easy bleeding or bruising

MAJOR CAUSES OF LIVER DISEASE

Hepatitis A Virus (HAV)

This disease is usually contracted by eating food or drinking water contaminated with fecal matter that contains the virus. Fruits, vegetables, shellfish, and even ice cubes contaminated with sewage-polluted water can carry HAV. The virus can live on a utensil or piece of food for three to four hours. It can also be transmitted through kissing and oral/anal sex. Symptoms of HAV include fatigue, jaundice, fever, nausea, abdominal pain, light-colored stools, and dark-colored urine.

There is no cure for HAV, though its symptoms can be treated. The virus usually runs its course and clears up on its own—in a month or two. In some cases, symptoms can last for up to a year.

This disease is completely preventable if you get a vaccine for hepatitis A. The Centers for Disease Control and Prevention (CDC) recommend the vaccine for those at high risk of contracting the virus.

Hepatitis B Virus (HBV)

This virus affects more than a million people in the United States. In fact, according to the CDC, some 4,000 to 5,000 people in this country die each year from HBV-related liver failure or liver cancer. Most new cases occur in teens and young adults (particularly homosexual men), since sexual contact is the most common form of transmission of the virus. It's also spread through infected needle-sticks in intravenous drug users. Over 90 percent of cases resolve after the acute infection with jaundice clears up, usually after several weeks. Once the infection is gone, people generally develop an antibody that protects them from being infected with this virus again. About five percent of those exposed to the virus as adults become chronically infected, which means they carry the virus for longer than six months. These patients have a higher risk of developing cirrhosis of the liver and liver cancer.

Hepatitis virus can also be spread quite easily from mother to infant during delivery. Persistent infection is more common in infants and children who are exposed to the virus. Studies show that the transmission rate to infants is as high as 70 percent if the mother is infected with HBV. This risk to the infant can be reduced to less than five percent if the baby receives protective antibodies and the vaccine at birth. For this reason, all pregnant women are given a blood test during their first prenatal visit to see if they carry HBV. *If you're pregnant or are planning to get pregnant, it's vital to have an HBV test to ensure that your baby receives preventive medication at the time of delivery.*

The good news is that there's a very effective vaccine that can prevent HBV—and it's the first vaccine that can prevent a form of cancer by preventing the acquisition of infection. This vaccine (given in a series of three shots: at one to two weeks old, one month, and six months) is recommended for all children under age eighteen and for adults at high risk.

Three treatments—interferon, lamivudine (Epivir), and adefovir (Hepsera)—can help keep HBV from seriously damaging your liver and occasionally can eradicate the virus completely. Doctors generally speak of controlling HBV rather than curing it, since the medications are not very effective at getting rid of HBV for good. However, they can keep the virus at bay and reduce liver damage. Not every person with chronic HBV infection needs treatment, but it is important to discuss this issue with your doctor.

Hepatitis C Virus (HCV)

This virus affects more than four million people in the United States, according to the CDC. If left untreated, between 55 and 85 percent of HCV cases become chronic (infection lasting longer than six months), which can lead to scarring of the liver, liver cancer, and liver failure. HCV is currently the leading cause of liver transplantation in the United States.

A HARMLESS LIVER DISORDER

Three to seven percent of Americans have an elevated bilirubin level without liver disease. This common condition is called Gilbert's (pronounced jill-*bare*) syndrome and is a benign, hereditary liver disorder. Having this condition simply means that the body produces excess bilirubin or that there's some interference in excreting bilirubin out of the body. It does not, however, indicate liver disease.

Symptoms of Gilbert's are virtually nonexistent. Occasionally mild jaundice may appear, especially after fasting or lack of sleep. Gilbert's usually shows up during a routine blood draw and is diagnosed when bilirubin is elevated but all other liver readings from the blood are normal. Gilbert's doesn't require treatment and won't interfere with a normal lifestyle.

Transmission of HCV mainly occurs through the exchange of contaminated blood. Intravenous drug users are at high risk, but transmission can also occur through unsterilized tattoo or body-piercing equipment, manicuring tools (those used to trim cuticles and remove calluses), and even razors at the barber shop. These items may become contaminated by microscopic amounts of blood without you knowing it. (One study found that the blue juice containers in beauty salons where razors, scissors, and combs soak provide an environment where HCV can thrive for three months.) Blood transfusion was the number-one cause of hepatitis C before more reliable donor screening began in 1992. Those who had a blood transfusion prior to this date are at risk for chronic HCV infection. Health care workers who get stuck with contaminated needles also are at risk. HCV can be sexually transmitted, but the risk is low and nowhere near as high as with HBV. Women with a sexual partner who has or had hepatitis C should be tested for HCV. Unlike HBV, this virus is passed from mother to fetus only five percent of the time, which is why pregnant women aren't screened for HCV. Up to ten percent of cases of HCV have no identifiable cause.

Unfortunately, there is no vaccine for HCV because the virus mutates easily into new variations. Six different genotypes and thirty different subtypes of HCV are currently known—each is unique, and several respond differently to the available treatments.

Newer treatments for HCV are now available. Overall, some 55 percent of people treated for HCV will have eradication of the virus long term. Pegylated interferon plus ribavirin is a standard therapy. Ribavirin, however, is teratogenic, which means it can cause birth defects, and it stays active in the body for six months after therapy is stopped. *Women who are treated with ribavirin should not become pregnant during treatment and for six months after taking the drug because of the risk of birth defects. A woman's partner must also be off ribavirin for six months before they try to conceive.*

Alcohol-Induced Cirrhosis

Alcohol takes a far greater toll on a woman's liver than on a man's. Women tend to weigh less than men, so

SHOULD YOU GET A HEPATITIS VACCINE?

VACCINATION GUIDELINES FOR HEPATITIS A VACCINE

The CDC recommends that the following people be vaccinated against hepatitis A:

- people traveling to or working in countries with high or intermediate rates of hepatitis A, including Mexico. (The CDC website, www.cdc.gov, has a list of these countries.)
- children over two years old in communities that have high rates of hepatitis A or periodic outbreaks. In this country that means American Indian and Native Alaskan populations.
- those who engage in homosexual sex
- illegal drug users
- people with chronic liver disease, including hepatitis B and C
- workers with an occupational risk for infection (health care workers, researchers who use HAV in their labs, those who work with primates)
- people with clotting-factor disorders who are given clotting-factor concentrates

Although the CDC does not specifically recommend vaccination for those on hemodialysis or with HIV/AIDS, they do say it is safe and effective for these groups. Discuss this issue with your doctor.

fewer drinks can have a more toxic effect. Even if we compare a woman and a man of the same body weight, pound for pound alcohol does more damage to the woman's liver. One possible reason is that women have

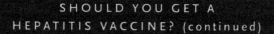

SHOULD YOU GET A HEPATITIS VACCINE? (continued)

VACCINATION GUIDELINES FOR HEPATITIS B VACCINE

The CDC recommends routine vaccination for hepatitis B for the following people:

- everyone under eighteen years of age
- all health care workers
- anyone older than eighteen who is at risk for the disease: those with multiple sex partners, homosexuals, injection drug users, anyone who may come into contact with infected blood or body fluids

lower levels of alcohol dehydrogenase, an enzyme that helps to break down alcohol in the stomach before it reaches the liver.

Imbibing too much can damage the liver by causing a condition called *alcoholic hepatitis*. This acute injury to the liver (if women continue to drink) can progress to scarring, called fibrosis, which can in turn lead to cirrhosis and end-stage liver failure.

My rule of thumb on alcohol consumption for women is: Don't drink more than two drinks a day. (Men may be able to tolerate up to four drinks a day without significant liver damage, more than twice what a woman can drink.)

Note: If you have chronic liver disease of any type (caused by viral hepatitis, a genetic disorder, obesity, etc.), you should not drink any alcohol at all. Even a little

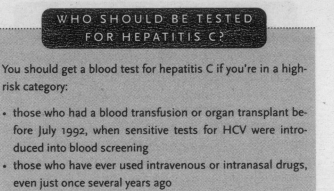

WHO SHOULD BE TESTED FOR HEPATITIS C?

You should get a blood test for hepatitis C if you're in a high-risk category:

- those who had a blood transfusion or organ transplant before July 1992, when sensitive tests for HCV were introduced into blood screening
- those who have ever used intravenous or intranasal drugs, even just once several years ago
- health care workers who suffer needle-sticks
- infants born to a hepatitis C–infected mother
- sexual partner of person with hepatitis C

alcohol can be extremely damaging to your liver if it's already diseased. Alcohol combined with acetaminophen can be a particularly dangerous combination and can cause a severe, acute liver injury and even liver failure. If you are using acetaminophen on a regular basis for any reason (flulike illness, arthritis, headaches, etc.), you should avoid alcohol.

Nonalcoholic Fatty Liver Disease

As I mentioned in Chapter 3, being obese can dramatically increase your risk of liver problems. Nonalcoholic fatty liver disease (NAFLD) affects 10 to 24 percent of the general American population, but the incidence increases to as high as 74 percent in obese individuals. Obesity, especially in the abdominal area, is the most common risk factor. About three-quarters of those with NAFLD are women, and those with adult-onset diabetes and elevated triglyceride levels have an even greater risk.

NAFLD encompasses a spectrum of disorders ranging from a mild condition called simple fatty liver (steatosis) to life-threatening cirrhosis. In the middle of this spectrum is a condition called nonalcoholic steatohepatitis (NASH), inflammation and liver injury related to the presence of the fat. Like liver problems caused by excess alcohol consumption, NASH can lead to scarring and progress to cirrhosis and eventually liver failure and even cancer.

NAFLD is believed to be the most common cause of *cryptogenic cirrhosis,* which has no symptoms and no apparent cause. Patients are counseled to lose weight and exercise and to abstain from alcohol. Newer therapies are currently being studied in clinical trials. These include antioxidants (such as vitamin E or S-adenosyl methionine), insulin sensitizing agents (such as metformin [Glucophage]), ursodeoxycholic acid or ursodiol (Actigall), probiotics, and lipid-lowering agents (such as gemfibrozil [Lopid] or one of the statins).

Medications

Nearly every drug out there can cause you significant injury if your liver is not able to properly handle the medication. In fact, one of the most common causes of liver disease among elderly people is one or more of the medications they're taking on a regular basis. Usually the hepatitis reverses itself once they go off the medication. Ibuprofen products (like Advil and Motrin) as well as other nonsteroidal anti-inflammatory drugs are common offenders. Healthy people who take these medications on a regular basis can have elevated liver enzymes and not even be aware of it. Excessive doses of vitamin A found in some vitamin supplements can also cause liver damage.

Prescription drugs that are more likely to cause liver damage include:

- "statins" to improve cholesterol levels: lovastatin (Mevacor), simvastatin (Zocor), pravastatin (Pravachol), and others
- high blood pressure medications: lisinopril (Prinivil), captopril (Capoten), labetalol (Trandate)
- antibiotics: ciprofloxacin (Cipro), erythromycin (ERYC, EES), nitrofurantoin (Macrobid, Macrodantin), isoniazid (Laniazid), and tetracycline (Sumycin, Achromycin)
- diabetes medications: glipizide (Glucotrol), troglitazone
- antifungal drugs, used to treat nail, skin, and systemic fungal infections: ketoconazole (Nizoral), fluconazole (Diflucan), itraconazole (Sporanox), and terbinafine (Lamisil)

When it comes to medications, liver injury is usually rare but is also unpredictable. Your doctor may take particular care to prescribe a medication that isn't associated with liver injury, but sometimes you simply can't avoid a medication that's needed to combat other health maladies. If risk to your liver is a concern, consult your physician about performing regular blood tests to monitor your liver enzyme levels while you're on the medication.

Autoimmune Disorders and Genetic Diseases

Occasionally, liver disease can be caused by an autoimmune disorder (like rheumatoid arthritis or lupus). Autoimmune hepatitis is far more common in women than in men, as are autoimmune diseases in general.

Genetic diseases usually run in families, and you may want to discuss this possibility with your doctor if you have a family history of liver disease. One genetic condition called *hereditary hemochromatosis* occurs when your liver stores too much iron. The excess iron can set up an inflammatory hepatitis in the liver that can ultimately lead to cirrhosis. This condition often isn't diagnosed until after a woman goes through menopause since she loses iron every month with menstruation. Many women may be carriers of this gene or have the condition without even knowing it. It usually requires two abnormal genes (one from both parents) to develop the disease. The disease is very common, present in as many as one in a hundred Caucasians worldwide. There is a genetic test to screen for this condition. If hereditary hemochromatosis is diagnosed and treated before the development of cirrhosis, long-term liver complications can be avoided.

LIVER DISEASE IN PREGNANCY

A small percentage of women develop liver disease for the first time during pregnancy. These liver problems are

TOXIC TYLENOL?

Many seemingly innocuous medications can cause significant injury to the liver if the liver isn't able to properly process them. Acetaminophen (Tylenol) can cause severe liver damage if taken with alcohol. The product label now contains a warning alerting those who regularly consume three or more drinks a day to consult their physician on the use of this medication. In those with pre-existing liver disease (such as chronic hepatitis), a rule of thumb is that the maximum dose of acetaminophen should be 2000 milligrams (four extra-strength tablets or six regular-strength tablets) per day, but you should check with your doctor to determine what's safe for you.

Ibuprofen and other NSAIDs can be dangerous, too. People with liver disease should avoid these products altogether since they can cause significant liver injury in susceptible individuals. They should also avoid dietary supplements containing high doses of vitamin A or iron since these can damage a diseased liver. Additionally, all women should stay away from herbal supplements containing valerian root, chaparral leaf, and comfrey—all of which can cause liver damage and even liver failure.

pretty rare, but they can be quite serious and require immediate medical attention. Additionally, women with chronic liver disease may experience a change in their symptoms during pregnancy.

If you experience abdominal pain in your right upper abdomen or other symptoms such as jaundice, fever, persistent nausea and vomiting (especially after the first trimester of pregnancy), swelling in your arms and legs, unusually large weight gain, light-headedness, easy bruising, or persistent itchiness, you may have a liver problem. Some of these symptoms occur normally in pregnancy, but you should still alert your doctor. He

DID YOU KNOW?

Liver transplantation has made some amazing advances in the past few years. Adults can now be living donors to other adults who are in need of liver transplants. (There is a huge shortage of livers from deceased organ donors, and many patients with cirrhosis and liver failure die before receiving a new liver.) Living donors have been used in children for over a decade with excellent results. For children, a smaller portion of the liver is donated (usually the left lobe or part of the left lobe). Living donor liver transplantation for adults is still fairly new and involves healthy donors giving up the right lobe (about 60 percent) of their liver to the recipient. Since a healthy liver can regenerate itself, both the donor and recipient "halves" can grow to full size and full liver function in a matter of weeks.

Donors and recipients must match blood types, and donors must undergo a very detailed evaluation to ensure that they do not have any health problems that would make donation less than safe for them. About four hundred right lobe living donor procedures have been performed in adults in the United States, as this book goes to press. The healthy donors must undergo invasive surgery, and their risk of dying has been estimated at 0.3 percent. This new technique has been life saving for many patients with liver failure and represents an important step forward in liver transplantation.

or she may want to do additional blood tests to evaluate your liver. Here are some rare but serious conditions that can occur.

- **Hepatitis:** Acute viral hepatitis is the most common cause of jaundice in pregnancy.
- **Hyperemesis gravidarum:** This condition can occur in women who have severe morning sickness where constant nausea and vomiting lead to dehydration and electrolyte imbalances. Some women can become slightly jaundiced in the first trimester as a result of not getting enough nutrients into their body. Specific treatment isn't usually necessary for this liver problem. Treatment aims at controlling vomiting and replacing fluid and electrolytes and keeping up nutrition.
- **Preeclampsia-induced liver disease:** Preeclampsia is associated with pregnancy-induced high blood pressure and occurs in five to ten percent of pregnancies, often during the third trimester. Your doctor tests for preeclampsia by taking your blood pressure during every prenatal exam and checking for protein in your urine. Among other problems, preeclampsia can cause liver problems and can, in extremely rare cases, lead to liver failure. It can also cause premature delivery or poor growth in the fetus. The good news is that preeclampsia and the liver problems associated with it clear up after childbirth. Sometimes early delivery is recommended if the life of the mother or fetus is in danger.
- **Acute fatty liver of pregnancy (AFLP):** This condition most often occurs during the third trimester and is

often associated with preeclampsia. Although it's very rare (occurring in just one in thirteen thousand pregnancies), AFLP can be very serious. Symptoms include headache, nausea, vomiting, malaise, jaundice, abdominal discomfort, and confusion. Once the condition is diagnosed, the pregnant woman should be hospitalized and delivery undertaken to help ensure a favorable outcome in both mother and baby. Early delivery is the most effective treatment for this condition, which usually resolves after childbirth.

13

IRRITABLE BOWEL
SYNDROME—IT'S NOT
ALL IN YOUR HEAD

IRRITABLE BOWEL SYNDROME (IBS) is epidemic in this country, affecting as many as 25 million Americans. Nearly 70 percent of IBS sufferers are women, which is why I think this is a particularly important chapter. In the United States the condition (previously called spastic colon, spastic colitis, or mucus colitis) accounts for 12 percent of visits to primary care doctors and 28 percent of visits to gastroenterologists. Yet IBS has no single cause and no single cure.

This fact can be perplexing both to doctors who treat IBS and to patients who suffer through its symptoms. I can tell you that I spend a lot of time reassuring my IBS patients that their symptoms are caused by a real medical problem but one that, thankfully, isn't life threatening.

Sadly, many women suffer silently with IBS symptoms because they're too embarrassed or afraid to talk about their symptoms or because they believe "that's just the way it is. I just have to live like this." Only 10 to

20 percent of IBS sufferers actually seek medical attention. The rest self-treat with over-the-counter remedies and endure chronic bouts of diarrhea, abdominal pain, gassiness, constipation, and nausea—all of which can occur with IBS.

Gina, a woman who recently came to my clinic, is a perfect example of this second group. After turning forty last year, Gina started taking stock of her health. She went to her family practitioner for a general physical and had some screening tests, which included a mammogram and a bone density exam.

Gina came to see me because she wanted to make sure she was covering all her bases. "Every time I'm stressed, I develop diarrhea and severe abdominal cramps," she told me. "I've had this problem for twenty years, but I just want to make sure it's not anything I need to worry about."

In college, final-exam week always triggered Gina's symptoms. When she went to work at an advertising firm, she found herself running to the bathroom right before she had to give a big presentation to a client. Gina also noticed that certain foods made her symptoms worse. She avoided pizza and leafy salads during her episodes. She also found that sometimes her diarrhea and cramps became excruciating right before menstruation.

I asked Gina, "Why are you coming to me now? Why didn't you see a doctor years ago?" She told me that her symptoms had recently become almost unbearable. She was afraid of going out to social events during an attack for fear of spending the whole night in the bathroom. I immediately suspected IBS because Gina's symptoms always improved after she got through a particularly stressful time. She was never awakened at night with diarrhea and never had blood in her stool—symptoms that can indicate inflammatory bowel disease or possibly cancer.

In fact, although Gina could have been helped much earlier, women with IBS are far better off today than they were ten years ago. First of all, there's an increased awareness among doctors that IBS is a real medical disorder with real symptoms that can be treated. Second, women themselves are much more knowledgeable about IBS. Most of us have heard of this medical problem, know a friend or relative who has it, and are familiar with its symptoms. Last, researchers are also finding new causes for IBS and are beginning to distinguish potential triggers for this condition. By pinpointing specific culprits (like increased sensitivity in the gut, a motility problem, a brain-gut interaction, or a gastrointestinal infection) that may set the stage for IBS, we may be able to develop more specific treatments. And we have far more effective ways to treat IBS than ever before. Two prescription drugs designed exclusively for use in women have entered the market as I write this book. Tegaserod (Zelnorm) is a new drug used to treat constipation in women with IBS. Alosetron (Lotronex), used to treat diarrhea in women with IBS, was reintroduced in the market in 2002. Both of these drugs have given doctors more medical options in treating IBS in women. (See "Medications for IBS" on page 406.)

Before I give you more details on effectively managing IBS, let's first explore what's happening in your GI tract to trigger IBS.

WHAT IS IBS?

IBS is a common disorder of the intestines that leads to crampy pain, gassiness, bloating, and changes in bowel habits. Some women with IBS have constipation, whereas others have diarrhea, and still others experience both. The most common definition used today for IBS is called the Rome II Criteria (see box, page 378). Not all people with IBS fit these criteria, as they were developed for research purposes. But they are helpful as a guide for physicians and lay people to understand the most common symptoms of IBS.

IBS is referred to as a functional disorder, which means the abnormality is caused by an altered way in which the body works rather than by a structural or biochemical problem. Symptoms result from some sort of disruption in the communication between the colon and the brain via the complex system of nerves linking the two. Since IBS is a functional disorder, it can't be diagnosed like other GI problems—that is, through a blood test, scoping procedure, X-ray, or ultrasound. In fact, with IBS, there are no signs of disease when the colon is examined.

THE BRAIN IN YOUR GI TRACT

Research is homing in on the exact causes of IBS, but at this point what we know is that the culprits lie somewhere in the nervous system of the brain and gut. Just

ROME II CRITERIA

Within the past year you've had twelve weeks (not necessarily consecutively) of abdominal discomfort accompanied by two of three of the following features:

- pain or discomfort relieved by having a bowel movement
- onset of pain or discomfort associated with more frequent or less frequent bowel movements
- onset of pain or discomfort associated with a change in stool appearance or form (for example, looser stools or hard, lumpy stools)

Additional symptoms, which are also IBS related, include abnormal stool frequency (less than three per week or more than three per day), abnormal stool passage (straining, urgency, feeling of incomplete evacuation, passage of mucus, bloating, or feeling of abdominal distension).

as your brain has a network of nerve cells, called the central nervous system (CNS), that enables it to communicate with the rest of your body, your GI tract has its own nervous system called the enteric nervous system (ENS). Often called the "minibrain" of the GI tract, the ENS performs a multitude of functions: It coordinates the wavelike movements of the GI tract muscles as they push food through; it determines when digestive chemicals are released into the stomach and intestines; and it triggers the reflex that makes you feel the urge to defecate.

The ENS also passes messages back and forth to the CNS along a network of connections called the brain-gut axis. Thus, your brain gets a full status report on how well your GI tract is working, and your GI tract gets a status report on whether you're feeling anxious or relaxed.

The ENS helps your six-foot-long colon process two quarts of liquid matter each day. It coordinates the rhythmic pulses of muscles that move food through your small intestine into your colon and the timed secretion of digestive fluids. The ENS also plays a role in triggering the reflexes that initiate the excretion of stool out through the rectum. Movement of food through the colon (called *colonic motility*) is controlled by chemicals like hormones and neurotransmitters that coordinate the electrical activity within the wall of the colon. The electrical activity serves as a "pacemaker" similar to the mechanism that regulates your heartbeat. With normal colonic motility, stool contents move slowly back and forth in the colon, edging closer and closer toward the rectum. A few times each day strong muscle contractions move down the colon, pushing fecal material ahead of them. Some of these strong contractions or reflexes result in a bowel movement.

As you can see, the orchestration of moving food through your colon is quite complex and really requires all systems to be in full-functioning order for everything to run smoothly. Lucky for us, the ENS functions at an involuntary level, which means we can't consciously control the workings of our GI tract. This is convenient because, as great as women are at multitasking, we'd be extremely overloaded if we had to think about the proportion of digestive chemicals needed to handle the latte and biscotti we just ate!

Being stressed, nervous, depressed, angry, or anxious can cause the brain to send a message along your brain-gut axis, which can trigger an alteration in the functioning of the GI tract. Colonic motility may increase or decrease or establish a pattern of out-of-sync contractions. Secretions of digestive enzymes or stomach acid may increase. Or the sensitivity of the nerves lining your colon may be heightened, so you feel pain from the normal movements of food through your colon.

After reacting to your brain's distress signal, your GI tract transmits a message back to your brain, which is how you become aware of abdominal pain, nausea, or the sudden urge to move your bowels. Sensory nerves around the colon usually send "pain" signals to the brain only when the colon gets full and stretches (from excess gas or stool) or when the colon spasms and squeezes tight. Your brain is highly astute at distinguishing the type of pain (burning, sharp, squeezing, bloating, crampy) and severity (wrenching, intolerable, mild).

Your GI tract doesn't, however, have the same fine sensory nerves as your skin, so it can't sense things like a temperature change or a light tickle from food particles moving through. In fact, many of my patients can't feel me snipping off polyps during a colonoscopy.

Even if you don't have IBS, you can experience GI changes during times of extreme mental distress. For instance, you may experience the sensation of "butterflies in the stomach" when you're about to speak in front of a group of five hundred people. Or you may get cramps or diarrhea. One of my friends spent two hours before her wedding ceremony vomiting in the bathroom. Yet she felt perfectly fine the moment after she kissed the groom and went into the reception.

THE FAULTY WIRING BEHIND IBS

With IBS, there's a breakdown somewhere along the brain-gut axis. Stool or gas may move spastically instead of smoothly through the colon, causing pain or bloating. Motility may be too quick, causing diarrhea, or too slow, causing constipation. Or there may just be a miscommunication between your brain and your gut, causing you to feel pain when all systems are actually operating without a hitch. Sometimes nerves surrounding your GI tract send pain signals to the brain even when stool contents are moving through normally.

Pain and other IBS symptoms may also be caused by overactive muscles in the wall of the colon or by a heightened sensitivity to distention. Researchers have found that the colon in a person with IBS will begin to spasm even after only mild stimulation (such as placement of a small balloon into the rectum). They've also found that IBS patients feel more pain when the colon is distended with gas or when air is introduced into the colon during a colonoscopy.

People with IBS are acutely aware of the workings of their GI tract. They may be more sensitive to gas after a meal, or they may feel cramps or bloating triggered by the motility of their colon as it moves food through. They usually have a heightened sense of their body's digestive processes and know that these processes can be easily disrupted if they veer from their normal eating habits or lifestyle activities. Miscommunication between the ENS and the CNS is the reason symptoms can occur in IBS patients not just during times of severe stress or emotional mayhem but from a tiff with a co-worker, missing a few hours of sleep, or the onset of a menstrual period. Unlike those without IBS who pretty much take their GI tract for granted, those with IBS regularly have their digestive tract on their mind.

IBS can manifest in different degrees of severity. In its milder form, symptoms occur intermittently and are closely related to your food intake, bowel movements, or stress. In its severest form, symptoms occur daily and are unrelenting and at times incapacitating. If you have IBS, you'll likely have good colon days and bad colon days. Often a trigger sets off the symptoms. Learning to identify the triggers that cause your IBS symptoms, which I explore in this chapter, can help immensely in avoiding attacks.

WHY ARE WOMEN SO VULNERABLE?

Until recently, gastroenterologists were at a loss to explain why women make up such a disproportionate number of IBS sufferers. A dearth of women in research studies left a lot of unanswered questions. Since the National Institutes of Health set up its Office of Research on Women's Health in 1990, an increasing number of studies suggest that gender differences in pain perception, physiological response to stress, and gastrointestinal function may partly explain why women are more susceptible to IBS.

Women with IBS often find that their symptoms are linked to their menstrual cycle. One review study from Great Britain found that almost 50 percent of women with IBS report an increase in symptoms during menstruation. What's more, one-third of healthy women say that they experience GI symptoms (a change in bowel habits, bloating, harder or looser

IS DIETARY FAT THE CULPRIT?

Many IBS sufferers say their symptoms often occur just after they begin a meal. Certain meals, however, can trigger more acute symptoms than others. Researchers are just beginning to find clues as to why this occurs.

Eating causes contractions of the colon. Normally this response, called the *gastrocolic reflex*, may cause an urge to have a bowel movement within thirty to sixty minutes after a meal. In people with IBS the urge may come sooner, with cramps and diarrhea. The strength of the response is often related to the number of calories and especially the amount of fat in a meal. Fat in any form (animal or vegetable) is a strong stimulus of colonic contractions after a meal. In fact, many IBS sufferers find that their symptoms are excruciating after eating out at their favorite restaurants. Restaurant fare is notoriously high in hidden fat and calories that come from cream, butter, whole milk, and oils that are used generously in many dishes to give them flavor and mouthfeel.

stools) during their periods. The study also found that women with IBS tend to have more abdominal pain with their periods (known as *dysmenorrhea*).

A study conducted by Sunanda Kane, M.D., and her colleagues at the University of Chicago found that IBS patients reported diarrhea more often during menstruation than healthy women and were more likely to experience a cyclical pattern to their symptoms. Women with IBS in this study tended to experience an aggravation in their symptoms, premenstrually or during the onset of menstruation. The researchers also found that women with IBS were more likely to suffer from premenstrual syndrome and painful menstrual periods than women without IBS.

As I discussed in Chapter 2, the sex hormones estrogen and progesterone may play a major role in your digestive tract functioning—especially if you have IBS. We don't know exactly how these hormones alter GI function. For instance, is it the drop in estrogen and progesterone levels just before menstruation that triggers symptoms? Or is it the body's response to the fluctuation in hormone levels that sends the digestive tract into a tailspin? Other chemicals, called *prostaglandins,* that are released to prevent hemorrhaging during menstruation may also play a role in triggering diarrhea or loose stools.

The role of hormones was further confirmed by research showing that having a hysterectomy could alter the course of IBS. Six months after a hysterectomy 60 percent of women with IBS found that their symptoms had improved, while 20 percent found that their symptoms had gotten worse. And 10 percent of hysterectomy patients who did not previously have IBS reported that they had developed IBS symptoms following the surgery.

A significant percentage of women also find that their bowel habits change significantly once they hit perimenopause or after their periods cease altogether—once again probably due to an alteration in sex hormones.

However, IBS isn't only a matter of having two X chromosomes or female sex hormones. In the United States and in western Europe, IBS is more common in women. But in other parts of the world—for example, in India— IBS is more common in men. And in other countries the gender breakdown is fifty-fifty. So the cause of the female predominance in the United States is uncertain. It may come from gender differences in seeking out a health care provider or from other triggers, such as sociocultural norms and expectations. For instance, in the corporate workplace, it may be more accepted for a woman to take sick days for cramps or diarrhea than for a man. I know my eight-year-old daughter will be more likely to seek out the school nurse for a stomachache than my eleven-year-old son, who might be worried that he'll miss his soccer game.

IS STRESS EXACERBATING YOUR SYMPTOMS?

Research suggests that people with IBS are more likely to be depressed or have anxiety, but I want to emphasize that having IBS doesn't automatically mean you have a mental disorder. Yes, you may be experiencing more stress in your life than someone who doesn't have IBS. But more important, your body is handling the stress in a different way.

Those with IBS have a malfunction in their colon that makes it more vulnerable to the detrimental effects of stress. A fight with a spouse or the loss of an important client at work can trigger crushing abdominal pains and diarrhea in an IBS sufferer, whereas it might trigger an excruciating migraine in someone else.

A patient named Suzanne, a thirty-six-year-old attorney, told me that she always develops diarrhea and cramping whenever she's under stress or run-down. "I have a stressful case, my IBS gets worse. I'm exhausted from traveling on a business trip, my IBS gets worse. Whenever my routine gets a little tripped up, I know my IBS is going to rear its ugly head," she says.

Stress is a huge aggravator of GI problems. A recent survey of college students at a major university found that 70 percent suffered from temporary bowel problems when they were under stress. Most suffered from diarrhea or constipation, and about half of the students also mentioned abdominal pain. So even for those who don't have IBS, normal bowel function can become uncomfortable during times when they feel anxious.

For women who suffer from IBS, recurrent episodes of stress can enhance their sensitivity to even normal GI stimuli and also escalate that response over time, even when the stimulus remains the same. For example, studies in patients with IBS showed that they subjectively felt more pain when a balloon was inflated in their rectum. When the balloon stayed inflated for more than a few minutes, the IBS patients described a larger area of pain and increased severity of pain. Healthy people, in contrast, experienced no additional discomfort, regardless of how long the balloon was distended. A conclusion to be drawn from this study is that prolonged stress not only prolongs IBS symptoms but can actually make them worse over time.

The cause of this heightened sensitivity is unknown. Some researchers theorize that it involves chemicals such as hormones or neurotransmitters that the GI tract, brain, or glands release during periods of stress. This complex cascade of events still isn't completely understood. Researchers are working to answer the remaining questions in an effort to develop better IBS treatments. Other researchers are studying the microenvironment of the colon. All of us have normal colonic bacteria, but some researchers postulate that increased stress may change the way we eat or depress our immune systems. Both of these things can alter the delicate balance of bacteria, which may be linked to IBS.

DID YOU HAVE A GI INFECTION?

Evidence is mounting to suggest that IBS may be triggered by a bacterial or viral infection. My colleague Anthony Lembo, M.D., an IBS expert at Beth Israel Deaconess Medical Center in Boston, estimates that 20 to 30 percent of IBS patients had an acute gastrointestinal infection that preceded their IBS. It could have been a case of traveler's diarrhea, salmonella poisoning, or intestinal virus, but in general the more severe the infection and the longer it lasted, the greater the likelihood of developing IBS.

Experts haven't yet mapped out the exact connection between intestinal invaders and IBS. In most cases, the infection does not remain the cause of IBS symptoms. Our own immune system can generally take care of the infection, but what remains may be an increase in motility, an increase in gut secretions, or a decreased ability of the gut to absorb water, all of which can result in cramping and diarrhea. It's not uncommon for a woman to come to my clinic with IBS symptoms and, after some reflection, recollect that the diarrheal symptoms all began after an episode of "Montezuma's revenge" or some other GI "bug."

Some patients may have a bacterial overgrowth in their small intestine that was spurred by an infection or by antibiotics used to treat the infection. In a study conducted at the Cedars-Sinai Medical Center in Los Angeles, researchers performed a lactulose hydrogen breath test on two hundred IBS patients to detect the presence of a bacterial overgrowth in the small intestine. They found excessive bacteria in 78 percent of the patients and treated them with a ten-day course of antibiotics. Treatment with antibiotics reduced or eliminated the bacteria in more than half of these patients, leading to significant improvements in their symptoms and even curing IBS in some.

Perhaps some infections leave a lasting impact on the immune cells that surround the GI tract. This intriguing area of IBS research has spurred a number of new studies looking at different oral antibiotics and even probiotics to change the colonic bacterial flora.

Antibiotic therapy is certainly not the mainstay of IBS treatment, but I'm definitely going to keep an eye on the research as it comes out, and your doctor should as well.

GETTING THE CORRECT DIAGNOSIS

Let's face it: When you go see your doctor, you're looking for the right diagnosis and then some kind treatment to alleviate your symptoms. In order to help your doctor make an accurate diagnosis, you need to provide a clear, accurate, and perhaps even chronological description of your IBS symptoms.

When I was training as a gastroenterology fellow, I was struck by how many women with incredibly different symptoms were lumped into one diagnosis of IBS. Some women had bloating and a sense of incomplete evacuation after they went to the bathroom, while others had so many episodes of diarrhea, they knew the location of every toilet in town. How could all these women have IBS?

Today we know a lot more about IBS than we did a decade or two ago. In the past, conditions like microscopic colitis and lactose intolerance were labeled IBS. We now distinguish between these various disorders and IBS. We also distinguish between IBS patients. Some women have more constipation, and these women have different needs and probably a different treatment regimen than a woman who has IBS that manifests itself as abdominal pain.

The questions your doctor will ask and the tests he or she will recommend will vary based on whether your dominant symptom is constipation, diarrhea, alternating diarrhea and constipation, abdominal pain, or some other variant of IBS. (You can find descriptions of the medical tests and treatments that pertain to each symptom in Part II.)

Your evaluation will be individualized and will depend on many factors, such as your age, sex, family history of gastrointestinal disease, presence of stress or other psychological factors, and specific symptom predominance. If you have "alarm signs" like unexplained weight loss, frequent awakening by symptoms, fever, blood in your stools, anemia, chronic severe diarrhea, or a family history of colon cancer, you may have a condition other than IBS that needs to be evaluated. If your IBS is linked to your menstrual cycle, you may need to see a gynecologist to be evaluated for endometriosis or some other gynecological condition.

An experienced physician's judgment is very important in determining which diagnostic tests you need. Many women with IBS are very concerned they might have inflammatory bowel disease, colorectal cancer, or an infectious diarrhea. The good news is that fewer than one percent of IBS patients without alarm symptoms, like blood in the stool, have these diseases. In fact, a recent review study found that a thorough medical history and a physical exam may be enough of a workup for most IBS patients. The study concluded that "the routine use of endoscopic, radiologic or microbiologic tests to rule out organic disorders cannot be endorsed" in all IBS patients, especially those without alarm symptoms. Here are some of the tests I may do in my clinic depending upon these factors.

DIAGNOSIS OF EXCLUSION?

Practically every week at least one patient walks into my clinic and tells me she is frustrated with her diagnosis of IBS. She tells me she saw her physician for her GI symptoms and was referred for some medical tests. When all her results came back normal, she was given a "diagnosis of exclusion": IBS. She'll then ask, "Just what is a diagnosis of exclusion? I think it means that my doctor has no idea what's wrong with me. But I still have these symptoms, and I need you to find what's being missed."

Personally, I very much dislike the term "diagnosis of exclusion." As a doctor, I believe it breeds distrust in our patients. The "well, we can't find anything, so you must have..." conclusion just doesn't cut it as a scientific approach.

Getting the message that your tests show nothing wrong with you can be maddening if you're experiencing acute pain or debilitating bouts of constipation or diarrhea. Think of it this way: People who have crushing migraines usually have completely normal brain scans with no evidence of a tumor. Their pain is still very real, even though there's no apparent culprit, and they must take steps to prevent migraines by avoiding certain foods or reducing stress and taking medications when the pain sets in.

IBS is like a migraine of the colon. The condition may cause a great deal of discomfort and distress, but it doesn't damage your colon and isn't life threatening. It doesn't raise your risk of colorectal cancer or any other GI cancer.

I avoid the "diagnosis by exclusion" approach at my clinic. If a woman has symptoms that fit the Rome II criteria and if her physical examination is normal, I usually start by

DIAGNOSIS OF EXCLUSION? (continued)

telling her that I believe that she has IBS. Making the diagnosis depends on ruling out other disorders, so I may order tests like blood work or endoscopy, if appropriate. I then explain that IBS is a disorder of gut function with increased gut sensitivity and perhaps a change in the motility—things we can't "see" on an X-ray or endoscopy—so I expect that if she has IBS, these test results will be normal. And if the results come back normal, we all breathe a sigh of relief and work on managing the IBS symptoms.

- **Blood Tests:** A complete blood count can be done to check for anemia and other abnormalities. In patients with diarrheal symptoms, I generally test for celiac disease. Other tests may be performed, including thyroid function tests or an erythrocyte sedimentation rate (which may indicate if tissue damage or inflammation is present).

- **Stool Tests:** The most common fecal examinations check for an intestinal infection by bacteria or parasites. I may also test for lactoferrin or white blood cells in the stool that can signal bowel inflammation, which is not associated with IBS. I can also check for occult (hidden) blood in the stool. (See Chapter 15 for more details.)

- **Sigmoidoscopy or Colonoscopy:** These examinations give doctors a direct view into the rectum and sigmoid portion of the colon (sigmoidoscopy) or the entire colon (colonoscopy) using the endoscope. These tests are recommended for all women with IBS over the age of fifty who have not had prior colorectal cancer screening. (See Chapter 15 for more details.)

- **Breath Testing:** Lactose tolerance breath tests can identify a deficiency in lactase, the intestinal enzyme necessary for the digestion of the milk sugar, lactose. Lactose intolerance may be the cause of increased gassiness, bloating, and diarrhea. Hydrogen breath testing may also be useful for identifying small-bowel overgrowth.
- **Anorectal Manometry:** This test measures neuromuscular function of the anus and is used in certain patients with predominant constipation or fecal incontinence. Colon transit studies may also be performed in these patients.

WHAT TO BRING TO YOUR DOCTOR APPOINTMENT

Of all GI conditions, IBS is the one whose management is most dependent upon a positive working relationship between patient and doctor. You both need to communicate effectively about the course of treatment that's most appropriate in your particular case. Your doctor needs to know about the kind of lifestyle you lead—your dietary habits, family relationships, stress levels, working environment—because it can play a big role in triggering symptoms.

Some typical questions your doctor may ask are listed below. Answer these questions and fill in the Daily Snapshot that follows, and bring both to your next doctor appointment.

1. What specific symptoms are you suffering from? _____
   _____

2. How long have you been suffering from these symptoms?
   _____

3. Does having a bowel movement relieve your abdominal pain?
   _____

4. How many bowel movements have you had this week, and
   what was their consistency (i.e., hard, lumpy, loose, watery)?
   _____
   _____

5. Do your symptoms get worse after you eat certain foods? If
   so, which foods?   _____
   _____
   _____

6. Are you currently taking fiber supplements? _____
   _____

7. How many servings of dietary fiber do you eat per day? (Some
   examples of fiber servings are: a piece of fruit, a cup of carrots,
   a bowl of bran cereal, a piece of whole-grain bread.) _____

8. Does fiber help relieve your symptoms? _____

   _____

9. How much water do you drink per day? _____

10. How often do you exercise? _____
    _____

11. How effectively do you manage stress? _____
    _____

12. What medications are you currently taking? _____
    _____

DAILY SNAPSHOT

If you're experiencing IBS symptoms, it's a good idea to keep a short journal of what you eat, how often you have a bowel movement, and when you experience symptoms. This information can help you and your physician gain a better understanding of your condition. I use journals a lot in my clinic. What I don't want is a twenty-page running commentary of your life with GI symptoms. I often just tell patients to use their monthly calendar. If you're having constipation or diarrhea, put an X for every time you have a bowel movement. And if there's anything important symptomwise about that date, write it on the calendar.

Another option is to copy the sample chart on page 397, filling it in with your own information. Chances are you'll soon see a pattern emerging. You'll also be able to track the effectiveness of the therapies you take or the lifestyle changes you've made.

MANAGING YOUR IBS

A diagnosis of IBS can be seen as a blessing or a curse. The blessing is that you don't have a life-threatening condition that will require strong medications or multiple surgeries to treat. The curse is that you have a chronic condition that is largely controlled by the type of lifestyle you lead. Manage your diet and stress levels correctly, and you'll most likely experience fewer flare-ups and more manageable symptoms. Allow your life to spin out of control by eating or sleeping erratically, and you'll probably pay the price with diarrhea, constipation, or abdominal pain. For many women, reassurance and lifestyle changes are all that is needed to improve their symptoms.

There are, of course, medications that can help control IBS symptoms, but taking a pill should not be a panacea for treating IBS. Most women who require medications find that combining them with lifestyle changes provides the most effective therapy. I usually discuss several lifestyle issues with my patients: diet modifications, exercise, stress levels, and sleep habits. It's vital to keep a regular sleep schedule—going to bed and waking up at the same time each day and aiming for about eight hours a night. Lack of sleep causes an increase in stress hormones like cortisol and can have the same negative impact on your colon as any other stress in your life. With stress, I have to be practical and realize that you can't necessarily quit a high-stress job or afford to hire a housekeeper to relieve you of some household responsibilities. I just ask that you set aside twenty minutes a day to get your body into a state of relaxation in a plan I describe on pages 399–403.

MANAGING YOUR DIET

When we get to the treatment phase, the first question nearly every woman asks me is "Dr. Yoshida, tell me what I can and can't eat." I wish it were that simple and that I could provide a single IBS diet plan that would relieve the symptoms of IBS. The trouble is, such a diet

Day	BREAKFAST	LUNCH	DINNER	SNACKS	BOWEL MOVEMENT	CONSISTENCY	SYMPTOMS EXPERIENCED	STRESS LEVEL
Mon	Bran cereal and coffee	Turkey sandwich and soda	Grilled chicken, string beans, roasted potatoes, and wine	Potato chips and chocolate chip cookies	One, but incomplete	Hard	Constipation, bloating, and abdominal pain	High

plan doesn't exist because different foods may aggravate symptoms in some people and not in others. A
food that triggers your symptoms may not be the same
food that triggers your friend's IBS symptoms.

Some women believe that spicy food and lettuce
are their worst offenders; others can eat all the salad
they want but need to stay away from fried and fatty
foods. And what may be more frustrating is that you
can eat pizza on a "good day" but don't dare try it on a
"bad day." And sometimes you don't know if it's a
good day or a bad day until after you've eaten the
pizza.

That's why keeping a simple food diary can be so
helpful. It will clue you in on which foods are most
troublesome. You can start by cutting back on these

RED FLAG FOODS THAT CAN AGGRAVATE IBS

- alcohol
- carbonated beverages
- caffeine beverages
- whole-milk dairy products
- dried beans, peas, and lentils
- cruciferous vegetables (broccoli, cauliflower, brussels sprouts)
- refined sugar (pastries, candy, cookies)
- baked goods made with white flour
- red meat
- fatty or greasy foods (fried foods, high-fat meats, butter, salad dressings, etc.)

foods or avoiding them altogether. I recommend avoiding the worst dietary offenders and then perhaps adding a little at a time back into your diet to see how much you tolerate. For instance, if you find that red meat is a trigger, see how you feel after skipping red meat for a week. If you find you miss your steaks and burgers, switch to a smaller portion size and leaner cuts of meat. Top round, sirloin, and extra-lean ground beef have less fat and may be easier to tolerate.

A high-fiber diet certainly isn't a cure-all for IBS, but it seems to help many of my patients, especially those with constipation. In some people a high-fiber diet can make IBS worse, but this usually doesn't happen if high-fiber foods like vegetables and whole grains are introduced into the diet slowly. In Chapter 6 I provide more information on switching to a high-fiber diet.

In general, eating smaller meals or smaller portions at meals can help ease symptoms. You should also avoid high-fat foods and base your diet on lean protein choices like fish and chicken breast and on unprocessed carbohydrates like brown rice, whole-wheat bread, whole-grain cereals, fruits, and vegetables.

DEALING WITH STRESS

For some IBS sufferers, stress triggers painful spasms or contractions in the colon. For others, stress causes an increased sensitivity of the nerves within the bowel, causing even normal bowel contractions to result in pain. For still others, the problem may lie in their brain's interpretation of the signals coming from the bowel. Your brain may interpret these signals differently when you're anxious.

It doesn't really matter, though, why your particular symptoms may get worse when you're under stress. The important thing is to focus on finding effective ways to manage your stress. Stress management can mean many things to many people. Some find that taking a kick-boxing class at the gym helps them unwind. Others find that staring out the window at the leaves for five minutes restores peace of mind. Obviously, you need to find what works for you.

Relaxation elicits a distinctive physiological response: decreased blood pressure, heart rate, and breathing rate. This, in turn, decreases your body's production of stress hormones, like cortisol and adrenaline. Some research suggests that it also boosts your brain's production of feel-good hormones like serotonin. This powerful calming effect is called the "relaxation response," a term coined by Herbert Benson, M.D., author of *Timeless Healing* and president of the Mind/Body Medical Institute at Harvard's Beth Israel Deaconess Medical Center.

Eliciting the Relaxation Response

Traditional Way: Sit comfortably, and pick a focus word or short phrase that's meaningful to you. Close your eyes, and relax your muscles. Now breathe slowly and naturally, repeating your focus word or phrase silently as you exhale. Throughout, assume a passive attitude.

Don't worry about whether you're performing the technique correctly. When other thoughts come to mind, simply let them pass without pondering them. Gently return to your repetition and continue for 15 to 20 minutes. When you finish, sit quietly for a minute or so, first with your eyes closed and then with your eyes open.

Progressive Muscle Relaxation: Sit in a comfortable chair with back and head support, or lie on a lightly cushioned mat on the floor. (A bed is too soft and will make you more likely to fall asleep.) Tense each of your muscles one at a time; inhale and slowly exhale as you release the tension from your muscles. Begin with your face by wrinkling your forehead and shutting your eyes as tight as you can. Exhale and release. Then tense your neck and shoulders by drawing your shoulders up into a shrug. Exhale and release. Work your way down to your arms and hands, pressing your palms together with elbows pointing outward and push as hard as you can. Exhale and release. Contract your stomach. Arch your back and release. Now tense your hips and buttocks, pressing your legs and heels against the surface beneath you. Exhale and release. Point and flex your toes and release.

Now tense all your muscles at once. Take a deep breath, hold it, and exhale slowly as you relax the muscles. Feel your body at rest and enjoy this state of relaxation for several minutes.

Meditation: The focused awareness that comes with meditation can let you appreciate the interconnectedness of all living things. Sit comfortably in an upright position with your head, neck, and back erect but not stiff. You can sit in a straight-backed chair or cross-legged on the floor. Choose a single object of focus, like your breathing or a portion of a prayer. Concentrate on the qualities of that object, the sounds, sensations, and thoughts, as they enter into your awareness.

You can also practice meditation in a natural setting, such as an outdoor garden or while sitting by a window. Watch the sun set, clouds drift, or stars twinkle, and focus on the air flowing into and out of your body as you breathe. Appreciating the beauty of nature takes your mind off your own problems and reminds you of how vast the world really is.

Many of my patients swear by other relaxation techniques. Some get acupuncture, while others find that weekly massages help to reduce stress. Yoga can also be a great stress reliever—yoga classes and videos seem to be everywhere these days. I also recommend relaxation tapes to my patients. A website called www.healthjourneys.com has a tape specifically for IBS.

Letting Go of Some of Your Stress

I realize it can be very hard to relax when you've got a million things to do and no time to do them. While I was working on revisions for this book, I was struggling with a full workload, two bored children at home who had finished summer camp, and a sick family member in the hospital for cancer treatment. I realized something had to give. I told my boss I needed to cut back my hours for several weeks, and I explained to my kids and husband that we'd be eating takeout for a while. My house was messier, and my kids learned to fold and put away their own laundry. I also leaned heavily on my friends. They took my kids to the beach for a few days and arranged playdates.

I know I can't be superwoman, and I think if more women understood this, we'd all be a lot better off. Yes, we must multitask and constantly juggle, but we also have to realize our limitations.

A Word About Professional Counseling

Some patients with IBS can greatly benefit from psychological counseling. I'm not talking about "talk therapy" alone but a wide range of behavioral therapies to help you control and manage stress or anxiety. Studies have shown that behavorial therapy is far more effective than a placebo at relieving individual IBS symptoms. In some cases, IBS patients also have depression or an anxiety disorder that requires a psychiatrist's intervention.

Recent research suggests that relaxation therapy, hypnotherapy, biofeedback, cognitive therapy, and psychotherapy may improve individual IBS symptoms. A professional psychologist can help you choose the therapy that's appropriate for you, based on your individual case and personal preference.

- **Relaxation Therapy:** Patients learn techniques (like the ones I outlined on pages 399–402) to release tension and relax. Relaxation therapy is based on the theory that stress sets off a chain of physiological events

COULD YOUR FEARS ABOUT IBS BE MAKING IT WORSE?

Marla came to see me during her fourth month of pregnancy because her obstetrician warned her that her IBS would probably get worse as her pregnancy progressed. She lived in constant fear that she wouldn't be able to care for her child. "What if I'm on the toilet and the baby is crying hysterically?" she asked me. "What if I pass this condition on to my child?" Marla had all kinds of negative thoughts running through her head and had convinced herself that she wasn't going to be a good mother. I referred her to J. Kim Penberthy, a psychologist who works with patients at the Women's GI Clinic.

Using a classic cognitive therapy technique, Dr. Penberthy challenged Marla's fears and actually was able to induce symptoms in Marla by having her conjure up her negative thoughts. Marla kept a symptom journal and found that at times when her anxieties about becoming a mother increased, so did her IBS symptoms. Marla spent several months in therapy, exploring why she was having such negative feelings and determining which fears were justified, based on reality, and which were not. Dr. Penberthy also employed behavioral therapy techniques, showing Marla that she held her breath and tensed her muscles whenever she became anxious: "I taught her some deep abdominal breathing exercises and monitored her breathing and heart rate to show her when she was doing it properly."

Marla ended her therapy about a month before her due date. She sent me a picture of herself and her adorable baby a few months later. I still see Marla occasionally to help her manage her IBS, but she said having a baby and having IBS is much more manageable in reality than in the scenarios she had built up in her mind during her pregnancy.

(increased heart rate, rapid breathing, etc.) that exacerbates IBS symptoms.

- **Biofeedback:** Patients learn to sense changes in rectal distention and to regulate bowel habits using biofeedback sensors that record which muscles you're tensing when you're under stress or trying to have a bowel movement. I go into more detail about this therapy on page 208.

- **Hypnotherapy:** This procedure can be self-induced and is associated with a deep state of relaxation. It may positively affect gut motility and intestinal smooth muscle contraction.

- **Cognitive Therapy:** This therapy is based on the theory that a person's usual pattern of responding to stressful events exacerbates their IBS symptoms. In cognitive therapy, patients learn how certain thinking patterns or interpretations of situations contribute to or worsen their IBS symptoms. The therapy trains you to utilize more effective coping strategies such as problem-solving or assertiveness training to better manage the stress.

- **Psychotherapy:** Some psychologists recommend long-term therapy if they believe a patient's IBS symptoms are a manifestation of traumatic life events. Psychotherapy provides insight about these life events and the association between these events and IBS symptoms. Through this insight, patients may experience lasting resolution of IBS symptoms.

Therapy is very helpful to many of my patients. We use it in conjunction with lifestyle changes and sometimes medications. We have a licensed psychologist in our clinic to whom I refer patients. Your doctor should be able to refer you to a counselor or therapist in your area. You can also contact the American Psychological Association for a referral at (800) 964-2000.

MEDICATIONS FOR IBS

Medications for IBS can't cure the condition, but they can help get symptoms under control. The most common types of drugs used to treat IBS are laxatives (for constipation), antidiarrheals (for diarrhea), antispasmodics (for pain), and antidepressants (for pain). Traditional therapies for IBS are symptom specific, which means that doctors frequently need to prescribe a combination of medications to bring relief.

Two new medications, specifically designed for women, may alleviate the need for multiple medications in some women. Alosetron (Lotronex), used for diarrhea-predominant IBS, and tegaserod (Zelnorm), used for constipation-predominant IBS, both appear to relieve a combination of symptoms associated with IBS. However, both medications may also have side effects. Your doctor will no doubt weigh these risks along with the benefits when determining which medication is appropriate to treat your symptoms. Here's what you need to know about the various treatments.

Laxatives

There are four main types of laxatives: fiber, osmotic laxatives, stimulant laxatives, and emollients (stool softeners). Dietary fiber should be the first treatment method if you have constipation-predominant IBS. A recent review of several studies found that fiber improves bowel function in IBS patients by easing the passage of stool and increasing satisfaction with bowel movements. It doesn't, however, help alleviate pain. What's more, fiber supplements (such as psyllium) can cause flatulence, distension, and bloating during the first few weeks of therapy, which is why I recommend adding fiber gradually—a few grams a day over several weeks until your body adjusts. (See Chapter 6 for more information.)

Osmotic, stimulant, and emollient laxatives have stronger effects, and I usually consider them to be a second line of treatment if fiber supplementation doesn't help. Check out page 203 for more details on the benefits and drawbacks of these types of laxatives. You can also try the various techniques I recommend for constipation in Chapter 6. They can be effective for managing symptoms if you have constipation-predominant IBS.

Antidiarrheals

Antidiarrheal medications are commonly used to treat IBS. They bind certain cells (with opioid receptors) in the intestines, resulting in decreased motility of the gut. Diphenoxylate (Lomotil) and loperamide (Imodium, Pepto Diarrhea) are frequently recommended antidiarrheals. Loperamide helps reduce stool leakage in IBS patients, especially at night. Diphenoxylate crosses into the brain and can, in rare cases, be habit forming.

Lomotil, though, has an additional ingredient, atropine, which further slows gut motility by a different mechanism. All of these antidiarrheal drugs can reduce the urge to defecate (especially in social situations or at important events). They should, however, be used cautiously because they can lead to constipation. They should be discontinued if constipation becomes significant.

Antispasmodics

These medications reduce abdominal pain associated with IBS by inhibiting smooth-muscle contractions in the GI tract. They are divided into three major types: anticholinergics, peppermint oil, and direct smooth-muscle relaxants (which are not currently available in the United States). Anticholinergics reduce spasms or contractions in the intestine and thus have the potential to reduce abdominal pain. But medical evidence that these medications work to improve IBS symptoms is not definitive. I usually prescribe them short term, to see if they work to improve my patient's pain.

The most commonly prescribed antispasmodics in the United States are dicyclomine (Bentyl), hyoscyamine (Anaspaz, Levsin), and clidinium. Hyoscyamine comes in oral spray form or in tablets that can be swallowed or rapidly dissolved and absorbed beneath the tongue. This dual availability can be very beneficial to some patients. If taken under the tongue, this medication is effective within minutes but may last for only 15 to 30 minutes. If swallowed, you may not get relief for 15 to 30 minutes, but the drug will last for several hours. Hyoscyamine may benefit women with occasional IBS symptoms who don't want to take a medication every day.

A long-acting form of hyoscyamine (Levbid) can be taken twice daily. The benefit of this medication is that it provides more long-term, "constant" relief of symptoms than the more symptom-driven shorter-acting hyoscyamine (Levsin). Donnatal is a combination of anticholinergic and phenobarbital. A significant side effect is drowsiness; thus it should be used cautiously.

The most common side effects of antispasmodics are headache, dizziness, blurred vision, difficulty urinating, decreased sweating, nasal congestion, stuffiness, rash or itching, and a dry mouth.

Peppermint oil works as an antipasmodic by relaxing the intestine and preventing calcium entry into intestinal smooth-muscle cells. Since calcium triggers a cascade of events that leads to muscle contraction, inhibiting calcium's entry into cells causes intestinal smooth-muscle relaxation. A recent meta-analysis of research found that in three of five studies peppermint oil was an effective IBS treatment. I think, though, that more research needs to be done before we can say for certain that peppermint can truly reduce abdominal pain associated with IBS.

In rare cases, peppermint oil can cause skin rash, headache, muscle tremor, loss of muscle coordination, slow heartbeat, and heartburn. Many physicians recommend using enteric-coated peppermint oil tablets because they decrease the side effects of nausea and heartburn. Health food stores and local pharmacies often carry these tablets over the counter.

Smooth-muscle relaxants are another type of antispasmodic, but they're not available for use in the United States. Studies performed in other countries, however, show that these drugs may improve IBS patients' overall well-being, pain, and abdominal distension. Further studies are needed to see if they are safe and beneficial.

Antidepressants

You may be surprised to learn that antidepressants may be prescribed for pain associated with IBS. These types of drugs are effective in relieving pain in a variety of chronic pain syndromes, including IBS. The benefit of antidepressants in chronic pain conditions appears to be independent of improvement of mood or decrease in anxiety. The most commonly prescribed medications are tricyclic antidepressants such as amitriptyline (Elavil), nortriptyline (Pamelor), and desipramine (Norpramin). They are thought to work by blocking the reuptake of the neurotransmitters serotonin and norepinephrine by nerve cells in the body's internal pain inhibitory system. Usually low doses of these medications are given for the treatment of IBS. A recent review study found that tricyclic antidepressants are effective at reducing symptoms in about one-third of IBS patients. The drugs appear to work best in those with pain-predominant IBS.

Researchers are studying the use of selective serotonin-reuptake inhibitors (SSRIs), which include sertraline (Zoloft), fluoxetine (Prozac), and paroxetine (Paxil).

PROBIOTICS: DO THEY WORK?

As evidence builds that bacteria and other microorganisms may be the culprit of IBS in some sufferers, researchers are trying to determine if probiotics can help alleviate IBS symptoms by restoring a healthy balance of bacteria to the GI tract. Probiotics are dietary supplements that contain live beneficial bacteria that help keep dangerous GI invaders—like viruses, infectious bacteria, and yeast—in check. You can buy probiotics over the counter in health food stores and pharmacies. One yogurt manufacturer, Stonyfield Farms, adds live bacteria to the yogurt after it's been pasteurized.

Probiotics certainly aren't harmful, but are they effective against IBS? Probiotic manufacturers would have you believe the answer is yes. Many claim on their websites that their supplements will help reduce diarrhea and abdominal pain associated with IBS. At this point, however, no solid research has been able to establish these claims as true. One randomized controlled trial involving thirty-four patients found that the probiotic *Saccharomyces boulardii* decreased diarrhea but didn't relieve other IBS symptoms like abdominal pain and constipation. One noted probiotic researcher, Jon Vanderhoof, M.D., a gastroenterologist at the University of Nebraska in Omaha, conducted two separate studies on IBS using various probiotics and found that none worked to relieve symptoms.

On the other hand, studies on dietary supplements are usually scant because of a lack of funding to conduct this research. So you can test these out for yourself and try probiotics for a few weeks to see if they work to alleviate your symptoms. At worst, you'll find the supplements have no beneficial effects and all that you've wasted will be your money. If you do opt to try probiotics, choose a brand that contains live bacteria cultures. Be sure to check the dose on the label. Doses should be in the hundreds of millions—not thousands.

These may work to relieve pain and other IBS symptoms, particularly for those who also have mood disorders like anxiety or depression. A major selling point is that SSRIs have fewer side effects than tricyclics, but evidence is lacking that SSRIs work in IBS patients who don't have a mood disorder.

Tricyclic antidepressants can cause a wide range of side effects that differ significantly from patient to patient. These side effects include drowsiness, increased appetite, weight gain, urinary retention, blurred vision, and constipation. They can't be taken if you have heart disease, bladder control problems, narrow-angle glaucoma, or dementia. The most common side effects of SSRIs are nausea, headaches, insomnia, and sexual dysfunction.

The Newest Treatments

There are several new kids on the block that could alter the way doctors treat IBS in women. Tegaserod (Zelnorm), approved by the FDA in 2002, has been shown to be effective against abdominal pain, bloating, and constipation. It works on specific serotonin receptors (known as 5-HT4 receptors) that are found in the GI tract and that regulate gastrointestinal motility and pain sensitivity. Clinical studies show that the drug stimulates the peristaltic reflex to increase colonic transit and decreases pain sensitivity. Tegaserod is the only FDA-approved agent for the treatment of female IBS patients with constipation. Patients taking this medication experienced less bloating and abdominal discomfort and improved satisfaction with their bowel habits in clinical trials conducted by the drug manufacturer.

At the present time, tegaserod is meant for short-term use—up to twelve weeks. This seems appropriate given the often-episodic and fluctuating course of IBS. Longer-term studies to determine the effectiveness and safety of this drug are currently under way. Diarrhea is the most common side effect, but it generally wanes over longer use of the medication, and very few patients in clinical trials actually discontinued the medication because of this problem.

Alosetron (Lotronex) was reintroduced in the market in 2002. This medication inhibits 5-HT3 serotonin receptors in the gut and is used to treat diarrhea-predominant IBS in women. This drug slows colonic transit and decreases pain caused by distension of the colon from gas or stool. Alosetron is the only FDA-approved agent for the treatment of IBS patients with diarrhea. It can be highly effective, and some of my patients consider it a miracle drug. In November 2000 its manufacturer halted distribution of the medication because of concerns that it caused severe constipation and ischemic colitis, an inflammation of the colon caused by decreased blood flow to the gut. By March 2002 the FDA had received reports of 84 cases of suspected ischemic colitis and 113 cases of suspected serious constipation. The risk of developing this form of colitis while taking alosetron is about one in a thousand—not large but still significant. In June 2002 the FDA approved restricted marketing of alosetron for the treatment of "women with severe, diarrhea-predominant IBS who have failed to respond to conventional IBS therapy."

Gastroenterologists are using caution when prescribing alosetron, yet for those of us who do prescribe it, we know that it is extremely useful to many of our patients with diarrhea-predominant IBS. If you're considering taking alosetron, my advice to you is to discuss all the pros and cons with your doctor. Certain restrictions apply to the prescribing of this drug. (See the FDA website, www.fda.gov, for more information on alosetron.)

FUTURE TREATMENTS

Several other IBS treatments are currently under development and may receive FDA approval in upcoming years. These include cilansetron (similar to alosetron), M3 receptor antagonists, zamifenacin, and darifenacin, which are being studied for diarrhea-predominant IBS. These antispasmodic drugs decrease motor activity in the GI tract and may help alleviate diarrhea and pain.

Rifaximin, a new nonabsorbable antibiotic, can help alleviate bloating and flatulence and can reduce the overall severity of IBS symptoms, according to a small clinical trial of the drug involving twenty IBS patients. Nonabsorbable antibiotics may become a new generation of IBS drugs that work by altering the microorganisms (like bacteria) that live in the colon and that may be causing symptoms in some IBS patients. Another treatment making its way through clinical trials is asimadoline, a pain reliever in the opioid family that is being tested in men and women with pain-predominant IBS.

IBS RESOURCES

AMERICAN GASTROENTEROLOGICAL ASSOCIATION
4930 Del Ray Avenue
Bethesda, MD 20814
tel. (301) 654-2055

www.gastro.org

The AGA offers a patient brochure on IBS and updated information on treatment, at www.gastro.org/clinicalRes/brochures/ibs.html.

INTERNATIONAL FOUNDATION FOR FUNCTIONAL
GASTROINTESTINAL DISORDERS
P.O. Box 170864
Milwaukee, WI 53217-8076
tel. (414) 964-1799
www.iffgd.org
The foundation has a site specifically devoted to IBS that provides publications, links to other IBS sites, and advice on coping with traumatic events and talking with your doctor: www.aboutibs.org.

NATIONAL DIGESTIVE DISEASES INFORMATION
CLEARINGHOUSE
2 Information Way
Bethesda, MD 20892-3570
tel. (800) 891-5389 or (301) 654-3810
digestive.niddk.nih.gov
The clearinghouse's information sheet (at digestive.niddk.nih.gov/ddiseases/pubs/ibs/index.htm) describes IBS causes, symptoms, and tests to rule out more serious intestinal diseases. It also offers lifestyle and medical approaches to symptom management.

UNIVERSITY OF NORTH CAROLINA CENTER FOR
FUNCTIONAL GI AND MOTILITY DISORDERS
Bioinformatics Building, CB #7080
Chapel Hill, NC 27599-7080
tel. (888) 964-2001
www.med.unc.edu/medicine/fgidc/
This website offers up-to-date information on IBS for patients and provides information on IBS research and

clinical treatment. It has a chat room that allows you to talk with the experts—including Dr. Doug Drossman, a leading authority on IBS—on the second Tuesday of every month from 8 to 10 P.M. EST.

IBS VILLAGE
www.ibsvillage.com
Run by the drug company Novartis, which makes Zelnorm, this site offers a questionnaire to evaluate your IBS symptoms and information on maintaining a healthy lifestyle to combat IBS. It also has a symptom checklist and treatment options.

All too frequently, IBS is referred to as a disorder that's "all in your head." By now you should know that it's not in your head. If you are suffering from IBS symptoms, I urge you to see your doctor rather than trying to self-treat with over-the-counter remedies. Far too many women put up with these symptoms for years and think they just have to learn to live with them. I can reassure you that IBS isn't as ominous as other GI conditions like colon cancer or inflammatory bowel disease. There are things you can do to alleviate your symptoms and prevent them from destroying the quality of your life. You can have a large measure of control over your IBS. Put yourself in the driver's seat, and learn to navigate your condition smoothly.

14

INFLAMMATORY BOWEL DISEASE—MEETING THE CHALLENGES

Y OU HAVE CROHN'S DISEASE," your doctor says. It's your worst nightmare come true. In a sense, you're relieved to know that you finally have a diagnosis for the intense waves of abdominal pain that literally take your breath away. But you're also afraid of what happens next. Will you need surgery? Will you be on steroids for the rest of your life? Can you safely become pregnant? Are you headed for colon cancer?

Unfortunately, these are very real concerns for the one million American women who suffer from inflammatory bowel disease (IBD), a term that refers to both ulcerative colitis and Crohn's disease. Ulcerative colitis is an inflammation of the lining of the large intestine, or colon. Crohn's disease most often is an inflammation of the lining and entire wall of the large and/or small intestine. In truth, Crohn's disease can involve any part of your GI tract from mouth to anus. When inflamed, the lining of the intestinal wall is red and swollen and can become ulcerated or bleed.

Yes, IBD can be a harrowing illness, and multiple surgeries may be needed to remove diseased portions of the intestine. It can increase your risk of colon cancer. Major symptoms of Crohn's and ulcerative colitis include rectal bleeding, abdominal pain, and diarrhea. These can be extraordinarily difficult diseases to discuss, and many women feel alone in their struggle to find support from friends, family members, and physicians.

Entire books have been written about IBD, and I encourage you to seek out additional resources because I don't have room to cover this topic in depth in this book. (See page 444.) But I do want to focus on particular areas that are of specific concern to women. I've been amazed at the new research findings that show the link between IBD and a woman's menstrual cycle. And more and more information is coming out about the effect of IBD on pregnancy and which medications are safe to take while you're pregnant and nursing.

As with other GI health concerns, with IBD, women are often given short shrift. On the whole about an equal number of men and women suffer from IBD. Studies that have looked at gender differences don't show a difference in the manifestation of symptoms or where the disease is found. However, my colleague Dr. Sunanda Kane, a gastroenterologist at the University of Chicago and a member of the advisory board for this book, found in her research that women who present with abdominal pain that is later found to be caused by Crohn's often took a lot longer to get a proper diagnosis than their male counterparts who also presented with abdominal pain caused by Crohn's.

Women with IBD may go undiagnosed for many

years because their doctors attribute their symptoms to irritable bowel syndrome. Several women have been referred to me (sometimes by fellow gastroenterologists) with unresolved abdominal pain and diarrhea, only to discover via colonoscopy that they have ulcerative colitis or Crohn's disease. Many of these women have been prescribed various antispasmodics and antidiarrheals with little improvement in their symptoms. And many were never referred for colonoscopy or small-bowel X-rays.

A case in point: A patient named Bernice, a forty-two-year-old accountant, recently came to see me following stomach bypass surgery. The surgery cured her obesity problem, but now she was losing weight too quickly and was on her way to becoming emaciated. She said her lifelong problem with diarrhea had gotten worse, and her surgeon said it was probably a side effect from the surgery. I decided to perform a small-bowel study and a colonoscopy. Although the colonoscopy did not reveal any abnormalities, the small-bowel study showed that a large segment of her small intestine was inflamed. Bernice had classic signs of Crohn's disease.

I gave Bernice a prescription for mesalamine (Pentasa), an anti-inflammatory drug that's milder than steroids, which is used as a first line of treatment for Crohn's. Within a few weeks she began to feel better. She regained about ten pounds and got into a healthy weight range. She also told me that she experienced loose stools every few days rather than six times a day. "I'm finally able to enjoy my new body," Bernice told me excitedly during our most recent appointment. "I'm even ready to join a gym, and I never thought I could tolerate exercise before because I was always running to the bathroom."

Bernice had been written off by her doctors in two ways. Because of her history of obesity, they assumed that her diarrhea was caused by her eating patterns or by the radical surgery she had to fix her weight problem. No one considered the possibility that Bernice could have Crohn's disease. I also think Bernice had her gender working against her. Research has shown that women are far less likely than men to be referred for a colonoscopy when they complain about lower-GI symptoms.

If you suspect you have IBD, you need to educate yourself about the condition, how it manifests, what you need to do to get a proper diagnosis, and various treatment options you should consider. This is one GI problem that can't be ignored. If left untreated, IBD can do irreversible damage to your small intestine or colon. This damage can increase your risk of cancer and requires you to have periodic cancer screening.

FAST FACTS ABOUT IBD

Like all diseases, IBD varies in severity from person to person. Sometimes the disease is mild and can be controlled with drugs and diet. Other cases are so severe they require frequent hospitalization, numerous surgeries, transfusions, or intravenous feeding. (Patients with severe cases are usually the ones who have trouble gaining and maintaining a healthy weight. They often have nutritional deficiencies and are severely underweight.)

Both Crohn's and ulcerative colitis involve inflammation of the intestinal wall. Ulcerative colitis affects only the inner layer of the large intestine (colon). It usually starts in the rectum and may involve variable amounts of the colon in a progressive fashion. Ulcerative proctitis is a disease limited to the rectum. Patients may also have left-sided disease (generally limited to the rectum and left side of the colon) or pancolitis (involving the rectum and the entire colon).

Crohn's involves the full thickness of the bowel wall. It usually does not involve the rectum but can affect the small intestine and/or colon, generally with normal areas of bowel in between (called skip lesions). As I said earlier, Crohn's can, in rare cases, involve inflammation in the mouth and stomach as well. Crohn's is also more likely to be associated with complications like abscesses (collections of pus) or fistulas (abnormal connections between the bowel and other areas of inflamed tissue). These connections may be from the bowel to bowel or to other areas such as the skin, vagina, or bladder.

The main GI symptoms of both Crohn's and ulcerative colitis are:

- abdominal cramping
- rectal bleeding
- diarrhea and loss of bowel control
- decreased appetite and weight loss (in some people)
- occasional nausea and vomiting

IBD may also be associated with other symptoms, including:

- eye diseases like iritis and uveitis
- skin rashes such as erythema nodosum or pyoderma gangrenosum
- arthritis or joint pain

- kidney stones
- osteoporosis
- liver disease

Unfortunately, IBD isn't curable. Once people are diagnosed with it, they have it for the rest of their lives. They need to take medications on a permanent basis to keep the disease in check. Most IBD patients experience periods of acute symptoms, called flare-ups or active disease; they also have periods where they have mild symptoms or are symptom free, called remissions or quiescent disease. During remissions patients take an anti-inflammatory drug, like 5-aminosalicylic acid (5-ASA), to keep inflammation in check. During flare-ups patients often need to take more potent medications like corticosteroids, antibiotics, or other anti-inflammatory agents. In severe cases, surgery may be needed to remove the diseased portion of the intestine or colon.

No one knows exactly what causes IBD. It primarily strikes in developed Western countries. Within those countries Jews of eastern European origin are five times more likely than non-Jews to develop IBD. The single biggest risk factor is having a first-degree relative (parent or sibling) with the disease. An estimated five percent of people whose parents have IBD develop it themselves.

I also want to emphasize that neither diet nor stress causes or triggers the disease, although both can exacerbate existing symptoms. Certain drugs like antibiotics can cause a flare-up; so can contracting an intestinal illness like traveler's diarrhea. There aren't any particular foods that must be avoided, but people find that certain foods may be more likely to cause pain and diarrhea. Common offenders are lactose-containing foods, alcohol, fatty foods, or foods high in roughage. But this varies so much from person to person that I don't have a particular IBD diet plan that I recommend.

The general consensus of the medical community is that IBD is caused by a combination of genetic predisposition, an environmental triggering stimulus, and an immune system that acts inappropriately to this stimulus. Unfortunately, no one knows what that triggering event is, and it may be different in different people. Several theories have considered infectious agents such as bacteria, as well as toxins or pollutants that people are exposed to in industrialized countries. IBD is currently thought to be a type of autoimmune disorder in which the body sees its own tissues as foreign and sends an army of immune cells to attack and destroy them. This results in inflammation and damage to the intestinal lining.

IBD may be progressive, causing more and more damage to the intestinal lining over time. Or it may cause mild inflammation that remains fairly constant over the years. When I first diagnose a patient, I usually can't predict how her disease will progress over time. Careful monitoring over the first few years after the disease is diagnosed will usually give me some indication whether a patient has mild disease that can be handled with medications or more severe disease that will require repeat surgeries.

GETTING THE PROPER DIAGNOSIS

If you came to my clinic with any of the symptoms I just mentioned, I'd take a very thorough medical history to determine if you had other symptoms that suggested IBD. As I said earlier, these may include the classic symptoms of IBD but also other symptoms that don't involve the GI tract (fever, weight loss, fatigue, etc.). I would also do a very thorough physical exam. I would evaluate your abdomen, but I'd also look closely at your eyes, mouth, joints, skin, and bones. I would do extensive perineal and rectal examinations. This is a standard way that most gastroenterologists would proceed.

You should also expect to have some blood tests. Your doctor will be checking your blood counts (to look for anemia), markers of inflammation, serum chemistries (to look for electrolyte imbalances from diarrhea and for evidence of malnutrition), liver enzymes (to look for concomitant liver disease occasionally associated with IBD), vitamin levels (to look for deficiencies in vitamins such as B_{12} and D), and a urine test (to look for blood that may signal inflammation or a kidney stone). You'll probably have a bone scan as well to see if you have bone loss associated with osteoporosis.

If your doctor suspects you have ulcerative colitis (whose hallmark symptoms are urgent, bloody diarrhea with abdominal cramps), you'll probably be referred for a colonoscopy. Since ulcerative colitis is confined to the colon, a colonoscopy can show the full extent of the inflammation if you do have this condition.

If your doctor suspects you have Crohn's disease

(whose hallmark symptoms are intense abdominal pain, bloating, and diarrhea with or without bleeding), you'll probably need to have both a colonoscopy and a small bowel follow-through. In about one-third of Crohn's patients the diseased portions occur only in the small intestine; in another third they occur only in the colon; and in another third they occur in both. For this reason I don't think you can get an accurate diagnosis unless you have a colonoscopy to evaluate your entire colon and a small-bowel follow-through to evaluate your small intestine.

Colonoscopy

This test involves the insertion of a lighted flexible tube into your rectum, which is used to examine the entire colon. The physician can get a close look at any area of inflammation and identify the location of the inflammation as well as other complications such as obstruction. During a colonoscopy your gastroenterologist will generally take a small biopsy from the diseased area to see if the tissue is inflamed or, in rare cases, cancerous. Before having a colonoscopy, you must take a laxative prep to clean out your colon. (I discuss what to expect during a colonoscopy and how to prepare for one in Chapter 15.)

Small Bowel Follow-Through

A small-bowel follow-through is an X-ray exam that looks at your entire small intestine. You drink several cups of liquid barium, and X-rays are obtained at different time intervals. The X-rays can reveal diseased segments of the small intestine and identify complications of Crohn's.

Starting at midnight the night before the exam, don't eat or drink anything until after the procedure, and abstain from smoking. Don't chew gum or take mints or any medication.

Fifteen minutes after you start drinking the barium, the technologist will take an X-ray. You'll continue to have an X-ray every fifteen minutes for a period of an hour. You will be asked to drink additional cups of barium in between these X-rays. After one hour the technologist will take an X-ray every thirty minutes until the barium passes through the entire length of your small intestine, which is about twenty-five feet long.

When the barium has passed through your small intestine, the radiologist will come into the X-ray room and take several pictures and may press on your abdomen to get a better "picture." The radiologist will look over all the X-rays that have been taken. If no more are needed, you'll be free to go. The whole process can take up to three hours.

The small-bowel follow-through will indicate whether you have inflammation in your small intestine, a sign of Crohn's disease. It can also show if you have an obstruction or a fistula, complications unique to Crohn's disease. Since Crohn's affects the entire thickness of the intestinal wall, an obstruction can occur if a section of the wall swells and becomes inflamed enough to block the hollow center of the intestinal tube. Patients with intestinal obstruction develop severe crampy pain, frequently associated with vomiting.

Anti-inflammatory drugs can reduce inflammation, but surgery may be required to remove the obstruction.

A fistula is the abnormal passage from one loop of intestine to another structure, such as another loop of intestine, skin, urinary bladder, or vagina. As the intestinal wall becomes thicker, it can sometimes adhere to an adjacent structure. A small passage may develop through the intestinal wall into the other structure, resulting in leakage of stool into that area. Large or multiple fistulas may require surgery if they are associated with intractable symptoms such as fever, weight loss, or abdominal pain.

MEDICATIONS

You may think that a diagnosis of IBD means that you need steroids or surgery to treat your condition. I want to dispel this notion and tell you that many women with ulcerative colitis and Crohn's can be managed with milder medications and regular monitoring. Yes, unfortunately, some with IBD have severe cases that are much more difficult to manage. They may need repeat surgeries and multiple rounds of steroid treatments. But they are at one end of the spectrum. Complications from IBD are by no means inevitable or even frequent, especially if you get the appropriate treatment.

5-ASA Agents

If your tests results show inflammation but no signs of an obstruction or fistula, your doctor will probably recommend medication as a first line of treatment. The most popular type of drug prescribed is the 5-ASA agent. These anti-inflammatory drugs have been shown to be effective at controlling inflammation and intestinal wall damage associated with both ulcerative colitis and Crohn's. Their effect is topical, which means most of the medication remains in the intestine to treat the inflamed area. For this reason, these medicines are generally well tolerated and are associated with less severe side effects than other IBD medications like steroids. The drug comes in enema and suppository forms to deliver the medicine directly to the end of the colon, as well as in oral preparations that deliver 5-ASA to specific areas of the intestine.

A patient who remains in remission on a 5-ASA agent generally has to take the drug permanently to prevent a flare-up or recurrence of the disease. The biggest downside to these medications is the number of pills required: as many as 8 to 16 tablets daily. Like all drugs, 5-ASA agents have some side effects, including rash, fever, hair loss, exacerbation of colitis, diarrhea (especially with olsalazine [Dipentum]), pancreatitis, and, rarely, kidney damage. The table on page 431 outlines the various 5-ASA agents and how they're prescribed.

Corticosteroids

Unlike 5-ASA drugs, corticosteroids aren't used for maintenance when the disease goes into remission. They are used primarily for flare-ups or when a severe case of IBD is initially diagnosed. These potent medications suppress immune system function to shut

THE OSTEOPOROSIS LINK

Patients with IBD—both men and women—are at greater risk than others for osteoporosis. There are several reasons for this increased risk. Inflammatory proteins that are produced during active disease can circulate in the bloodstream and cause destruction of the cells that build bone, or activate those cells that break down bone. What's more, Crohn's disease often interferes with the absorption of bone-building nutrients like vitamin D and calcium. Bones can become deficient in these nutrients, which causes them to become brittle and less dense. People who are particularly debilitated by Crohn's may be less physically active, which can also lead to bone loss. Last but not least, chronic use of steroids (even if only intermittently, when attacks occur) can cause bone loss—one of the side effects of steroid use. Approximately 40 percent of women with IBD over the age of fifty will experience a fracture due to osteoporosis during their lifetime.

I firmly believe that everyone who has Crohn's or ulcerative colitis who is treated with steroids needs to have a bone mineral density test once they reach age forty. You may want to have this test when you're first diagnosed with IBD just to get a baseline measurement. Insurance companies will cover routine bone density screenings only if a woman is taking steroids or is postmenopausal. The most common test, dual energy X-ray absorptiometry (DEXA), utilizes X-rays and a harmless radioactive isotope to measure bone density. DEXA can cost a few hundred dollars if you have to pay for it out of pocket. You definitely need a bone density scan if you take steroid drugs periodically. If your doctor finds that you've lost a lot of bone, you may need a yearly bone density test.

A number of treatments are available if you have significant bone loss. These include bisphosphonates such as alendronate (Fosamax) and risedronate sodium (Actonel), which can increase bone mass. Other medications are calcitonin, hormone replacement therapy, and compounds known as selective estrogen receptor modulators (SERMs). Your doctor may also recommend calcium and vitamin D supplementation. Your doctor can help you decide which treatment is best for you.

down the inflammatory process that leads to IBD. Steroid (hydrocortisone) suppositories, foams, and enemas are effective in treating active ulcerative proctitis and ulcerative proctosigmoiditis but have been studied less extensively in Crohn's disease. They may, however, be effective when Crohn's disease involves the lower colon.

Oral forms of corticosteroids (prednisone, methylprednisolone, and prednisolone) are given when the disease progresses far enough to warrant therapy with these potent drugs. Most patients who require steroid therapy have not responded to 5-ASA agents. Oral steroids have been shown to be effective against active ulcerative colitis and active Crohn's (either in the colon or the small intestine). I try to reserve these drugs for patients who are in the throes of a serious attack of pain and diarrhea.

THE 5—ASA AGENTS

DRUG	HOW DISPENSED	INDICATIONS DURING A FLARE-UP OF DISEASE	INDICATIONS FOR MAINTENANCE THERAPY
Topical mesalamine enema (Rowasa)	4 gm unit dose	active proctosigmoiditis (inflammation in the rectal and sigmoid tissue)	quiescent proctosigmoiditis (rectosigmoid)
mesalamine suppository (Rowasa, Canasa)	500 mg suppository	active proctitis (inflammation of the rectal tissue)	quiescent proctitis (rectum)
Oral sulfasalazine (Azulfidine) enteric coated and plain	500 mg tablet	active ulcerative colitis (UC) active Crohn's disease (colon)	quiescent UC (colon)
mesalamine (Asacol)	400 mg tablet	active UC active Crohn's	quiescent UC or Crohn's (small bowel, colon)
mesalamine (Pentasa)	250 mg capsule	active UC active Crohn's	quiescent UC or Crohn's (small bowel, colon)
olsalazine (Dipentum)	250 mg capsule	active UC	quiescent UC (colon)
balsalazide (Colazal)	750 mg capsule	active UC	quiescent UC (colon, especially left side)

In the most serious cases, a patient may require hospitalization and is treated with high doses of steroids delivered intravenously or through an injection. This therapy can reverse and calm the inflammatory disease in 50 to 75 percent of patients, helping them avoid surgery.

Although very effective at treating painful IBD attacks, steroids used in high doses over the short term commonly cause adverse reactions, including insomnia, alterations of mood, voracious appetite, night sweats, and altered glucose metabolism (which can lead to high or low blood sugar). Prolonged usage can cause a rounding of the face, acne, excessive hair growth, cataracts, osteoporosis, muscle weakness, and hypertension. Your doctor should discuss these side effects with you before you begin taking steroids.

Some newer types of steroids, called rapidly metabolized steroids (such as budesonide [Entocort EC]) are now being used in Crohn's patients. They have potent anti-inflammatory actions in the intestine, but once absorbed they clear rapidly from the bloodstream. These new drugs may help people avoid the side effects often associated with steroid use.

Immunomodulators

Several drugs can inhibit specific components of the immune system that are thought to play a role in the inflammatory process in IBD. Six-mercaptopurine or 6-MP (Purinethol) and azathioprine (Imuran) inhibit the effects of T-helper lymphocytes (CD-4 cells) that are thought to cause inflammation in the intestinal wall. These drugs are usually reserved for patients who haven't responded to 5-ASA drugs or who have responded to steroids but can't remain on them long-term. They are potent anti-inflammatory agents that can also heal fistulas.

Stronger drugs are usually associated with more side effects, and you should know that these drugs are no exception. In about ten percent of patients these drugs cause reversible side effects, including allergic reactions, fever, rash, nausea and headache, inflammation of the pancreas, and bone marrow depression with lowered white blood cell count.

Cyclosporine (Neoral, Sandimmune), another immunomodulator, is also helpful in alleviating active IBD and has proven effective in inducing remission in patients with Crohn's who haven't responded to other medications. Cyclosporine is best known as a medication that prevents immune rejection in transplant patients. It also has various short- and long-term side effects such as excessive hair growth, numbness of the hands and feet, hypertension, and seizures. Other immunomodulators that may be used include injectable methotrexate and infliximab (Remicade), which is given intravenously. In Crohn's, the body overproduces a substance known as tumor necrosis factor alpha (TNF-alpha), which contributes to the inflammation. Remicade works by neutralizing this substance.

A number of new immunomodulatory drugs are in the research stages, which may offer effective relief with fewer side effects. The Digestive Health Center of Excellence at the University of Virginia Hospital is currently doing research on some of these drugs. You may be eligible to participate in a clinical trial in your local area; ask your doctor for information on such trials.

WHY YOU NEED TO STAY ON YOUR TREATMENT REGIMEN

I cannot emphasize enough how important it is for you to take your medications for IBD. I rarely have to convince women to take medications during a flare-up because they're feeling so desperate for symptom relief. But when symptoms abate, many women become skeptical about why they need to continue taking medication. Some maintenance medication regimens require you to take 8 to 12 pills per day—not easy to swallow when you're feeling "just fine."

But as I explain to my patients, maintenance medications are extremely important for preventing flare-ups and keeping any flare-ups that do occur to a minimum. They give you a better chance of avoiding complications and even cancer. I can't tell you how many times I've seen patients with really major problems from IBD that occurred because they stopped taking their maintenance medications.

One patient, Felicia, a forty-seven-year-old mother of two, came to the clinic with severe Crohn's symptoms. She had stopped taking her medications because she didn't think she needed them when she had no symptoms. When Felicia came to see me, she was in the throes of an IBD attack. She was so bloated and nauseated that she couldn't eat. She was malnourished and continuing to lose weight. I did a colonoscopy and found that Felicia had three areas of stricture with severe scarring that caused bowel obstruction. She needed immediate surgery. Now Felicia's disease is under control, and she finally realizes that she needs to be on lifelong medication to keep her disease under control.

Whenever you see your doctor for IBD follow-up, it's imperative for you to tell him or her if you don't like the way a medication makes you feel or, more important, if you stop taking your medication. Also, don't forget to tell your doctor about any new medications you may be taking—either prescription or over the counter. Medications that you may think are benign may have a big impact on your disease. For instance, nonsteroidal anti-inflammatory drugs—ibuprofen (Advil, Motrin, Nuprin), naproxen sodium (Aleve), and ketoprofen (Orudis)—are a big no-no because they can trigger a flare-up by harming the lining of the intestines.

Antibiotics

Various antibiotics like metronidazole (Flagyl), ciprofloxacin (Cipro), and other broad-spectrum antibiotics appear to be useful in inducing remission in active Crohn's and in treating the fistulas and abscesses that complicate Crohn's disease. They haven't proven as useful in treating active ulcerative colitis.

SURGERY

When IBD is particularly severe, I may recommend surgery. I am very fortunate to work with two exceptional colorectal surgeons who regularly see patients with IBD. A colectomy (removal of the large intestine) cures ulcerative colitis. Initially following a colectomy, the patient will be left with an ileostomy. Here the last part of the small intestine is attached to the skin of the abdominal wall; the patient eliminates waste into a plastic colostomy bag attached to the skin. The trend nowadays is to follow this procedure with another operation in which the small intestine is reattached to the rectum or anus so the patient can eliminate waste normally. Patients who have this procedure may experience softer, more frequent bowel movements.

Surgery for Crohn's disease usually involves removal of only that portion of the bowel that is significantly diseased. In general, surgeons try to remove as little of the bowel as possible. Surgery may be indicated when a section of the intestine becomes so inflamed that it must be removed or when certain complications (obstruction, perforation, or fistula) do not respond to medical treatment. If possible, only the diseased portions of the bowel are removed and the healthy ends are resewn or stapled back together. Crohn's disease can recur after surgery, and when it does, it commonly happens at the site where the sutures or staples are. A good number of patients with Crohn's require multiple surgeries over time to keep the disease at bay.

The Cancer Link

I don't want to scare you, but I do need to warn you. Having IBD predisposes you to colon cancer. After ten years of having the disease, your risk of colon cancer goes up by one percent per year compared to someone your age without IBD. For example, if you were diagnosed at age twenty and you're now fifty, your risk of getting colon cancer is three to five times higher than the average woman your age. To put this into perspective, the average woman has a six percent risk of developing colorectal cancer over the course of her lifetime. A woman who has had ulcerative colitis involving her entire colon for thirty years may have an 18 to 30 percent risk of getting colorectal cancer at some point during her life.

I don't want you to obsess about the numbers. My point is that IBD patients do have a very real increased risk of colorectal cancer. Because of the elevated risk, most gastroenterologists recommend relatively frequent colonoscopies to screen for colon cancer (every one to two years), particularly for those who have had IBD for eight years or more.

MENSTRUAL FLARE-UPS

Research suggests that IBD symptoms can follow the ebb and flow of a woman's menstrual cycle. This is not the case for all women who have IBD, but it certainly applies to some. Many female IBD sufferers feel their worst symptoms of diarrhea and abdominal pain during the week before and the week of their period. They feel their best during the middle two weeks of their menstrual cycle. One study conducted by Dr. Sunanda Kane found that 65 percent of female patients with active ulcerative colitis and 63 percent of those with active Crohn's noticed a correlation between their symptoms and their menstrual cycle.

In my practice I may treat "cyclical" IBD differently than normal flare-ups. I sometimes recommend an oral contraceptive, though I usually refer the patient to a gynecologist to determine which formulation would work best for her. U.S. studies indicate that oral contraceptives may help alleviate or reduce IBD symptoms that are linked to a woman's menstrual cycle. That's because they help reduce the hormonal fluctuations (especially monophasic preparations that have the same dose of estrogen/progesterone in every pill) that normally occur throughout the month. Research conducted in Europe found that oral contraceptives didn't work to relieve IBD symptoms, but that may be because they used formulations with higher doses of estrogen than are typical of U.S. formulations.

The truth is, we just don't know for certain if oral contraceptives work. However, if you have menstrual flare-ups, you may want to consider them to see if they

SMOKING AND CROHN'S

Research indicates that women are more likely than men to have complications from Crohn's if they smoke. Now, I'm certainly not advocating that men smoke, but I do want to stress that smoking is particularly dangerous for women with Crohn's. They are more likely to have aggressive Crohn's disease that is more difficult to control, and if they need surgery to remove diseased portions of their intestine, their disease is more likely to recur faster than in male Crohn's patients who smoke and have surgery.

So are male smokers with Crohn's better off than female smokers with Crohn's? Perhaps, but both genders are playing with fire if they smoke with Crohn's. See page 142 for tips on quitting smoking.

work in your particular case. Some of my IBD patients swear that going on the pill helped their flare-ups, while others have told me that the pill made no difference or gave them minimal relief at best.

CAN YOU GET PREGNANT AND HAVE A HEALTHY BABY?

You certainly can. You do have to take some precautions and plan ahead. The best advice I can give you is to get your disease in remission before pregnancy. According to the latest research, women with either ulcerative colitis or Crohn's who get pregnant when they have no active disease do better and generally have fewer flare-ups during pregnancy. They also have a higher chance of carrying the baby to term and fewer problems at the time of delivery. Women who get pregnant in the middle of a flare-up, however, are taking a roll of the dice. For about a third of them the flare-up will subside during pregnancy; for another third the flare-up will stay its course; and for a third it will get worse.

Several months ago I treated a twenty-year-old woman, Kaitlin, who got pregnant during a flare-up of her ulcerative colitis. Kaitlin needed to be hospitalized for several weeks, and we agonized together over which medications she should take to treat her ulcerative colitis and not harm her baby. "I'd rather take a milder medication than put my baby at risk," she told me. I told her I understood completely but explained that she probably needed stronger medications, like corticosteroids, to get her into remission. "Having your flare-up continue or get worse can harm your baby, to say nothing of the agony that it will put you through," I said.

Kaitlin finally decided to have surgery, a colectomy, to remove the diseased portions of her bowel. It was a risky procedure that carried a small chance of miscarriage, but it worked. Kaitlin no longer had active disease, and she was able to carry her baby to term. She delivered a healthy baby girl and was ecstatic. "I'm so happy that my disease is in remission because I really want to nurse her without worrying about medications passing into the breast milk," she told me. As I held baby Trina and saw her little fist squeeze my finger, I took comfort in knowing that Kaitlin had made the right decision.

The good news is that having ulcerative colitis or Crohn's that's in remission doesn't affect a woman's fertility. Men with IBD, though, may experience a decrease in fertility, and women with a flare-up of Crohn's run a greater risk of premature delivery, stillbirth, or miscarriage.

Can you continue to take your medications during pregnancy? That depends. Medications are usually forbidden during pregnancy, but certain categories of IBD drugs appear to cause no ill effects to the fetus. Mesalamine and other 5-ASA compounds, as well as prednisone and other steroids, are very safe. If you take a more potent immunosuppressive drug, like 6-mercaptopurine, you should discuss the pros and cons of continuing it with your doctor. Methotrexate can cause birth defects and is not recommended during pregnancy.

If you have IBD, you need to discuss your plans with your doctor at least three months before you try to become pregnant. Make sure that whatever medication you're taking is safe for your fetus. Some drugs should be discontinued several months before conception since they can remain active in the body for a time after you stop taking them. Obviously, it's a personal choice whether to take a medication when you become pregnant. No medication is 100 percent safe, but you have to weigh any risk against the danger of your suffering a flare-up. A flare-up may be worse for your fetus than a medication that's considered to be generally safe. I can only tell you that you and your doctor need to look at your own individual case to make the decision that's best for you.

CAN YOU HAVE IBD AND IBS?

As I mentioned, many women with IBD are mistakenly misdiagnosed with IBS, until they have the proper diagnostic tests to evaluate their symptoms. Further complicating the picture, a significant percentage of IBD sufferers also have IBS. So yes, it's possible to have both conditions. This is especially true for women.

Alison was diagnosed with Crohn's disease at the age of twenty-two. When I first met her, she was a thirty-year-old single mother of a two-year-old daughter. Her previous doctor had prescribed a number of different and progressively stronger IBD medications with no success. Her diarrhea and abdominal cramping were getting out of hand. She had a hard time making it through the workday and was seriously considering quitting her job as a medical secretary and applying for disability.

Alison had recently separated from her husband and was struggling financially because of her lost workdays and mounting medical bills with medicine trials for her IBD. She was stressed, which she told me worsened her GI symptoms. Instead of just treating her symptoms as a flare-up of her IBD, I ordered a colonoscopy and a number of lab tests and actually found that Alison's Crohn's

FINDING A SUPPORT SYSTEM

IBD isn't caused by stress or other emotional factors, but it can be an emotionally wrenching illness at times. One of the best things you can do for yourself is to establish a strong support system. Call on friends and family members if you're having difficulty coping during a flare-up. Find a doctor you can talk to and trust. You may also want to join a support group to make contact with other IBD sufferers. For instance, the support group at the University of Virginia Hospital is sponsored by the Digestive Health Center of Excellence and the Crohn's and Colitis Foundation of America (CCFA). This group provides an excellent resource for patients and families.

Ask your gastroenterologist about a local support group that might be sponsored by your hospital. Or join an online group. I did a search on the Web and found several online support groups for IBD such as Chronnies Chat at www.tinkertech.net/crohns/. The CCFA (www.ccfa.org) can also provide you with information on groups meeting in your local area.

ACUPUNCTURE: IS IT WORTH A TRY?

Research suggests that acupuncture can cause changes in the immune system. Some studies have shown that it can suppress immune function in lab animals that have overactive immune systems. IBD is believed to result from an autoimmune disorder in which the body attacks the intestinal mucosa, seeing it as foreign tissue. So it seems reasonable to theorize that acupuncture might help reverse the effects of IBD by suppressing immune function in the GI tract.

No well-designed clinical trials of acupuncture in IBD have been performed. Asian researchers published an article of case reports describing thirty-nine IBD patients who responded favorably to acupuncture. A second case study of sixty-one patients also found beneficial effects. I want to emphasize that these select case reports can't provide strong evidence that acupuncture works. However, if you're eager to minimize the use of medications, you may want to give it a shot. There is some scientific basis for the theories, and it can't cause you any harm. It's important to find an acupuncturist who knows the acupuncture points that are associated with the intestinal mucosa. (One of the case report studies used the acupuncture points ST-25, ST-36, CV-6, and CV-1.)

For information on finding a reputable acupuncturist, contact the National Certification Commission for Acupuncture and Oriental Medicine at (703) 548-9004 or log on to www.nccaom.org.

was in remission on her maintenance Crohn's medications.

What, then, was the problem? We explored the idea that her symptoms might be caused by IBS. She was surprised to hear that she could actually have both conditions at the same time but was also relieved to know that she could take steps to relieve her symptoms. Instead of adding more IBD medications to her regimen, I worked with Alison to modify her diet—increasing her intake of fiber and cutting down on caffeine. I prescribed some very mild antispasmodics. Alison also worked on reducing stress by identifying her stressors and finding ways to get a break. She asked her sister to babysit her daughter twice a week so she could get to the gym to exercise, and she hired a housekeeper to come once a week to clean the house. Yes, Alison still has to contend with IBD, but she also has IBS, and understanding that connection has helped her get control of her GI symptoms.

IBD RESOURCES

THE CROHN'S AND COLITIS FOUNDATION OF AMERICA
tel. (800) 343-3637 or (212) 685-3440
www.ccfa.org
The foundation provides information on recent research and news topics on IBD; allows you to order books and other resources; and gives information on becoming an advocate and joining a local chapter of a support group.

MEDLINEPLUS
www.nlm.nih.gov/medlineplus
If you do a search of Crohn's disease or ulcerative colitis on this website, you'll find a wealth of information about the two conditions, such as drug information and clinical trials. The Crohn's page has an interactive tutorial as well. You'll also find a medical encyclopedia on this site.

**NATIONAL DIGESTIVE DISEASES INFORMATION
CLEARINGHOUSE**
tel. (800) 891-5389 or (301) 654-3810
digestive.niddk.nih.gov
The clearinghouse's website provides complete background
information on Crohn's and ulcerative colitis; click on
"Digestive Diseases." It also provides links to other government sites and to information on clinical trials.

A wide variety of books about inflammatory bowel
disease are on the market. Here are two books
recommended by the Crohn's and Colitis Foundation of
America. You can buy them on the CCFA website; check
out your local bookstore or www.amazon.com for others.

Stanley H. Stein, ed. *Inflammatory Bowel Disease: A Guide
for Patients and Their Families,* 2nd ed. Philadelphia:
Lippincott Williams and Wilkins, 1999.

Penny Steiner-Grossman. *The NEW People ... Not
Patients: A Source Book for Living with Inflammatory
Bowel Disease.* CCFA, 1997.

There are many issues involved with managing IBD.
First and foremost you need to educate yourself as
much as possible about your condition. Being prepared
is the best way to be in control of your illness. This is a
chronic disorder, but it doesn't have to be debilitating,
and it doesn't have to control your life. Sure, there are
some aspects of the disease, like flare-ups or complications, that can sidetrack you temporarily. But you can
gain back control by staying on your maintenance
medications and knowing what to expect in terms of

treatment. You also need to remember that you did nothing to cause this disease.

I think the most important thing you can do is to find a physician whom you can trust and put your faith in to treat your IBD. You need to feel that your doctor is a real partner who takes your concerns into account when devising a treatment plan. Remember, you are not alone. Others are going through similar experiences, and you can lean on them through support groups or your loved ones to help manage this condition and continue with the active life you've always led.

COLORECTAL CANCER—
THE NUMBER-THREE
CANCER KILLER OF WOMEN

I TALK TO MY PATIENTS AND women friends about cancer scares all the time. I know what women are most concerned about: breast and ovarian cancer—and sometimes even brain tumors (as rare as those are). Colorectal cancer isn't on most women's minds, yet it's the third-leading cancer killer of women, right behind lung and breast cancers. Contrary to popular belief, colon cancer afflicts as many women as men. Yet many women still think of colon cancer as a "man's disease."

In recent years colon cancer in women hit the national spotlight. In memory of her husband who died of colon cancer, TV journalist Katie Couric led the campaign to promote colonoscopies by actually having hers performed on her morning news show. Sharon Osbourne, star of the MTV show *The Osbournes*, announced in 2003 that she had been treated for colon cancer. Yet even with all this recent publicity, the vast majority of women aren't getting screened for the disease.

According to 2000 data from the CDC, just 41 percent of women over age fifty get regularly screened for colorectal cancer. Fewer women get screened than men. Yet screening could prevent half the deaths from this disease in the United States.

The good news is that the incidence and death rate for colorectal cancer are falling. This trend has probably come about from our improved ability to catch colon cancer early, even in a precancerous stage. But it may also have to do with certain lifestyle factors. Taking a daily baby aspirin (which many of us take to prevent heart disease) appears to protect against colon cancer. So, too, does getting enough calcium in the diet.

In nine out of ten cases, colon cancer arises from growths called polyps. They're common (a third of adults over fifty have them) and usually benign (noncancerous), and they can show up anywhere along the large intestine. Most polyps are either one of two types: hyperplastic or adenomatous. Hyperplastic polyps are benign, with zero cancer potential. I tell my patients that they are just bumps of tissue like pimples that have no risk of turning into cancer. Adenomatous polyps are precancerous, but not all adenomatous polyps will turn into cancer. In fact, only a minority of adenomatous polyps will become cancerous over time, generally the large polyps—those bigger than one centimeter.

Since gastroenterologists can't predict which adenomatous polyps will become cancerous, we usually remove any we find during a colonoscopy. Polyps go through a number of mutations before they change into cancer. These genetic changes take time, and it is estimated that in many cases over a decade passes between the inception of a polyp and the development of colon cancer. This is why you only need to get a colonoscopy every ten years if you're healthy and at average risk for colon cancer.

The vast majority of polyps occur in men and women over age fifty. For this reason nearly every major health organization in the country recommends that healthy people get regularly screened for colon cancer from fifty onward. If colorectal cancer runs in your family, you need to begin screening at a younger age, generally ten years before the age when your family member was diagnosed. As is often the case with cancer, *colorectal cancer frequently causes no symptoms until the tumor is large or has spread.* By the time a colon growth causes a symptom like abdominal or rectal pain, rectal bleeding, or a change in bowel habits, it's often more difficult to treat. Major surgery may be required to remove the cancerous portion of the colon, and the cancer may have spread beyond the colon, increasing the risk of mortality.

Colorectal cancer screening saves lives the way Pap smears do. Just as a Pap smear screens for precancerous lesions in the cervix, screening for colorectal cancer screens for polyps before they become malignant. Yes, I'll be the first to admit that a colonoscopy is more invasive, expensive, and uncomfortable than a Pap smear. But it's a one-step process that screens for polyps and removes them on the spot. And if you're at average risk, you need to be screened only once a decade. Just as Pap smears have the potential to banish cervical cancer, regular colon cancer screenings have the potential to *prevent* the vast majority of colon cancers.

I recently saw a patient who underscored the importance of having routing screening colonoscopies. Ellen, a fifty-two-year-old third-grade teacher, came to see me for a screening colonoscopy. She told me she was missing school that day and had left her students with a substitute teacher. "I hate leaving the kids with a substitute to get a medical exam, but my gynecologist told me that I *had* to have this test before my next birthday." Ellen told me she had no symptoms and felt perfectly fine. "This should be a breeze," I assured her.

As I was performing the colonoscopy, my heart sank as I turned the corner to her right colon and saw a large mass near the cecum, in the uppermost portion of the colon. Immediately after the colonoscopy, I spoke to her and her husband about the mass and explained that it was too large to be removed by colonoscopy. I told them to prepare for the possibility that it might be cancer. I could see Ellen's face go pale. "What will I tell the kids?" she asked me. I knew she meant both her own teenage children and her third-grade students.

After our appointment I introduced Ellen to our colorectal surgeon, and the next day she had surgery to remove the mass and a portion of her colon. We were all thrilled to learn that the growth was a large precancerous polyp. Given its size, it's highly probable that it would have turned into cancer, and by the time she developed symptoms, the cancer might have spread. Ellen was lucky. Her family and her third-grade students were lucky. "Your gynecologist saved your life," I told her.

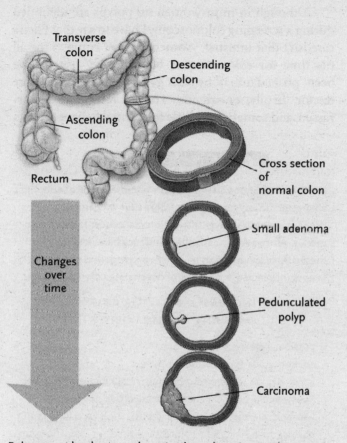

Polyps can develop anywhere in the colon. As a polyp grows, genetic changes occur that can increase its potential to become cancerous. This process can take several years. The goal of screening colonoscopy is to detect polyps at an early stage and to remove them before they become malignant.

Although in most women no polyps are identified during a screening colonoscopy, I have to say that Ellen's case isn't that unusual. Women like her come to me all the time for colonoscopies because they feel they've been "pushed into it" by their gynecologist, primary care doctor, family, or friends. They're reluctant, embarrassed, and sometimes a little frightened to have the test.

WHAT IS YOUR RISK?

In the United States an individual's lifetime risk of developing colorectal cancer is six percent. More than 90 percent of cases occur in individuals over fifty. Colorectal cancer is more common in African Americans than in Caucasians and in both of these ethnic groups than in Asians or Hispanics. Certain risk factors may increase your risk of developing colorectal cancer.

YOU'RE AT INCREASED RISK FOR COLON CANCER IF YOU HAVE ANY OF THE FOLLOWING . . .

- previous colorectal cancer
- adenomatous (precancerous) polyps
- a first-degree relative (mother, father, sibling, or child) who has had colorectal cancer or precancerous polyps
- two or more distant relatives (aunt, uncle, cousin, grandparent) who have had colorectal cancer or precancerous polyps
- inflammatory bowel disease
- any of the colon cancer genes (Genetic tests are available to test for familial polyposis and hereditary nonpolyposis colon cancer genes.)
- a history of breast, ovarian, or endometrial cancer

Note: If you're at increased risk, you may need to begin screening at a younger age and may need a colonoscopy more frequently than an average-risk person. If you fit into any of these categories, talk to your doctor about when you should start screening and how often you should be screened.

YOU'RE AT AVERAGE RISK FOR COLON CANCER IF YOU . . .

- don't have any of the above risk factors, and you're fifty or older.

But I can tell you that they're always happy after they have the screening test. Most women find that the colonoscopy isn't as bad as they expected. In fact, they usually have little recollection of the experience once the sedative wears off. More important, they never regret gaining the knowledge that the test gives them. Either they get a clean bill of health, which is a big relief, or the test finds a suspicious growth that would have continued to grow had the colonoscopy not been performed.

COLORECTAL CANCER SCREENING RECOMMENDATIONS

For years U.S. medical societies have debated the merits of various screening tests for colorectal cancer. In 2003 the American Gastroenterological Association, the American Cancer Society, and several other health organizations endorsed updated guidelines for colorectal cancer screening. These are the following:

Colorectal cancer screening in average-risk patients should begin at the age of fifty. Recommended screening options include:

- colonoscopy every ten years

  or

- fecal occult blood test annually

  or

- flexible sigmoidoscopy every five years

  or

- annual fecal occult blood testing plus flexible sigmoidoscopy every five years

  or

- double-contrast barium enema every five years

The reason for these multiple recommendations is a practical one: Specific colorectal cancer screening procedures may not be available in some areas or appropriate for all patients. Moreover, these recommendations give patients and physicians a choice of screening options. Your choice should be based on the test that is most acceptable to you, given your concerns about cost, safety, and comfort, as well as which tests are available to you in your geographic location. The next section gives you some information about the various tests available and can help you to choose which one is right for you.

Whichever option you choose, be assured that it is right for you. The most important message I can impart is that colorectal cancer screening can save your life and that any screening is better than none.

WHICH TEST TO HAVE?

All medical tests have their advantages and disadvantages, and colon cancer screening tests are no exception. The ones that are the least invasive are the least specific, which means they cast a wide net and may pick up many suspicious findings that turn out not to be cancer. Ultimately, the decision about which screening test to have may lie in your hands. Your doctor may make a recommendation, but you'll probably have some say in the decision. Here's what you need to know about the pros and cons of all the screening tests.

Colonoscopy

Colonoscopy is the accepted gold standard test for colon cancer screening. It enables physicians to see the entire length of the colon, and polyps can be removed during the procedure—which, in essence, can prevent the vast majority of polyps from ever turning into cancer. It involves the insertion of a lighted flexible tube into the rectum, which is advanced upward to examine the entire colon. Any polyps detected are usually removed and biopsied to determine if they are cancerous, precancerous, or harmless. Two high-quality studies, the National Polyp Study and the Veterans Cooperative Study, have confirmed that colonoscopy is the most accurate way to detect colon polyps. Like the Pap smear for cervical cancer, colonoscopy can drastically reduce your risk of getting colon cancer, and most of my colleagues agree that it's the most effective way to prevent the disease.

Colonoscopy, though, has its drawbacks. It's the most invasive, inconvenient, and risky screening test. Most women prefer to be sedated for the procedure, which means you'll need to have someone to drive you home afterward and you may feel groggy for a few hours. Colonoscopy also requires you to completely clean out your colon beforehand, since any stool contents can make polyps harder to detect. There are several different preparations for this cleaning procedure, but basically all involve taking strong laxatives and spending a fair amount of time on the commode emptying your bowels. Most women tell me that the preparation is inconvenient and unpleasant and that the test itself is much easier.

Colonoscopy is the most expensive of the screening tests if your insurance plan doesn't cover it. (Most plans now provide coverage for all or part of the cost.) Colonoscopy also carries a very small risk of serious side effects. When I go over the informed consent for the procedure, I tell all of my patients that there is a risk of infection, bleeding, perforation (poking a hole through the bowel wall), and reaction to the medications given for sedation. The likelihood of these complications is low (a risk of one in a thousand for serious bleeding and perforation requiring surgery and a risk of three in a thousand for bleeding that requires hospitalization, according to one study). Legally, your doctor is required to make you aware of these possibilities, however remote they may be.

The truth is, colonoscopy is a complicated procedure that must be performed by a well-trained physician. Ask your family physician to refer you to a qualified gastroenterologist to perform your colonoscopy, or see Chapter 8 for guidelines on finding the right physician.

Colonoscopy Prep: Various Options for the Big Clean-Out: Everyone passes around terrible tales of their colonoscopy prep. "I had to drink gallons and gallons of a vile-tasting liquid" is a complaint I hear often from patients after they've had their procedure. I'm sympathetic to this problem. I really am. I want to make the colonoscopy experience as tolerable as possible, so that my patients will come back for follow-up screenings. Every doctor has his or her preferred method of prep. But each method also has both benefits and drawbacks. If you prefer one method over another, you should discuss your preference with your doctor. Here's a quick

---

Katie Couric on Colonoscopy:

"It's a minor inconvenience, but it's a lot less inconvenient than premature death—believe me. Maybe you're frightened of [having a colonoscopy], but it's much more frightening to get a diagnosis of colon cancer. I didn't feel a thing when I had mine. I said, 'When are you going to start?' and he [her physician] was already halfway up."

—**Katie Couric,** whose husband died of colon cancer at age forty-two

run-down. (*Note:* I don't provide specific instructions here. Your doctor will hand you a list depending on the prep you choose.) The preparation itself begins on the day before the procedure and may follow one of the three following protocols:

Colyte (pronounced co-light) *or Golytely (pronounced* go lightly), *or polyethylene glycol:*   Colyte/Golytely is a powder packaged in a gallon-size plastic container that you fill with water. Refrigerating the solution overnight usually makes it more pleasant to drink. Many preparations come with flavor packets (pineapple, cherry, lemon lime, etc.), or you can add a few drops of lemon or vanilla extract to the unflavored preparation to make it taste better. Starting the evening before your procedure, you need to drink an 8-ounce glass about every ten minutes to finish the entire gallon in two to three hours. Drinking the entire preparation in this short time span is essential for it to be effective. I have to warn you, though, that most patients tell me drinking such a large amount of liquid in such a short period of time is often difficult. If you feel nauseated, take a break for about a half hour and start again.

You'll begin to have loose stools one to three hours after you begin drinking the Colyte/Golytely. Upon completion, the bowel movement should be liquid and clear (like tea). That's a sign that you've done a good prep.

Fleet's Phospho-Soda: This is my preferred method because you don't need to drink as much liquid and you can mix the Phospho-Soda into the clear liquid beverage of your choice. I've been told that this prep is much more palatable than others. In my experience the prep with Phospho-Soda is as good as that with Colyte/Golytely (which means that the colon is clear and easy to view), especially if the patient drinks *plenty of liquids the day before.*

A 3-ounce (90-milliliter) bottle of Fleet's Phospho-Soda can be purchased over the counter at your local drugstore. It can be mixed with the clear, chilled beverage of your choice. My patients tell me that ginger ale, a lemon-lime soft drink, or apple juice dramatically improves the taste. You will take the prep in two stages, generally half the night before, and the other half several hours before your colonoscopy.

Note: Patients with heart or kidney problems may not be able to take the Phospho-Soda since this can cause a dangerous rise in sodium and phosphate in their blood.

Visicol: The newest kid on the block, Visicol tablets are laxatives in pill form. But don't be fooled—you'll still need to drink a large amount of liquid to dissolve these tablets. And there are a total of forty large pills. You need to drink about a gallon of clear liquid—most people will naturally drink this much in order to swallow the pills.

Some patients prefer the Visicol prep; others have called me in the middle of the prep to ask me if they could switch to Phospho-Soda because they couldn't force down another pill. So I'd have to say that this newest prep has about the same tolerance rate as the other two. Finally, some doctors don't like this prep because it can leave a white film coating on the lining of the colon at the time of the colonoscopy.

These are the three most common types of preps, though some doctors may do a combination of laxatives like Phospho-Soda, magnesium citrate, two or three Dulcolax tablets, and/or a suppository. No matter what prep you use, you should expect to be in the bathroom for a good portion of the evening and into the night. Be prepared with a good book or magazine and some soft toilet tissue. Some of my patients experience irritation or an aggravation of their hemorrhoids with the frequent bowel movements and wiping. You may choose to use Vaseline around this area to relieve irritation or to gently pat the area clean with soft moist tissues, baby wipes, or Tucks Medicated Pads, which contain witch hazel.

Some people have trouble abstaining from solid food for a day or two. If you're really hungry for some food with texture, a company called E-Z-Em just began offering colonoscopy prep foods that are designed to pass through the system easily. They offer chicken noodle soup, nutrition bars, and rice cakes, to name a few. The food options are called Nutraprep, and you can find out more about them on E-Z-Em's website (www.ezem.com).

Flexible Sigmoidoscopy

When I first began practicing as a gastroenterologist about fifteen years ago, flexible sigmoidoscopies (a.k.a.

flex sigs) were the routine screening method for colorectal cancer. In this test a flexible lighted tube, with a tiny camera attached, is inserted into the lower third of the colon to check for polyps or cancer. It takes about ten minutes and can be performed in your doctor's office without sedation. You don't need to go through the hassle of the colonoscopy prep, although you'll need to take a few enemas before the procedure.

The problem? The sigmoidoscope can only reach about a third of the way up the colon, whereas the colonoscope can span the entire length. A colleague of mine, the current AGA president, Dr. Dan Podolsky, puts it this way: "Relying on flexible sigmoidoscopy is

One Woman Peeks at Her Own Colon

"My mother was diagnosed with colon cancer in her sixties, so I was concerned about my own health risk. My doctor recommended that I get a colonoscopy when I turned forty-five. I had a hard time drinking a gallon of Colyte. Sitting on a toilet every ten minutes was no picnic, either, though I didn't have any abdominal pain or cramps. I have to admit, though, that I felt great once I was cleaned out, and I found that the actual procedure was a breeze. I didn't want much sedation because I wanted to see my colon on camera, since I'm an anatomy professor. My gastroenterologist found a few polyps that she removed and [she] told me I needed to be monitored every five years. I can't say I look forward to my colonoscopies, but I certainly don't dread them."

—**Sharon,** 56, grandmother of four, whose mother survived her bout of colon cancer as clinically logical as performing mammography on one breast to screen women for breast cancer. It is time to go the distance."

Yes, doctors can detect and prevent some colon lesions using "flex sig," but they'll completely miss all growths that are beyond the reach of the scope. Studies have shown that flex sig misses 20 to 30 percent of cancers and polyps. These are usually located beyond the reach of the scope, on the right side of the colon. What's more, polyps are generally not removed at the time of the sigmoidoscopy, so if your doctor finds any, you have to then undergo a colonoscopy to have the rest of the colon looked at and to have any polyps removed. There is still a slight risk of perforation with flexible sigmoidoscopy, but it is thought to be less than the risk with colonoscopy.

Still, flex sigs serve a purpose, especially in rural areas that don't have facilities that offer colonoscopy screenings. They are incredibly reliable for finding polyps and malignancies in the lower portion of the colon, where the majority of polyps occur. I'd rather have a patient go for a flex sig than have no colon cancer screening at all. Several health organizations, including the American Cancer Society, have endorsed flex sig as a screening option for colon cancer—especially if it's performed in conjunction with a fecal occult blood test. The latter screen can help detect malignancies in the upper reaches of the colon that are left unchecked by the sigmoidoscope.

Double-Contrast Barium Enema

In this screening test your colon is X-rayed after you are given an enema containing barium, a chalky solution that coats the colon, allowing polyps to show up on an X-ray. The test can miss small growths, though, so it's not as accurate as a colonoscopy. In fact, the landmark National Polyp Study found that double-contrast barium enema may fail to detect up to 30 percent of polyps that are larger than 1 centimeter. It has an even lower accuracy for lesions smaller than a centimeter.

The day before your exam you need to do a bowel prep (similar to what you do before a colonoscopy). During the procedure your colon is filled with a mixture of barium and air. You may feel crampy and very bloated. You may feel an urgency to move your bowels (a common feeling with any enema). The radiologist will take several X-rays of different areas of your colon, which takes 15 to 30 minutes. After the X-rays are complete, you'll be allowed to evacuate the enema in the restroom. The plus side to a barium enema is that the risk of perforation is very low. No sedation is required, so you are alert and able to resume your normal activities right afterward. The downside is that the barium enema may miss large polyps or even cancer, and you'll need to have a colonoscopy to remove any polyps that are found by this procedure.

Fecal Occult Blood Test

This test, which should be done each year, is by far the easiest to perform. In fact, you can do it yourself with a take-home kit that your doctor provides. You'll collect three stool samples and smear them on special cards that you seal and mail back to your doctor. The presence of blood can indicate polyps or colorectal cancer. Those who test positive are usually referred for a colonoscopy.

Annual screening with a fecal occult blood test can reduce your risk of dying from colon cancer by 33 percent—about the same reduction as a mammogram for breast cancer. The problem with the test is that it is not very reliable. Even the most accurate one misses cancer about 15 percent of the time (false-negative results) and wrongly signals polyps or cancer in some 6 percent of cases (false-positive results). Still, I think this test can be very useful, especially if you have no family history of colon cancer or other risk factors (see the box "What Is Your Risk?" on page 452) and you're reluctant to have a colonoscopy. I'd rather you got a yearly fecal occult blood test than no screening at all.

To avoid a false positive, don't collect fecal samples during your period (or up to three days afterward) or if you have hemorrhoids that are bleeding. Depending on the type of test your doctor uses, you may have to avoid the following foods and drugs for three days beforehand: aspirin and other nonsteroidal anti-inflammatory drugs; undercooked meat (it can contain blood); certain fruits and vegetables—melons, radishes, and cherry tomatoes—that are high in the enzyme peroxidase (which can skew test results); and vitamin C supplements (which can cause a false negative).

This advice, however, is controversial. A recent analysis of five randomized trials found that the per-

SCREENING TESTS AT A GLANCE

Here's a quick reference guide to the various colorectal screening tests, so you can compare the differences among them.

COLONOSCOPY

- estimated reduction in risk of death from colorectal cancer in those who follow screening recommendations: 59 percent
- estimated reliability at detecting polyps (sensitivity): greater than 90 percent
- estimated accuracy at distinguishing polyps from normal colon tissue (specificity): greater than 99 percent
- anesthesia needed: light sedation
- patient preparation: liquid diet for twenty-four hours before test and oral laxative

FLEXIBLE SIGMOIDOSCOPY

- estimated reduction in risk of death from colorectal cancer in those who follow screening recommendations: 59 percent (for lesions in the left side of the colon)
- estimated sensitivity: 90 percent for areas within reach of scope; 50 to 70 percent for entire colon
- estimated specificity: 99 percent
- sedation required: none
- patient preparation: enema or oral laxative

FECAL OCCULT BLOOD TEST

- estimated reduction in risk of death from colorectal cancer in those who follow screening recommendations: 15 to 33 percent
- estimated sensitivity: 40 percent (misses 60 percent of polyps)
- estimated specificity: 96 to 98 percent
- sedation required: none
- patient preparation: dietary restriction of red meat, horseradish, and aspirin products before and during the test

Source: New England Journal of Medicine, vol. 346(1) (January 2002): 41.

centage of people who tested positive for fecal occult blood in their stool was the same regardless of whether they were told to follow dietary restrictions. Check with your doctor to see if you still need to follow these recommendations.

WHY FEWER WOMEN GET COLORECTAL SCREENING THAN MEN

The vast majority of women who should be getting screening for colorectal cancer aren't doing so. Yes, screening is on the rise, but far more women still get mammograms than get colorectal exams. Just 41 percent of women have had a colorectal cancer screening test of any kind, while 71 percent of women over forty have had a mammogram and 80 percent of women have had a Pap smear in the last two years. Here are some common reasons neither women nor men get tested, according to a 2002 study conducted by the National Cancer Institute:

- fear of pain or discomfort
- anxiety about potential test results
- embarrassment or unpleasantness of the test

Women, though, may have an even greater obstacle to getting tested: Their doctors often don't even refer them for colorectal screening. In one of many studies that evaluated gender bias, women were 6 to 19 percent less likely to undergo flexible sigmoidoscopy than men. Another study of patients who had polyps detected by sigmoidoscopy found that 80 percent of those who failed to go for a follow-up colonoscopy were women. I can only hope that with increased awareness of colorectal cancer in women, all doctors are finally seeing this cancer as both a "men's and women's" disease.

SCREENING TESTS
ON THE HORIZON

These next tests are on the horizon but are not yet ready for prime time. I tell my patients who are having their colonoscopies that these rapidly advancing, less invasive

DID YOU KNOW?

In 2001 Medicare (the U.S. government's health insurance program for people over sixty-five) began providing coverage for a screening colonoscopy every ten years for people at average risk. (They previously provided coverage only for those at high risk.) Most insurance companies and managed care organizations have now followed Medicare's lead.

Many people, however, still aren't aware that they have insurance coverage for colorectal screening tests. A recent survey of Medicare beneficiaries found that nearly 12 percent did not think that fecal occult blood tests were covered by Medicare, and another 16 percent didn't know whether it was covered. Nearly 28 percent of Medicare recipients weren't aware that they had coverage for flexible sigmoidoscopy, barium enema, or colonoscopy.

tests will likely be around soon, maybe even by the next time they have to undergo colorectal cancer screening.

Virtual Colonoscopy

Virtual colonoscopy is making its way out of the research world and into hospitals throughout the United States, but I wouldn't call it revolutionary. Basically, instead of inserting a colonoscope up through the expanse of your colon, it images your colon using a CT (computer tomography) scan. At this point in time you still have to undergo the colonoscopy prep to clean out your colon. But the procedure doesn't require sedation. What's more, it's far less invasive than colonoscopy and doesn't carry the same risk of complications.

Virtual colonoscopy sounds sexier than it actually is. Recent studies suggest that patients who have undergone both virtual and conventional colonoscopy actually prefer the conventional procedure. That's because virtual colonoscopy can sometimes cause discomfort when carbon dioxide is pumped into the colon to distend it before imaging. Most patients in these studies also felt that the nurses and gastroenterologists performing conventional colonoscopy were more knowledgeable about colorectal cancer screening and took more time and effort to care about their level of comfort than did staff performing virtual colonoscopy. The accuracy of virtual colonoscopy in detecting particularly smaller polyps is significantly lower than with conventional colonoscopy, and small pellets of stool seen during this examination may be confused for polyps. What's more, if a polyp is found during virtual colonoscopy, conventional colonoscopy must be performed to remove it. (We haven't yet figured out a way to do a virtual biopsy.)

Most facilities do not perform the two procedures on the same day, so if a polyp is found, it is likely that you will have to undergo another prep if you also need conventional colonoscopy. The most promising development for virtual colonoscopy may be an ability to accurately perform the examination without bowel preparation. This would likely make the test more attractive to patients than conventional colonoscopy. At this time virtual colonoscopy remains a subject of active research. To date no medical group has elected to endorse virtual colonoscopy as a colorectal cancer screening option, as it is still considered experimental. And the $500-to-$1,000 price tag is not reimbursed by Medicare or private insurers.

Fecal DNA Testing

Another technology on the horizon that is being actively researched today is fecal DNA testing. Scientists test a sample of stool for a number of different molecular markers to determine if genetic changes associated with colon polyps or colorectal cancer are present. PreGen-Plus, a simple, noninvasive stool DNA test, became available in August 2003. Completed studies suggest that this test detects between 65 and 70 percent of colorectal cancers. Although less accurate than colonoscopy, fecal DNA testing may be a useful screening option,

HIGH-TECH COLON SCREENING OF THE FUTURE?

In the 1966 science fiction movie *Fantastic Voyage*, a miniaturized submarine manned by a medical crew is sent into a man's body to annihilate a life-threatening blood clot. Within the next few years this capsule-size sub could become a diagnostic reality if upcoming clinical trials prove that it works.

As this book goes to press, a swallowable imaging capsule is being tested on GI patients throughout the country. Patients merely strap on a 3.5-pound fanny pack containing a wireless recorder, then swallow the capsule, which is the size of a large vitamin pill. The capsule hurtles down the esophagus into the stomach, and normal peristalsis propels it through the small intestine. Its video camera transmits an image of the inside of the gut, at the rate of two frames per second, to the recorder. Patients can perform their normal routines until they excrete the capsule six to eight hours later. They then return the recorder pack to their doctor's office, where the video is downloaded and viewed on a computer workstation. (The $300 capsule doesn't have to be recovered—a cost that will be factored into the total cost for the procedure.)

The question is: Can it work as well as a colonoscopy? At this time the answer is still unknown. For now the capsule is mainly used to image the entire 15-to-20-foot length of the small intestine, which is an important development since an endoscope can reach only through the first few feet of the intestine and the colonoscope can only look at the last six or so feet of the colon. Preliminary results so far seem promising. Researchers report that the capsule studies are better than standard barium studies of the small bowel, plus they can find bleeding lesions and precancerous tumors that are outside the reach of the endoscope.

The researchers are hopeful that the capsule will be used eventually as a first-line screening for colon cancer. Patients would still have to undergo the laxative prep to clear out the colon. And they would still have to have a follow-up colonoscopy if polyps were found, because the capsule can't remove polyps for a biopsy. I think it's too early to predict whether imaging capsules will replace more invasive GI tests. But if these capsules prove effective at finding polyps, many gastroenterologists and patients alike will be eager to try them.

particularly if you're reluctant to get a colonoscopy. It's still new, though, and more research on its effectiveness has to be completed. The cost of the new test on the market is about $800, and it is intended to be used once every three to five years.

Genetic Testing

Blood tests can detect inherited mutations in genes responsible for some rare forms of colorectal cancer, accounting for only one to three percent of cases. Those with specific genetic mutations (patients with familial adenomatous polyposis or hereditary nonpolyposis colorectal cancer) can have up to a 100 percent risk of developing colorectal cancer. You may be a candidate for genetic testing if you have a strong family history of colorectal cancer, especially if more than one generation is affected. Individuals suspected of having a genetic mutation that may increase their risk of colorectal cancer are usually referred to a genetic counselor, who studies their family tree and decides which genetic tests are appropriate.

Genetic testing can't replace traditional colorectal screening tests, but it can tell you whether you need to be screened more frequently. Those who do carry a colon cancer gene need to have frequent colonoscopies, as often as every one to three years instead of every ten. They also need to start screening earlier, in their twenties or thirties instead of in their fifties.

CAN YOU LOWER YOUR RISK OF COLORECTAL CANCER?

I'm always eager to read those women's magazine articles that promise to "prevent cancer" or "lower your risk by 30 percent," but I take them with a grain of salt. Like most cancers, colorectal cancer likely has multifactorial causes, some genetic and some due to things we're exposed to in the environment. And the "environment" of the colon has a lot to do with diet. Yes, studies come out all the time showing that some food or supplement can lower your risk of getting colorectal cancer. But don't get fooled into believing that changing just one thing (e.g., taking an aspirin a day) will prevent you from developing colorectal cancer. When I speak with a patient who's just had a colonoscopy where I've found polyps, I'm invariably asked, "What can I do?" to prevent polyps or cancer from growing.

Lifestyle changes alone can indeed decrease your cancer risk, but it's important to remember that what increases the risk for cancer in one person may not be the same in another. And what protects one person may not be as protective to another. Doing any one thing in a vacuum does no good. You need to look at the big picture and aim for an overall healthy lifestyle.

The following recommendations may decrease your risk for developing colorectal polyps or cancers, but I want to emphasize that *none* substitute for regular colorectal cancer screenings. So while it's fine to do these things, make sure to keep that appointment for your next colonoscopy! Here's what the latest research shows about minimizing your risk of colorectal cancer:

- **Reduce intake of red meat and certain fats:** Evidence suggests that eating red meat increases the risk of colorectal cancer. People who eat diets rich in saturated fat (found in whole-milk dairy products, fatty cuts of beef, chicken, and pork, and butter) or in trans fatty acids (found in margarine and partially hydrogenated vegetable oils) have a higher risk as well. Switching to monounsaturated fats (olive oil, nuts, avocados) and low-fat protein sources can help reduce risk.
- **Maintain a healthy weight:** Being obese (having a BMI over 30) doubles the risk of colon cancer in premenopausal women. And research has found a link between obesity and death from colorectal cancer. One study found that morbidly obese women (with a BMI of 40 or greater) who had

colon cancer were 62 percent more likely to die of the cancer than thinner women with colon cancer.

- **Eat folate-rich foods:** Folate, a mineral found mostly in fruits and vegetables, has been associated with a reduced risk of colorectal cancer. Research has shown that diets rich in folate are associated with a decreased relative risk of colon cancer, and conversely, a higher rate of malignancy is seen in those whose diets are lacking in folate. The Harvard Nurses' Health Study found that women who got more than 400 micrograms a day of folate had a 30 percent lower risk of colon cancer than women who ate less than 200 micrograms a day. Folic acid may protect genetic material, DNA, from getting damaged, which can turn a healthy cell into a cancerous one. Now that federal regulations require bread and cereal to be fortified with folate, you should have no trouble getting a healthy dose every day.

- **Stop smoking:** Smoking can ravage your body in numerous ways—and now here's another: Research shows that women who started smoking before age thirty and smoke a pack a day for ten years or more have twice the risk of colorectal cancer as nonsmokers. (Tips on quitting smoking can be found on page 142.)

- **Lower alcohol intake:** Drinking more than four drinks per week increases your colorectal cancer risk. If you imbibe a nightly glass of wine, however, studies suggest you can reduce this risk by taking supplemental folic acid.

- **Exercise:** The Harvard Nurses' Health Study found that women who ran for more than two hours a week had a 40 percent lower colorectal cancer risk than their sedentary peers. Walking briskly for three or four hours a week can produce the same benefit.
- **Eat fiber?** For years it was assumed that fiber—found in most fruits, vegetables, and whole-grain products—could lower the risk of colorectal cancer. Fiber was thought to have some protective effect against toxic colon by-products before it passed out of the body as waste. Scientists theorized that fiber could prevent the development of precancerous polyps. Recent studies, however, have failed to identify such a benefit. I'm not ready to discount the fiber theory, though. Often studies take ten to twenty years to find a real benefit on whether a dietary habit can prevent the progression of a polyp into cancer. Most of these studies have followed patients for only three or four years at most. I say, keep striving to get at least 25 grams of fiber in your diet each day. (See page 197 for more details on increasing your fiber intake.) Even if fiber-rich foods prove to have no effect against colorectal cancer, you're still eating the healthiest foods around and getting the other benefits of an increased fiber intake, like a lower cholesterol level and a reduced risk of diabetes.
- **Stock up on calcium:** Research has shown that those who consume more calcium have a reduced risk of developing colorectal cancer. One study found that consuming 3000 milligrams of calcium a day

(more than twice the RDA) reduced the chance of recurrence of adenoma, a type of colorectal tumor. I definitely recommend getting at least 1200 to 1500 milligrams of calcium a day. You may prefer to get this amount through low-fat dairy products and other calcium-rich foods, since supplements can cause GI problems like constipation or bloating.

• **Hormone replacement therapy/oral contraceptives:** Recent studies have supported evidence that hormone replacement therapy in postmenopausal women may be protective against colorectal cancer. Given all of the recent publicity about the health risks of HRT, however, I would strongly recommend that you have a frank discussion with your doctor about its pros and cons in your particular case.

   By the same token, several other studies suggest that using oral contraceptives may be protective against colon cancer. Protection appeared to be greater in women who had used oral contraceptives more recently, but those who used oral contraceptives in the past still had some protection. Researchers are now conducting studies to find the mechanisms by which female hormones protect against colorectal cancer.

• **Consider aspirin:** In a study of 90,000 women, those who took four to six aspirin tablets per week for twenty years had a 44 percent reduction in colorectal cancer risk. Two recent studies published in the *New England Journal of Medicine* suggest that taking an aspirin every day reduces the number and size of colon polyps. Aspirin may block an enzyme, cyclooxygenase-2 or COX-2, which appears to play a role in spurring cell growth that can lead to tumors. (Other nonsteroidal anti-inflammatory drugs like ibuprofen and naproxen sodium and COX-2 inhibitor drugs like Celebrex may confer the same benefits, but rigorous research studies haven't yet been done to test them.)

You might consider taking aspirin, especially if you have a family history of colorectal cancer. But deciding to try it isn't like resolving to eat more vegetables. Like all medications, aspirin has its risks, especially if you have a sensitive stomach or an ulcer, or you're taking an anticoagulant drug. You need to check with your doctor before you embark on this prevention strategy.

SYMPTOMS OF COLORECTAL CANCER

The majority of polyps and early cancers begin with no symptoms at all. Even after a polyp becomes cancerous, it may grow silently for up to five years before symptoms start to appear. Contact your doctor immediately if you have any of these signs:

- rectal bleeding or blood in the stool
- change in bowel movements (especially in the shape of the stool—e.g., narrow like a pencil)
- abdominal pain or cramping, or frequent gas pain

- weight loss and/or anemia
- discomfort in moving your bowels or the urge to do so when there is no need to

TREATMENT FOR
COLORECTAL CANCER

Colorectal cancer can be cured if it is detected early. Most colon cancers, when localized to the innermost layers of the bowel wall, can be completely removed by endoscopic resection of the diseased tissue or through surgery alone. Once the tumor has penetrated the full thickness of the colon wall, however, additional therapies such as chemotherapy or radiation may be required and the survival rate drops dramatically to less than 40 percent over five years.

With modern surgical techniques, permanent colostomy is required in less than five percent of colorectal cancer patients. Those with more advanced colorectal cancer have a better chance of surviving if they are given adjuvant therapy (chemotherapy or a combination of chemotherapy and radiation) in addition to surgery. Several interesting new therapies are making their way onto the clinical horizon. Here are some promising new treatments you should know about.

Irinotecan

Researchers from the Memorial Sloan-Kettering Cancer Center in New York have found that combining the drug irinotecan (Camptosar) with standard chemotherapy drugs used to treat stage IV colorectal cancer (that has spread throughout the body) can slow the progress of the disease and prolong patients' lives somewhat. This therapy may also prove useful in treating less advanced stage II and III cancers.

COX-2 Inhibitors

A study published in the *Journal of the American Medical Association* reported that colorectal cancer patients with high levels of the COX-2 enzyme in their tumor cells had a reduced chance of long-term survival. The five-year survival rate in patients whose tumors contained COX-2 was 40.5 percent. In those whose tumors did not test positive for COX-2, the survival rate was 91.6 percent. Research is under way to determine if COX-2 inhibitors, a new type of non-steroidal anti-inflammatory drug, may be helpful in the treatment of colon and other types of cancer. Studies have already shown that the inhibitors are capable of halting the growth of tumors in animals.

Elderly Do Benefit from Chemotherapy

A study has found that elderly people with colon cancer benefit from chemotherapy after surgery as much as younger patients, and elderly patients tolerate it just as well. Some doctors have been reluctant to prescribe chemotherapy to patients over sixty-five, and some patients reject it because they don't think they'll save enough years to make it worth it. The study from

the Mayo Clinic and six other centers in North America and Europe found that chemotherapy increased
the rate of those who survived for at least five years
from 64 percent to 71 percent, regardless of the patients' ages.

COLORECTAL CANCER RESOURCES

AMERICAN GASTROENTEROLOGICAL ASSOCIATION
4930 Del Ray Avenue
Bethesda, MD 20814
tel. (301) 654-2055
www.gastro.org
The AGA has brochures with details on colorectal cancer
screening and treatment options at www.gastro.org/-
clinicalRes/brochures/cc_screening.html. Its Foundation
for Digestive Health and Nutrition has additional
information on colorectal cancer screening for women at
www.fdhn.org.

CENTERS FOR DISEASE CONTROL AND PREVENTION
600 Clifton Road
Atlanta, GA 30333
tel. (800) 311-3435
www.cdc.gov
Detailed information on colorectal cancer screening
appears on the CDC's Screen for Life program website,
www.cdc.gov/cancer/screenforlife/fs_detailed.htm

AMERICAN CANCER SOCIETY
tel. (800) ACS-2345
www.cancer.org
The ACS is one of the best resources I know for all
information relating to cancer, including finding a

support group in your area. The website includes links to other cancer sites.

CANCER FACTS AND FIGURES
www.cancer.org/downloads/STT/CancerFacts&-
Figures2002TM.pdf
This site provides up-to-date statistics on all cancers, including colorectal cancer, and has survival figures for various stages of cancer.

NATIONAL COLORECTAL CANCER RESEARCH ALLIANCE
tel. (800) 872-3000
www.nccra.org
In 2003 Katie Couric launched a CD-ROM for patients called *Colorectal Cancer Education—What You Need to Know,* now available free at this website.

The strongest message I can convey in this chapter is that once you've gone through colorectal cancer screening, don't give up. Many patients will come to me for their first screening colonoscopy at age fifty because their gynecologist "strongly recommended this test." Nearly every week a woman tells me to "get a good look because this will be the last time" she'll have this test. And every week I tell these women to keep up with colorectal cancer screening. Like a trial lawyer, I lay out all the evidence. First, the risk of forming colon polyps and colon cancer increases with age. So having a one-time-only screening is as rational as having a one-time-only Pap smear—not likely to protect you overall. Second, newer technologies are being tested every day, and less invasive options are on the horizon and may even be available by the time they do their next screening. Third and probably the most convincing, the vast majority of women tell me that their expectations of the test were far worse than the actual experience. So if you take one piece of advice from me, make it this: Keep up with your colorectal cancer screening. It just may save your life.

CHAPTER 16

PROBLEMS "DOWN THERE"— HEMORRHOIDS, FECAL INCONTINENCE, AND MORE

So MANY WOMEN HAVE THEM, YET so few of us ever discuss them. We may mention them to our friends with a cursory "they got really bad during pregnancy." But we don't talk about how we deal with them. I'm talking about hemorrhoids, or swollen veins that appear in the anal canal (the last one and a half inches of the colon).

Ten to 25 percent of the population suffers from hemorrhoids, which occur most commonly in people ages forty-five to sixty-five. They also affect at least 50 percent of pregnant women. The pressure of the fetus in the abdomen, as well as hormonal changes, cause veins in the anus to enlarge. These vessels are placed under severe pressure during childbirth, and some women find that their hemorrhoids require medical treatment after delivery. For most women, however, hemorrhoids caused by pregnancy are a temporary problem that resolves following delivery.

You may be surprised to learn that gastroenterologists treat hemorrhoids. Usually women think of hemorrhoids as a gynecological problem even though they have nothing to do with the reproductive tract. Gastroenterologists also diagnose and treat other anal problems like fecal incontinence, anal fissures, and fistulas. Your anus, after all, is at the very end of your digestive tract; therefore other GI disorders can play a role in whether you have problems "down there."

If you have one of the following three symptoms, you have a medical problem that needs to be evaluated:

- bright red bleeding from your anus, blood in your stool, or even just blood on the toilet tissue after you wipe yourself after a bowel movement
- pain in the anal canal
- a problem with soiling your underwear because you just can't make it to the bathroom in time

Far too many women choose to suffer silently in pain or misplaced shame rather than discuss this sensitive subject with their health care provider. I hope this chapter will lessen any embarrassment you may feel and facilitate these discussions. I've divided it into four parts, dealing with the most common conditions that occur in the anus: hemorrhoids, fissures, fecal incontinence, and a number of other problems that can be mistaken for hemorrhoids, like fistulas and anal warts. Far too frequently, hemorrhoids are blamed for these problems and women go for years without relief because they've been misdiagnosed.

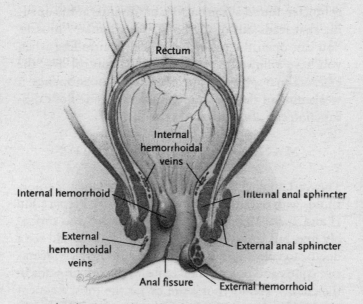

Rectum

Internal
hemorrhoidal
veins

Internal hemorrhoid

Internal anal sphincter

External
hemorrhoidal
veins

External anal sphincter

Anal fissure

External hemorrhoid

Hemorrhoids occur when blood vessels in or just outside the anus swell and become irritated. These engorged, fragile veins can cause itching, bleeding, and a sense of fullness at the anus. Anal fissures are small tears in the lining of the anal canal that can be painful or bleed during defecation.

WHAT'S GOING ON "DOWN THERE"?

Your anus is an inch-and-a-half-long ring of muscles that separates the rectum from the perineum. The muscles surrounding the anal canal are important for fecal continence. The internal anal sphincter, which allows stool to pass from the rectum into the anus, is an involuntary muscle controlled by the peristaltic contractions of the digestive tract. The external anal sphincter, found at the bottom of the anus at the opening that leads out of the body, is a voluntary muscle. You can open the sphincter at will, controlling when you have a bowel movement. Losing control over the external anal sphincter can lead to fecal incontinence. A weakening of the anal muscles due to pelvic floor dysfunction can also lead to this problem.

MANAGING HEMORRHOIDS

The vast majority of women self-treat their hemorrhoids with over-the-counter remedies like Preparation H and Tucks Medicated Pads. In general, this is probably fine, but if you have any bleeding, you should see a doctor to rule out more serious conditions like ulcerative colitis and polyps (cancerous or benign growths in the colon). Hemorrhoids are by far the most frequent cause of bright red bleeding from the colon. This bright hemorrhoidal blood is distinct from darker blood or *melena,* a black tarry stool that results from problems farther up in the digestive tract. Dark blood is usually mixed in with the stool, whereas hemorrhoidal blood is usually found on toilet paper or in the water in the toilet. Still, I wouldn't rely on a physical inspection to diagnose the source of your bleeding. You need confirmation by a medical professional.

Bleeding from hemorrhoids occurs when blood vessels in or just outside the anus swell and become engorged with blood. When the veins swell, the tissue or skin on top of the veins becomes thin and fragile. The friction from stool passing through can rub the overly-

WHEN IT'S NOT HEMORRHOIDS

As common as hemorrhoids are, they're mistakenly diagnosed far too frequently in women who actually have some other problem. This was the case with Tracy, a newly married twenty-five-year-old, who came to my clinic complaining of bleeding hemorrhoids. She had had episodes of bright red rectal bleeding for over two years. These episodes usually lasted a few weeks and gradually got better on their own. Tracy told me she saw her family doctor over a year ago for her bleeding, and he told her she had hemorrhoids and should use Preparation H.

Tracy finally came to see me because her latest bleeding episode began two months ago and still hadn't gotten any better. "My hemorrhoids must really be severe," she said. "I wonder if I need surgery." As I talked with Tracy a little more, I discovered that she was actually having bloody diarrhea with urgency. These were the same symptoms she had always attributed to "hemorrhoids." When I examined Tracy, I couldn't find any hemorrhoids. I did a blood test and found out that she was anemic, which meant she could be bleeding out somewhere along her digestive tract. I performed a colonoscopy on Tracy the next week and found evidence of ulcerative colitis. I took Tracy off the Preparation H and got her started on more appropriate therapy for her colitis.

ing tissue raw and cause a small break in the vein, which begins to bleed.

Hemorrhoids occur in two locations: inside the anus (internal hemorrhoids) and under the anal skin at the opening to the anus (external hemorrhoids). Be-

OVER-THE-COUNTER HEMORRHOID MEDICATIONS: A SHOPPER'S GUIDE

Here's a brief run-down of what you'll find in the hemorrhoid section of your local drugstore.

- **Anusol:** This product is available as an ointment or suppository. It contains an analgesic, pramoxine, to relieve the pain, soreness, burning, and itching associated with hemorrhoids. Mineral oil helps to lubricate swollen, irritated hemorrhoidal tissue, and zinc oxide forms a temporary protective coating over inflamed tissues to prevent drying. You should use this product in the morning, at bedtime, and after each bowel movement. Do not use it more than three or four times a day.

- **Preparation H:** This product is available as a suppository, ointment, or cream. Its active ingredient is a live yeast cell derivative that supposedly helps build collagen and increases the ability of the tissue to absorb oxygen to promote healing. It contains no analgesic but does have shark liver oil, mineral oil, and petroleum as lubricants. It should be applied whenever symptoms occur but no more than four times a day.

- **Dibucaine (Nupercainal):** This product is a topical anesthetic to relieve pain and itching. The cream, ointment, or suppository can be used whenever symptoms occur, up to four times a day for the cream or ointment and six times a day for the suppositories. This product may also be used topically for temporary relief of pain and itching associated with sunburn, minor burns, cuts, scrapes, insect bites, or minor skin irritation.

- **Hydrocortisone ointment, suppository, and cream (Anusol-HC, Anucort-HC, Hemril-HC, Cort-Dome, and others):** These products contain 0.5 percent hydrocortisone to decrease inflammation of the tissues and to relieve swelling and itching. They should not be used more than three or four times a day. Hydrocortisone suppositories should be used only when clearly needed during pregnancy. Discuss the risks and benefits with your doctor. This medication may be excreted into breast milk. Consult your doctor before breast-feeding.
- **Tucks Medicated Pads or Preparation H Medicated Wipes:** These wipes contain witch hazel, which is soothing to inflamed tissues. They temporarily relieve the external itching, burning, and irritation associated with hemorrhoids. They may be applied three to four times a day.
- **Bulking agents:** Metamucil, Citrucel, or some other bulking agent that contains fiber may be helpful in keeping stool soft and making bowel movements less painful.

cause of the interconnectedness of these groups of blood vessels, your doctor may find you have both types.

Experts aren't sure why hemorrhoids occur. Some people may be genetically predisposed to them. Hemorrhoids may also be triggered by a low-fiber diet, which causes harder stools that can be passed only with great straining. Having a job where you sit for long periods of time can also increase your risk, since sitting leads to increased pressure within the veins. Some experts contend that weak muscles within the bowels allow a downward slide of hemorrhoidal veins, resulting in swelling and bleeding. Pregnancy is notorious for causing hemorrhoids due to the weight and pressure of the growing fetus as well as changes in the body that occur from rising hormones.

Internal hemorrhoids become visible when they swell downward and out of the anus. Known as *prolapse,* these tender, bluish, soft bulging veins protrude when you strain and disappear when you relax. Internal hemorrhoids usually cause no pain, though they may bleed or discharge mucus. Hemorrhoids can remain in place or can project out of the anal canal while defecating but return after defecation.

External hemorrhoids are located closer to the anal opening and are covered with skin—unlike internal hemorrhoids, which are covered with more delicate rectal tissue. External hemorrhoids can cause mild discomfort but rarely cause pain unless they form a blood clot known as a *thrombus.* In that case they turn blue and may cause sudden, severe pain.

Symptoms

Internal hemorrhoids, which are not usually seen or felt unless they protrude out through the anus, can cause symptoms such as a feeling of fullness in the rectum, particularly after passing stool. You may also have an annoying deep-seated itching, known as *pruritus ani.* Internal hemorrhoid bleeding also produces the hallmark bright red blood, and you may feel an increase in symptoms if these veins prolapse or push out through the anus.

When you part your buttocks, you or your doctor can actually see external hemorrhoids around the opening of the anus. They look like big distended bluish veins outside the anal canal and can bleed when they become irritated. Old hemorrhoids may be skin tags or an extra buildup of skin that occurred from the veins continually swelling and shrinking. Skin tags do not bleed because the blood vessel within them has shrunk. External hemorrhoids occur most frequently in young and middle aged adults—especially pregnant women—and usually cause no symptoms. They can, however, become irritated by stool and cause itching or pain if the anal area isn't cleaned thoroughly.

External hemorrhoids can, as I mentioned, become quite painful when a blood clot forms, causing a thrombus. The level of pain varies from woman to woman, but typically the pain comes on suddenly and increases rapidly to a throbbing or burning sensation, accompanied by a new "lump" in the anal region. Sometimes the "lump" has a bluish discoloration caused by the clot. With time the body usually dissolves the clot on its own, and the thrombosis goes away. Unfortunately, patients may be in pain for days waiting for the thrombosis to heal. During this time people can have difficulty defecating and sitting and may have an increased likelihood of forming an ulcer at the area or an infection at the area.

Diagnosis

Your first step in dealing with hemorrhoids should be to make an appointment with your doctor to rule out other possible causes of bleeding. Your doctor will probably perform a visual examination of your outer anal skin first and then a digital rectal exam. Using a well-lubricated gloved finger, he or she will feel for hemorrhoids in your anal canal.

An anoscopic exam may follow. A small, usually clear plastic tube is inserted just into your lower anorectal canal. Using a light, your doctor will be able to see the anal canal, any internal hemorrhoids, and the opening to the rectum more clearly. The lubricated anoscope is inserted slowly as your doctor applies gentle pressure on the end of the instrument to push it in. (An anoscope is sometimes used to remove a low rectal polyp that cannot be removed through a flexible endoscope.)

Your doctor may ask for a stool sample to test for the presence of blood. You may also be referred for a colon cancer screening test like flexible sigmoidoscopy or colonoscopy, which I explain in detail in Chapter 15.

Treatment

Once the diagnosis of hemorrhoids is made, you and your physician can focus on treatment. For small hemorrhoids, your doctor will probably recommend increasing the amount of fiber in your diet to 25 to 30 grams per day and increasing your fluid intake to six to eight glasses of water a day to soften stool. Follow my plan for "What You Can Do to Get Things Moving" on page 196. If your job requires that you sit for prolonged periods, make a point of getting up more often.

The most important advice I can give: Don't strain when you're on the toilet. Often, swollen hemorrhoids can make you feel like there's still a little something left after defecating. Most women will strain just to get out a pea-sized piece of stool. That straining only exacerbates the hemorrhoids and sets up a vicious cycle of more swelling. So when it's time to go, just go. What you can get out, fine. Don't strain to get that last little bit out—it'll come out next time. Make sure you thoroughly wipe away all stool from around your anus, since stool can be extremely irritating. Dry toilet paper often doesn't do the trick. Try a Tucks Medicated Pad, baby wipe, or a wet tissue to completely clean that area. If your hemorrhoids are causing you particular discomfort, soak in a warm sitz bath several times a day. These baths will greatly help to reduce pain and swelling.

A number of medicated creams and suppositories are available to help reduce inflammation from hemorrhoids. Creams generally work better for external hemorrhoids and suppositories for internal hemorrhoids. If you choose a suppository, make sure it is firm. If the suppository is soft, you can chill it in the refrigerator for thirty minutes or hold it under cold, running water. To place the suppository in, lie down. If you're on your left side, then raise your right knee to your chest and insert the suppository in about one inch. Wait about fifteen minutes before standing up, then wash your hands. Check with your doctor about the proper use of any hemorrhoidal medication.

If self-help treatments aren't bringing you relief, you may need medical intervention. If you have internal hemorrhoids, there are several options that your doctor may suggest. The most common is a procedure called rubber band ligation. This technique uses endoscopy or anoscopy to apply one or two small rubber bands around the hemorrhoids to cut off the blood supply to the veins. This procedure generally causes only minimal discomfort, and the majority of patients don't require anesthesia.

The veins clot and wither, but because they are internal hemorrhoids, this is not usually painful. Within a week to ten days, the rubber band and excess tissue slough off into the stool. This procedure cures hemorrhoids in up to 75 percent of patients with first- and second-degree hemorrhoids, and 65 percent of those with third-degree hemorrhoids experience a major improvement. The risk of side effects like infection is very small.

Other effective options for hemorrhoid removal include *infrared cautery,* which uses a heating light to burn and seal the hemorrhoids. *Bipolar cautery* creates heat energy using electricity to cauterize the hemorrhoids. Both procedures can be done without anesthesia and have an 80 to 85 percent success rate.

If internal hemorrhoids bleed excessively or obstruct the passage of stool and are no longer relieved by the therapies already mentioned, your doctor may recommend surgery. You may also benefit from surgery if you have too many hemorrhoids, which can make the other techniques too time-consuming.

During surgery, which requires anesthesia, the surgeon lifts up and removes the hemorrhoids using a scope (a long, flexible tube). Any variety of techniques (blade, scissors, laser, or electrocautery) can be used to remove the hemorrhoid. You will need two to three weeks to recover from the surgery. You'll have some bleeding and pain for a few days afterward, but you shouldn't be bedridden.

Surgical complications include a very small risk of bleeding, infection, and fecal incontinence. This latter complication can occur because surgery can sometimes damage the anal muscles responsible for holding back stool and flatulence. Injury to these muscles can also heighten feelings of pain from the passage of stool or the development of new hemorrhoids.

Treatment for external hemorrhoids is far more limited than for internal ones. Doctors don't usually recommend medical treatment beyond over-the-counter remedies and lifestyle measures like proper anal hygiene. The best medicine for these hemorrhoids is not to let them get too severe by avoiding straining and preventing constipation. If you have acute, severe pain, it's very likely that you have a thrombosed external hemorrhoid.

Treatment of a thrombosed hemorrhoid generally requires a thrombectomy, a procedure done in your doctor's office. Your anal area will be cleansed with a cleansing ointment, usually Betadine, and the area anesthetized with local anesthesia. Using scissors, a small incision is made into the hemorrhoid, and the clot is removed. This generally results in relief of the pain, though the incision site may be sore for a few days. You may need antibiotics to avoid infection, but this area, because of its excellent blood supply, generally heals very quickly.

Surgery is hardly ever necessary for external hemorrhoids, but on occasion it's used to remove those that are very large or for excessive bleeding or pain. General surgeons at the University of Virginia Hospital usually perform this procedure at an outpatient surgery center. Resection can be painful, and complete recovery can take a few weeks. Most patients find themselves sitting on a soft pillow for a while.

ANAL FISSURES

Anal fissures are small tears—I think of them as paper cuts—in the lining of the anal canal near the entrance of the anus. This common condition occurs most often in young, otherwise healthy adults. Both women and men can develop anal fissures, and all too frequently their condition is mistaken for hemorrhoids. (See the figure on page 485.)

We don't really understand why anal fissures occur. Some say that straining to pass a hard stool causes these tears, but according to research, only one in four people with fissures has constipation. Along these lines, some experts speculate that a low-fiber diet increases the risk of fissures because it leads to hard, difficult-to-pass stools. Another cause of anal fissures may be trauma during pregnancy. About 11 percent of women with chronic anal fissures developed the symptoms immediately following childbirth. Pressure from the fetus descending into the birth canal can damage the tissue lining of the anus. In some people, anal fissures can be caused by an internal anal sphincter that shuts too tightly. This can result in a pulling or pressure on the anal lining that causes small tears in the tissue.

Symptoms of anal fissure include pain during or after a bowel movement, with bleeding (bright red blood) from the anus. The pain is often severe and may last for a few minutes or persist for several hours after going to the bathroom. Itching (pruritus ani) occurs in about half of cases. Anal fissures can occur with hemorrhoids, and the two conditions together can cause a significant loss of blood.

Diagnosing an anal fissure is relatively easy. Your doctor will part your buttocks to look at your anus, and you may be asked to bear down. Generally the fissure can be seen. Most anal fissures resolve on their own within a few weeks or with simple lifestyle changes along the lines of what I recommended for hemorrhoids: Don't strain; increase your fiber and fluid intake; use stool softeners if constipation is present. Using a hydrocortisone-containing hemorrhoidal cream around the external anal canal may also soothe things. Any fissure that lasts longer than six weeks is considered to be chronic and usually requires medical intervention to heal. Treatments include prescription drugs like organic nitrates (GTN nitroglycerin paste) or isosorbide dinitrate or ISDN (Isordil), which are applied as topical creams and work to relax the anal sphincter. Headaches are a common side effect of GTN and ISDN, and an anal fissure can recur once these medications are stopped.

I've had a lot of success with botulinum A toxin—yes, the very same toxin injected by plastic surgeons to make facial wrinkles disappear. Research has shown that injecting botulinum into the anal sphincter lowered resting anal pressure and healed 82 percent of chronic fissures. One study found that about six percent of patients, however, developed a recurrence of fissures in six months, ten percent developed a painful blood clot or thrombosis at the injection site, and seven percent developed fecal incontinence. Other studies found a much higher success rate (96 percent of patients had healed fissures) and much lower complication rates.

My husband, who is a plastic surgeon, laughs when I tell him where I inject BOTOX. Truth is, when medication fails to heal an anal fissure, a BOTOX injection can be a very effective treatment. The basic principle is the same as it is for fixing wrinkles—it temporarily "paralyzes" the muscles that cause the "spasm." After the anal area is carefully cleaned, BOTOX is injected through a tiny needle directly into the anal canal. After 24 to 48 hours the toxin usually works to relax anal spasm, and healing of the anal fissure is expected in one to two weeks.

Surgery is used as a last resort to heal an anal fissure. One of the most common and effective procedures is called a sphincterotomy, which involves making an incision into the internal sphincter to separate the fibers and reduce anal pressure. The main drawback to this technique is that the resulting scar from the procedure can stretch out over the years, causing a space in the muscle called a *keyhole defect*. This defect can result in fecal incontinence a decade or two after the surgery. Up to 30 percent of women who have this procedure develop some degree of incontinence over time.

To avoid this debilitating side effect—especially if you have a fissure that occurred from a severe tear or episiotomy during childbirth—your doctor needs to assess your internal anal sphincter using anorectal ultrasound and manometry before recommending surgery. If your sphincter is already damaged and resting anal pressure isn't too high, you're probably better off receiving a different surgical procedure called an *anal advancement flap*, which directly repairs the actual tear instead of altering the sphincter.

FECAL INCONTINENCE

We've all seen the commercials for Depends undergarments, but none of us actually think we're ever going to need an adult diaper—at least until we're well into old age. But I can attest to the fact that many women in their forties, fifties, and sixties do need some sort of protection because—to their dismay and horror—they suffer from fecal incontinence. Alyssa, a forty-two-year-old mother of three, developed fecal incontinence after giving birth to her third child. She had three "big" boys weighing over eight pounds each at delivery. She had a tear with her first delivery and episiotomies with the last two.

After her second son was born, Alyssa noticed a small amount of mucus leakage into her underwear. After her third delivery, however, she discovered to her shock and embarrassment that, as she put it, "I have absolutely no control of myself." She told me she couldn't believe she was changing her own diapers as well as her newborn son's.

When Alyssa saw her gynecologist for her first postpartum visit, she waited until she was almost out the door before she mentioned this problem. Her gynecologist then referred her to Dr. Kathie Hullfish, my colleague at the UVA Hospital, who specializes in fecal incontinence. She did a thorough pelvic examination, then referred Alyssa to me.

I performed an endoscopic ultrasound and found that, sure enough, Alyssa had a sizable defect in her sphincter muscle. What used to be a round, continuous muscle around the anus had now developed a three-centimeter keyhole defect. This gap, which can be caused by anal fissure surgery, can also be caused by stretching during pregnancy, tearing during delivery, or repeated episiotomies.

In Alyssa's case, I found that both her internal and external anal sphincter muscles were involved, which explained why her fecal incontinence was so severe. Alyssa had feared she would have to wear diapers the rest of her life. However, after Dr. Hullfish explained her options, Alyssa had surgery to correct her sphincter muscle defect. She's a lot better now and wears only a minipad on occasion. She also does Kegel exercises on a regular basis to keep her pelvic floor muscles strong.

Alyssa was lucky. She broke her silence and got treated. Too often this condition is simply swept under the carpet. No one wants to talk about it because it seems so shameful. Even urinary incontinence is far more acceptable (and far more frequently discussed) than fecal incontinence. A survey published in the medical journal *Lancet* found that fewer than 50 percent of patients with fecal incontinence report the symptom to their doctor unless directly asked.

Here are some disturbing statistics:

- Fecal incontinence is eight times higher in women than in men.
- Up to 17 percent of healthy women ages fifteen to sixty-four suffer from fecal incontinence, and this number reaches nearly 50 percent for women who are physically debilitated or in nursing homes.
- Fecal incontinence occurs in 35 to 50 percent of women with urinary incontinence.

The good news is that fecal incontinence is often treatable. You don't have to live with this debilitating and embarrassing problem.

Causes

Many women with fecal incontinence first assume they have diarrhea. I want to dispel the myth that diarrhea causes fecal incontinence—it usually doesn't. Even if you have severe, watery diarrhea caused by food poisoning or other intestinal virus, your external and internal sphincter muscles are generally tight enough to prevent fecal incontinence. Chronic fecal incontinence (even intermittent bouts) is almost always due to some other factor.

THE EPISIOTOMY PROBLEM

One study involving 127 women found that 35 percent of first-time mothers and 44 percent of mothers with multiple children developed defects in their internal anal sphincter after having an episiotomy during childbirth. (Fewer than six percent of women who go through labor without an episiotomy develop this injury, even if they've had vaginal tears from the delivery.) The study also found that 37 percent of the women who had sphincter defects experienced extreme urges to defecate, and 20 percent developed incontinence.

When I was training to be a doctor, episiotomies were performed in nearly all first-time mothers and in 80 percent of women giving birth on a repeat occasion. Now obstetricians are definitely doing this procedure less routinely, but about half of women still get them during delivery. The risk of future fecal incontinence is definitely something you and your doctor should take into consideration if you're planning a pregnancy. But the majority of women don't develop fecal incontinence immediately after delivery as Alyssa did above. Most women get their fecal incontinence ten or twenty years later. The reason is that what started out as a few-millimeter-wide keyhole defect, after increased pressure on the perineum—generally from sagging organs putting pressure on the pelvic floor—becomes larger, maybe a few-centimeter-wide defect, that results in incontinence.

Pelvic Floor Dysfunction. Both the internal and the external anal sphincters need to be functioning properly to prevent incontinence. You also, however, need to have a strong and well-functioning pelvic floor. The pelvic floor is made up of a group of interconnected muscles attached to the bones of the pelvis. Think of the pelvic floor as a trampoline. This thin layer of muscle is taut in younger women and able to support the bladder, uterus, and rectum. With aging and after repeated pregnancies, the pelvic floor sags and loses its tone. This process is perhaps worsened by chronic constipation or bad habits like putting off urination.

Having too much urine in your bladder, excess stool from constipation, or several periods of additional weight from carrying a baby can change the entire structure of the pelvis. Everything sinks—or sags. (And you thought the only things sagging were above the waist!) One particular muscle, the *puborectalis,* acts as a sling and provides support for your rectum and anus. With pelvic floor dysfunction (which I discuss in more detail in Chapter 2), your puborectalis muscle weakens and becomes slack. (See the figure on page 71.) This is a common cause of constipation—especially in older women—and may also contribute to fecal incontinence.

Surgical Procedures and Obstetrical Injury. Surgery for hemorrhoids or an anal fissure can sometimes cause this problem, as can surgery to repair a fistula. Having a tear or an episiotomy during childbirth (an incision that widens the opening between the vagina and the rectum) can be a direct cause of fecal incontinence. So, too, can having a baby delivered by forceps or giving birth to an infant who weighs nine pounds or more.

Medications.   Although medications themselves don't cause incontinence, if you have an anal sphincter defect, any drug that causes diarrhea can increase your likelihood of fecal incontinence. Certain medications are more likely to cause diarrhea and may be associated with fecal incontinence. Antibiotics, for instance, commonly have a side effect of diarrhea. This can be true for those taking potent antibiotics to wipe out *H. pylori,* the bacteria associated with ulcers. Those who abuse laxatives are also at risk for developing fecal incontinence, since this can bring on diarrhea and eliminate natural urges to defecate. Surprisingly, some medications that aggravate constipation (some antidepressants and antimotility drugs) can also lead to fecal incontinence by causing the buildup and impaction of stool. Liquid stool passes around the solid ball of impacted stool, causing increased pressure that results in a burst of incontinence. This most commonly occurs in the elderly or in nursing home patients who are bedridden.

Nerve Damage.   When stool is present and needs to be passed, nerves surrounding the anus and rectum normally signal the brain. This is called the *sampling reflex.* Your brain, in turn, signals the external anal sphincter, giving you some voluntary control over when to defecate. Some patients with stroke, dementia, or other brain or nervous system disorder develop fecal incontinence because these nerve pathways are damaged. Local nerve dysfunction can also be caused by radiation therapy to the pelvis, inflammatory bowel disease, or other medical condition like diabetes.

Diagnosis

As with any GI problem, diagnosing fecal incontinence depends largely on taking a thorough medical history. I always ask about fecal incontinence if a patient tells me she has a sense of strong urgency before having a bowel movement or has diarrhea, urinary incontinence, diabetes, or some neuromuscular disease like multiple sclerosis.

Once I determine that a patient has fecal incontinence, I try to gauge the severity of the problem. Does she have minor leakage from time to time? Or does she live her life as a recluse because she has at least one major accident a day? Is she generally okay if she's within range of a bathroom? Does it occur during sleep? Is it only with loose stools? The type and severity of incontinence will dictate the intensity of the workup and treatment.

If your physician suspects fecal incontinence, he or she will perform a physical exam that tests your anal reflex. Your doctor will examine your perineum (the region between your anus and vulva) and your anus to look for signs of a tumor, skin inflammation, infection, scars, skin tags, hemorrhoids, or other problem. You may be asked to bear down as your doctor checks for rectal prolapse (which means a portion of your rectum protrudes from your anus), leakage of stool, and swelling of the perineum—all of which suggest a weakness in the pelvic floor muscles. Your doctor will also evaluate a specific reflex, called the cutaneoanal contractile reflex, by stroking the perianal skin with a pin or probe. If the external anal sphincter doesn't contract as it should, this may indicate a nerve problem.

Your doctor will then perform a digital rectal exam (inserting a lubricated finger into the rectum) to feel the length of the anal canal and evaluate the tone of the internal anal sphincter. You may be asked to squeeze, as if trying to prevent defecation, so your doctor can feel the strength of the muscle contraction. During this exam your doctor will also check the strength of your puborectalis muscle (which can indicate pelvic floor dysfunction) and check for a rectal mass or impacted stool. Your doctor may also evaluate your perineal bar, the area of skin between your vagina and anus, for thinning, laxity, or evidence of a prior obstetrical tear or episiotomy. Occasionally your doctor may also perform a full vaginal examination as well to discern if there is evidence of a cystocele (bulging of the bladder into the vagina) or rectocele (bulging of the rectum into the vagina).

Other tests your doctor may choose include:

- **Endoscopic evaluation** of your rectum and colon to determine if there are any physical abnormalities that could be preventing the normal passage of stool.
- **Anal manometry** measures the pressure in your anal canal at rest and during a voluntary contraction of the external anal sphincter. The test also measures the response of the internal and external anal sphincters when the rectum is distended with a small balloon. To perform anal manometry, a tube is inserted into your anus and passed up into

your rectum. The tube is equipped with a small balloon at the end of it, which is filled with air. As the balloon is filled with air (simulating the presence of stool in your rectum), your doctor can determine how well your anal and rectal muscles work.

- **Imaging tests** such as *defecography*, an X-ray of the anorectal area and lower segment of the colon. This test evaluates the pelvic floor muscles, rectal muscles, and angle of the rectoanal canal. It also evaluates the completeness of stool elimination, identifies any anorectal abnormalities, and measures rectal muscle contractions and relaxation. During this test a small amount of barium is injected into the rectum, and you're then seated on the toilet as a videotape is made as you cough, bear down, and pass stool. Other imaging tests include *endoscopic ultrasound* (which uses a small ultrasound probe to look for a keyhole defect in the anal sphincter muscle) and *transvaginal ultrasound*. *MRI* may also be used to check for structural defects or anatomical abnormalities, but it's used less frequently than ultrasound because of its high cost and lack of availability.

Treatment

Treatment for fecal incontinence ranges from the conservative to the invasive and varies widely from patient to patient. If a specific cause is found, treatment can be targeted to that cause. For example, diabetic patients

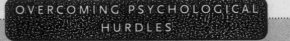

OVERCOMING PSYCHOLOGICAL HURDLES

A large part of managing incontinence involves dealing with psychological issues. A lot of my patients have a real fear of experiencing fecal incontinence in public. This fear may cause them to withdraw from get-togethers with friends or other social activities. "I've become a recluse, and I was always known as the life of the party," says Janet, a forty-year-old mother of two who recently came to see me. Fecal incontinence can also lead to depression if a woman feels her lifestyle has been unfairly curtailed. One book that my patients have found to be a helpful resource in dealing with the day-to-day management of incontinence is *Keeping Control: Understanding and Overcoming Fecal Incontinence* by Marvin M. Schuster and Jacqueline Wehmueller (Johns Hopkins University Press, 1994).

who have incontinence caused by nerve damage may have their condition improved by better management of their blood sugar levels. Those who have nerve damage due to pelvic floor dysfunction can help prevent their problem from becoming worse by avoiding excess straining and by strengthening their pelvic floor muscles through Kegel exercises. Or they might benefit from surgery if their problem is severe.

If a specific cause of incontinence is not found, certain measures can help prevent incontinence. Here are the most common approaches.

Bowel Retraining: Keeping your colon and rectum free of stool can help prevent incontinence. In order to do this, you need to "schedule" a bowel movement every day—if you don't usually go that often. That is, you should set aside a regular time every day to have a bowel movement. This should be within thirty minutes after a meal, to take advantage of the gastrocolic reflex, the "urge to go" reflex that kicks in after eating. For the first few days, at the end of the meal, if you don't normally feel the urge to go, you can try inserting a glycerin suppository laxative into your rectum. If you have a problem with diarrhea, you need to have this symptom evaluated and properly managed before you can deal with the incontinence.

Another important step you can take: Engage in pelvic muscle exercises. Strengthening your pelvic floor muscles through Kegel exercises can help improve fecal incontinence. One study found that 63 percent of women with fecal incontinence who failed to be helped with dietary therapy experienced an improvement in their symptoms or were actually cured of their problem after performing Kegel exercises on a daily basis. I give detailed instructions on performing Kegels on page 72.

Drug Therapy: If you have chronic diarrhea and fecal incontinence, bulking agents (fiber) and antidiarrheal drugs like loperamide (Imodium) or diphenoxylate (Lomotil) may be the treatments of choice. These help control the liquidity of stool, which in and of itself may significantly reduce incontinence. Loperamide may also improve the muscle tone of the internal anal sphincter. Those without diarrhea may benefit from low doses of these drugs, but the jury is still out on this possibility.

Biofeedback Training: This technique is a way to condition you to become conscious of a physiological process in your body that you're normally unaware of. With fecal incontinence, it teaches you to be aware of the contraction of your external anal sphincter in response to stool, air, or other distention in your rectum. In a typical session, a balloon manometry device is attached to a pressure monitor to show how pressure in the anal canal can be increased by contracting the external anal sphincter. You're then instructed to contract the sphincter every time the rectal balloon is distended. At first the balloon is filled with a lot of air to give you more of a sensation of distention. In later sessions the balloon is filled with just a small amount of air because you will have become more sensitive to feelings of distention.

This method may be most helpful in those who have fecal incontinence accompanied by constipation. In those who have reduced urges to have a bowel movement, stool builds up until an explosive and uncontrollable bowel movement occurs. Learning to feel just a small amount of stool and to move your bowels on a regular basis can help prevent these incontinent episodes. Studies suggest that about 70 percent of patients who learn to control their bowel movements through biofeedback experience a disappearance or significant reduction in their fecal incontinence.

Most major hospital and medical centers offer biofeedback, usually through their psychology department. I refer patients for biofeedback on a routine basis, and you can ask your doctor for a referral.

Surgery: Surgery is the last resort for those who don't respond to medical therapy for their incontinence. It's also an option for those who have a clearly defined anatomical problem, such as women who suffered an obstetrical injury to their anal sphincter during childbirth. A number of procedures are used, and the most appropriate method depends on the specific anatomical defect.

I want to stress that these operations are complicated and should be performed by a skilled surgeon and, even then, only after an extensive evaluation has been done with the appropriate medical tests. You should be aware that surgery isn't a cure-all. About 70 to 90 percent of women experience significant improvement, but many of them still have some incontinence, especially with more-liquid stools.

Those who have damage to the external anal sphincter caused by childbirth or some other trauma usually are treated with a procedure called *sphincteroplasty,* which involves making an incision into the scar and re-forming the sphincter to make a viable muscle. Studies show this procedure works in about 75 percent of patients who were suitable candidates—at least over the short term. Incontinence can return several years later in a significant number of patients.

When urinary and fecal incontinence occur together, cystocele and rectocele repair may be necessary. This operation lifts and tightens the tissue around the bladder and rectum so that these organs no longer push against the vagina. This repair can be combined with an elevation or suspension of the bladder, which will result in more effective and complete urination and

A MYSTERIOUS PAIN IN YOUR A— —

Usually doctors can locate the cause of severe pain in the anus or rectum, whether it's a hemorrhoid or a fistula or a fissure. Sometimes, though, we find absolutely nothing to explain a sudden intense pain in the region of the rectum and anus that hits with a wallop, lasts several minutes, and then disappears completely.

This pain may be caused by one of two conditions: proctalgia fugax or levator ani syndrome. These are fancy names for benign problems. *Proctalgia fugax*, occurring in 5 to 15 percent of the population, can cause very severe pain in the anal region that makes sufferers wonder "What the hell was that?!?" Some equate the sharp pain with labor pains or a gallbladder attack. Fortunately, the pain from proctalgia fugax is very brief. Some find it occurs in the middle of the night during deep sleep or following sexual activity. The pain is felt deep in the rectum and has been described as searing, cramping, stabbing, grinding, and gnawing. Attacks seem to average about six per year.

Unlike other anal conditions, this pain doesn't coincide with defecation. The attack, though, may end with a passage of a little gas or stool. At one point experts thought this pain was related to IBS or constipation, but now they think there's no link and no risk of serious complication associated with the pain.

Levator ani syndrome occurs predominantly in young women under forty-five. The discomfort is described as a vague tenderness or aching sensation high in the rectum. It can last twenty minutes or more and recur more frequently than proctalgia fugax. It's usually worse after having a bowel movement and with sitting. Walking around or lying down can relieve the pain.

Causes? We don't know for sure, but some believe these conditions are caused by a muscle spasm—a "charley horse" of the backside. Whatever the cause, you can take comfort in the knowledge that this pain is perfectly benign. If it occurs frequently, you should see your doctor to rule out other causes.

better bowel control. Bulging and pressure sensations in the vagina will also be relieved.

Women with fecal incontinence caused by nerve problems due to pelvic floor dysfunction can benefit from a surgery called *total pelvic floor repair*. In this operation the puborectalis is sutured together with two other sets of pelvic floor muscles. In one study, 41 percent of women achieved complete continence after this procedure, and another 55 percent experienced a substantial improvement.

A new technological advance has been the development of an *artificial anal sphincter*. This procedure involves the placement of a hydraulic ring around the anal canal with a reservoir and pump device to keep the ring inflated (which closes the sphincter) between bowel movements. The ring can be deflated (which opens the sphincter) when a bowel movement is desired. This technique is still experimental, and infection caused by the ring is still a problem that needs to be worked out.

OTHER PROBLEMS "DOWN THERE"

Quite a few other anal conditions can cause problems, including anorectal abscess, fistula, rectal prolapse, anal warts, and anal cancer. If you're experiencing certain symptoms, your doctor may want to rule out these other conditions. You should know that these problems are less common than hemorrhoids and fissures. They do, however, occur and are sometimes mistaken for more common anal problems before a proper diagnosis is finally made.

Anorectal Abscess

This is an infected sore that results from an untreated infection of the anal glands. Crohn's disease, fissures, and anal surgery can sometimes cause this type of abscess. Swelling, throbbing, and continuous pain are the most common symptoms. Treatment involves making a small incision and draining the abscess, then taking a course of antibiotics to clear up the infection. Abscesses can cause life-threatening infections if they're not treated properly.

Fistula

A fistula is an infected pathway that may develop from a sore or abscess in the anal skin that works its way down to the outside of the skin. A fistula can be painful or painless and usually involves a lot of drainage of blood or pus. About half of patients who undergo drainage of an abscess will develop fistulas. Fistulas generally have to be treated with surgery.

Rectal Prolapse

This condition occurs when the rectum bulges or protrudes into the anal canal. It can be caused by chronic constipation and overstraining, decreased pelvic muscle support of the rectum, or a long, floppy sigmoid colon that pushes down on the rectum. Rectal prolapse often occurs in older women along with bladder and uterus prolapse through the vagina—all of which are due to weak pelvic floor muscles. Many women experience rectal bleeding and fecal incontinence as a result of rectal prolapse. Although treatment of constipation and pelvic floor strengthening exercises can help somewhat, surgery is nearly always required to alleviate the condition.

Anal Warts

Like genital warts, anal warts are caused by human papillomavirus (HPV), a sexually transmitted virus that's also related to cervical cancer. About one percent of women who are sexually active have anal warts. (The vast majority of them, however, carry HPV because the virus is so common and easily transmitted.) The warts can itch or be painful but are fairly easily treated with topical therapies like podophyllin. Surgery or cryotherapy (which freezes the wart) may be necessary to treat large warts or warts that are resistant to topical treatments. Once the warts disappear, however, they can recur over time because HPV remains in the body and can't be cured.

Anal Cancer

Anal cancer is very rare, occurring in one in 100,000 people each year in the United States. Anal bleeding is the most common symptom; some people may also feel the sensation of a mass. Your risk of developing this cancer is increased if you carry HPV. Your doctor will feel for an anal tumor during your digital rectal exam, but keep in mind that chances are extremely slim that your anal symptoms are caused by this cancer.

A FINAL WORD

AFTER READING THIS BOOK, I hope you'll feel comfortable talking with your doctor about any digestive health issues, including anal or rectal problems. I refer to them as problems "down there," but I really want to give you the tools to speak specifically about your symptoms and sensations without using ambiguous references. If you communicate openly and prepare for visits according to the guidelines in Chapter 8, you will have done your part to establish a strong, trusting relationship with your doctor.

By now you know that there are few "magic bullet" cures for digestive woes. Getting relief may require time, patience, and perseverance. In many cases, I advise approaching symptoms and conditions with lifestyle changes first. You may need to embark on a weight-loss program, give up smoking, or find ways to reduce stress. You might also need to schedule time for exercise or switch to a healthier diet. My rule of thumb is that it's okay to self-treat for about two weeks if you have no "red flag" warning symptoms. If relief doesn't come during that time, seek medical advice.

Once you have a treatment plan and your symptoms are under control, remain vigilant about sticking to the lifestyle changes you've made. If shedding excess pounds helped to alleviate your reflux, be aware that regaining weight is likely to mean the return of symptoms as well. If certain foods aggravate your IBS symptoms, you'll probably always need to steer clear of them. (This may sound obvious, but I know from my patients that it's all too easy to slack off.) You and your doctor may also need to revise your plan from time to time.

Problems like IBS, Crohn's, and GERD must be managed over the course of a lifetime, and taking the time to focus on your overall good health will have enormous payoffs. Your GI tract will thank you by running smoothly and leaving you free to do the things you really want to do. Here's to your good health!

INDEX

ABOUT THE AUTHORS

CYNTHIA M. YOSHIDA, M.D., is a gastroenterologist in private practice in Charlottesville, Virginia. As an associate professor at the University of Virginia Health System in Charlottesville, she was the founder and director of the university's Women's GI Clinic. She is a frequent speaker at national and international medical conferences and a recognized media spokesperson on women's digestive health, and she has published numerous research papers.

DEBORAH KOTZ is a health journalist who regularly works with bestselling authors. She also writes articles for the *Washington Post, Good Housekeeping, McCall's, Parents,* and other magazines.

ABOUT THE AMERICAN GASTROENTEROLOGICAL ASSOCIATION

Founded in 1897, the American Gastroenterological Association is one of the oldest medical specialty societies in the United States. Its members include physicians and scientists who research, diagnose, and treat disorders of the gastrointestinal tract and liver. Representing almost 14,000 gastroenterologists worldwide, the AGA serves as an advocate for its members and their patients, supports gastroenterology practice and scientific needs, and promotes the discovery, dissemination, and application of new knowledge, leading to the prevention, treament, and cure of digestive and liver diseases. www.gastro.org

The Foundation for Digestive Health and Nutrition (FDHN) is the foundation of the AGA. It is separately incorporated and governed by a distinguished board of AGA physicians and members of the lay public. The foundation raises funds for research and public education in the prevention, diagnosis, treatment, and cure of digestive diseases. Along with the AGA, it conducts public-education initiatives related to digestive diseases. The foundation also administers the disbursement of grants on behalf of the AGA and other funders. www.fdhn.org